BIOCHEMICAL IMBALANCES in DISEASE

of related interest

Dietary Interventions in Autism Spectrum Disorders
Why They Work When They Do, Why They Don't When They Don't
Kenneth J. Aitken
ISBN 978 1 84310 939 6
eISBN 978 1 84642 860 9

Relating to Clients
The Therapeutic Relationship for Complementary Therapists
Su Fox
ISBN 978 1 84310 615 9
eISBN 978 1 84642 718 3

The Insightful Body
Healing with SomaCentric Dialoguing
Julie McKay
ISBN 978 1 84819 030 6
eISBN 978 0 85701 026 1

Body Intelligence
Creating a New Environment
Second Edition
Ged Sumner
ISBN 978 1 84819 026 9
eISBN 978 0 85701 011 7

A PRACTITIONER'S HANDBOOK

BIOCHEMICAL IMBALANCES in DISEASE

EDITED BY
LORRAINE NICOLLE and
ANN WOODRIFF BEIRNE

FOREWORD by DAVID S. JONES

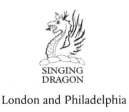

SINGING
DRAGON

London and Philadelphia

First published in 2010
by Singing Dragon
an imprint of Jessica Kingsley Publishers
73 Collier Street
London N1 9BE, UK
and
400 Market Street, Suite 400
Philadelphia, PA 19106, USA

www.singing-dragon.com

Library of Congress Cataloging in Publication Data
A CIP catalog record for this book is available from the Library of Congress

British Library Cataloguing in Publication Data
A CIP catalogue record for this book is available from the British Library

ISBN 978 1 84819 033 7

Printed and bound in the United Kingdom

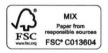

MIX
Paper from
responsible sources
FSC
www.fsc.org   FSC® C013604

CONTENTS

Chapter 8 Dysregulation of the Immune System: A Gastro-Centric Perspective 256

Michael Ash, Intergrative Health Consulting Ltd, UK

Chapter 9   Poor Energy Production and Increased Oxidative Stress   298

Surinder Phull, Thames Valley University, UK

Chapter 10   Dysregulated Neurotransmitter Function   325

Basant K. Puri, Imperial College London, UK and Helen Lynam, nutritional therapist, UK

LIST OF FIGURES, TABLES AND BOXES

Figures

Tables

Boxes

FOREWORD

Biochemical Imbalances in Disease will prove to be an important publication that adds to the expanding body of literature about functional medicine (FM).

During the last decade, significant FM textbooks have become available. Initially, FM practitioners celebrated the arrival of *Clinical Nutrition: A Functional Approach*, published by the Institute for Functional Medicine (IFM). This important textbook was followed by the first edition of *Laboratory Evaluations for Integrative and Functional Medicine*, published by the Metametrix Institute, revised and reprinted in a second edition in 2008. In 2005 the comprehensive and voluminous *Textbook of Functional Medicine* (IFM) provided the research and concepts behind the robust architecture and disciplined methodology of FM. Functional medicine is a systems medicine approach that addresses the primary challenge of the twenty-first century: *improving prevention and treatment for complex, chronic illness*. These textbooks together set the boundaries, evidence and methodologies for providing a new, comprehensive, clinically relevant medical paradigm shift for achieving this urgent goal.

What is the real importance, you may ask, of functional medicine and, in particular, of this latest text on its application? We currently have in place in the industrialised world (and elsewhere) a method of healthcare developed and based on the twentieth century acute-care medical model. Such a model is characterised by rapid differential diagnosis – with an organ system focus – aimed at prescribing a drug (or procedure) that will ameliorate the patient's presenting symptoms and avert the immediate threat (Ely 2000). It is a model that evolved in response to the primary causes of morbidity and mortality in the last century, namely acute infections and trauma. The experts within this organ systems model are the various specialists within conventional medicine, such as cardiologists, pulmonologists, endocrinologists, neurologists and orthopaedic surgeons.

Inherently, this methodology minimises the involvement of the patient, who functions mostly as a passive recipient of the procedure or prescription (Holman 2004). It is not a model that reimburses the practitioner for looking into why the patient became ill, or for reducing the probability of the patient later developing ramifications of the same underlying problem (American College of Physicians 2006). Instead, it prioritises immediate solutions to the most pressing problems. It is, of course, absolutely essential in emergency and hospital-based care of many kinds, but difficulties arise when this model is applied to ongoing, community-based care for the non-acute, chronic conditions that represent 80 per cent of the daily work of present day clinicians (Holman 2004).

This new book, *Biochemical Imbalances in Disease*, discusses the principles of functional medicine and shows how they can be usefully applied to frequently encountered clinical situations. In so doing, it illustrates the shift that will be required to enfold into twenty-first century medical practice the innovative clinical practises of patient-centred, personalised, systems-based medicine. A core principle of functional medicine maintains that diagnosis is the starting point for the clinician's primary set of responsibilities, not the last step before prescriptive interventions. The most complex of skills, *clinical decision making* and *medical judgment*, in the context of chronic, complex co-morbid illnesses, require:

- a persistent exploration of the accretion of scientific evidence, tempered by...

- the wealth of knowledge and judgment inherent in clinical experience, along with...

- the creation of a real partnership with the patient.

Clinical decision making, when exercised at the most efficacious level, drills deeply into the 'why' of every diagnosis. Pursuit of the elusive network of causality in the deeper intersections of genetic individuality, within each client's unique context of living, is an essential responsibility of the clinician. This clinical guide illustrates, using step-by-step examples, how to achieve more satisfying outcomes through an integrated clinical assessment and treatment programme using the *Functional Medicine Matrix Model*™.

Stepping out of the shadow of conventional poly-pharmacology and procedure-based interventions, into the bright sunlight afforded by twenty-first century breakthroughs in personalised medicine and systems biology, re-enchants and illuminates the practice of clinical medicine. The blending of the foundational sciences of genomics (unique genes in a unique environment) with the intellectual architecture of functional systems-thinking enables the creation of a more comprehensive portfolio of clinical services. The authors' careful explanations in this volume illustrate how clinical practice, coupled with skills learned through rigorous training in FM, can successfully bring to the therapeutic relationship real patient-centred answers for chronic, complex illnesses.

The most powerful motivator for changes in our behaviour as physicians is listening attentively to compelling stories brought to the clinic by our patients – stories that illustrate the angst of chronic pain and disability. The intense satisfaction of successfully resolving their hitherto unanswered questions, by applying a different lens for evaluation and assessment, is transformative. Functional, integrative, systems medicine provides such a lens, and the carefully documented clinical story narrated in Chapter 11 of this book is both evocative and educational.

Hence, *Biochemical Imbalances in Disease* will prove to be an important publication about functional and integrative medicine in clinical practice. I hope you enjoy the in-depth discussions and case presentation herein, as they so well exemplify the clinical application of this important medical model for the twenty-first century.

David S. Jones, MD, FABFP
President of The Institute for Functional Medicine
Director of Medical Education, IFM

References

American College of Physicians (2006) *The Impending Collapse of Primary Care Medicine and its Implications for the State of the Nation's Health Care: A Report from the American College of Physicians.*

Ely, J.W., Osheroff, J.A., Gorman, P.N., Ebell, M.H., Chambliss, M.L., Pifer, E.A. and Stavri, P.Z. (2000) 'A taxonomy of generic clinical questions: classification study.' *British Medical Journal 321*, 7258, 429–432.

Holman, H. (2004) 'Chronic disease – The need for a new clinical education.' *Journal of the American Medical Association 292*, 9, 1057–1059.

Chapter 1

THE HEALTHCARE FUTURESCAPE: HOW DID WE GET HERE AND WHERE ARE WE GOING?

Lorraine Nicolle and Ann Woodriff Beirne

Introduction

Since 2005, when the Prince of Wales-commissioned Smallwood Report (Smallwood 2005) called for a greater co-operative alliance between conventional and non-conventional healthcare practitioners in the UK, no serious discussion on the future of our healthcare system has seemed complete without reference to the need for more 'integrative medicine'. Similarly, in the USA, the need for a significant shake-up of current models of healthcare is now very publicly recognised, with key leaders and stakeholders emphasising the importance of an integrated system that is, 'participatory, preventive, predictive and personalized' (Hyman and Jones 2009).

In recent years this acknowledged need for a model of patient care that can bridge the current divide between conventional and complementary healthcare has led to the functional medicine (FM) model (Jones and Quinn 2005, p.17), attributed such a bridging ability because it is holistic, while also being grounded in the evidence base.

An overview of FM is outlined in section 3 of this chapter. The diagnostic and intervention approaches put forward in this book are guided by the FM principles. Written by UK nutrition researchers, educators and clinicians, the text consolidates information on identifying and nutritionally treating the key biochemical imbalances that are common to most of today's chronic health problems, thus helping the patient to better manage his or her situation. It should therefore prove to be a valuable resource for the nutrition practitioner, as well as the medical professional who is interested in working with nutritionally-oriented practitioners in the interests of providing an integrated service.

The FM model can be used for all patients, no matter what their current presenting symptoms or clinical diagnosis. Indeed, this approach is increasing in usefulness, as patients seem to have ever more complex aetiologies, for example in cancer or autoimmune disease. Many such patients find that a conventional, or allopathic, medical approach is limited in its ability to identify and treat the causes of their condition.

To put this new healthcare paradigm into context and to fully appreciate the logic of the FM approach it is helpful to understand its roots, as well as the ways in which modern medicine, as we know it, has taken shape over the last 2000 years or more.

1. Some key shapers of medicine

1.1 Hippocrates, Galen and humorism

HIPPOCRATES (BORN C.460 BC)

According to most medical historians, the Father of (clinical) medicine was Hippocrates. He was the first recorded physician to separate illness from religion, stating it instead to be the product of environmental factors, diet and living habits. His work was based in 'humorism' (see Box 1.1) and on *vis medicatrix naturae* (the healing power of nature). This suggests that the body contains within itself the power to rebalance the four humours (physis), which, when out of synchronisation (dysc(h)rasia) will lead to disease. Rest and immobilisation were of primary importance; as were keeping the patient clean and sterile, being gentle and undertaking no harsh interventions. This methodology led to a part of the Hippocratic oath (often (mis)interpreted as 'first, do no harm'): 'I will prescribe regimens for the good of my patients according to my ability and my judgment and never do harm to anyone.' Hippocrates was a firm believer in extending clinical observation into family history and environment and was therefore a detailed case history taker.

The groundwork for naturopathy was laid by Hippocrates, when he wrote in a treatise on epidemic diseases, 'Nature is the healer of all disease. Let foods be your Medicine and your Medicine your Foods' (National Association of Naturopathic Physicians 1970).

GALEN (AD 131–201)

Galen was a proponent of the humoral theory and believed that different foods would affect each humour differently – and that certain foods could be used to produce more of each type. The foods were based around the qualities of the humour involved, so if someone was suffering from a phlegmatic disorder (excess damp and cold) then warm and dry foods would help to rebalance the phlegm.

Box 1.1 Humoral theory or humorism

This consists of the concept that there are four 'humours' (from Greek *chymos*, meaning juice or sap or, metaphorically, flavour): blood, black bile, yellow bile and phlegm. To be healthy, all four humours should be in balance; when one or more goes out of balance, disease results.

The humours are also related to the four elements, earth, air, fire and water and, in excess, to personality types, as shown in this table.

Humour	Season	Element	Organ	Qualities	Personality
Blood	Spring	Air	Liver	Warm and moist	Sanguine
Yellow bile	Summer	Fire	Gall bladder	Warm and dry	Choleric
Black bile	Autumn	Earth	Spleen	Cold and dry	Melancholic
Phlegm	Winter	Water	Brain/lungs	Cold and moist	Phlegmatic

Humorism brought about the 'curative' measures of purging, bloodletting, cupping and emetics – all designed to bring the humours back into balance. These practices have been questioned throughout the ages but retained dominance until the mid-eighteenth century.

Humorism persisted throughout many centuries and different cultures, until Rudolf Virchow published his book on cellular pathology in 1858. It then fell out of favour in Western medicine and has remained in the background ever since. But humorism still has its legacy, in the name of the humoral immune system, and in blood dyscrasia (blood disease or abnormality).

1.2 The nineteenth century medical revolution

As biological sciences developed with, amongst other things, greater usage of microscopy, the nineteenth century saw humorism being replaced with newer philosophies of medicine.

1.2.1 THE *MÉTHODE EXPECTANTE*, THE NUMERICAL METHOD AND SCEPTICISM

Dr Pierre Charles Alexandre Louis (1787–1872) was against bloodletting and started moving away from humorism. He introduced the 'numerical method': the concept that knowledge about a disease, its history, clinical presentation and treatment could be derived from observations of the treatment responses of different groups of patients (the first clinical trials, perhaps). Like its precursors, this method also involved taking detailed case histories, so as to bring a complete picture to the final analysis (Louis 1844). Louis was also a proponent of the *méthode expectante*: that the physician's role is to do everything possible to aid nature in the process of disease recovery, and nothing to hinder it.

Oliver Wendell Holmes (1809–1894), also a supporter of the *méthode expectante*, published a paper in 1843 stating that puerperal fever was contagious and suggesting drastic measures to counteract the spread by physicians. These measures included burning all clothes worn at the time and allowing no further attendance at obstetric cases for six months. His theories were first ignored and then denounced. Holmes went on to become a noted therapeutic sceptic, causing uproar within the medical profession by pronouncing that 'if the whole materia medica, *as now used*, could be sunk to the bottom of the sea, it would be all the better for mankind – and all the worse for the fishes'. He is also quoted as saying 'no remedy is useful unless employed at the right moment' and was known for being distrustful of the seductive power of the marketplace, where profits influence treatment (Bryan and Podolsky 2009).

1.2.2 THE IMPORTANCE OF HYGIENE

Florence Nightingale (1820–1910) observed the unsanitary conditions of a barracks hospital while working as a nurse in the Crimea in 1854 and became convinced that the lack of sanitation directly contributed to the disease and death that was rife in the wards, killing ten times more soldiers than the war itself. She had got much of her inspiration from Elizabeth Fry, who had set up a school for nurses, teaching them about the importance of cleanliness and hygiene in recovery and health. Eventually, Nightingale was able to bring about improvements in sewers, sanitation and ventilation and this, coupled with adequate diet and activity, caused the mortality rate to drop markedly. 'She understood even then that the mind and body worked together, that cleanliness, the predecessor to our clean and sterile techniques of today, was a major barrier to infection, and that it promoted healing' (Neeb 2001, p.2).

Ignaz Semmelweis (1818–1865) managed to reduce the incidence of postnatal puerperal fever by the simple expedient of introducing handwashing to obstetric clinics in 1847; this was following his independent discovery that 'cadaverous particles' could be transferred from dead bodies undergoing post mortem to patients giving birth. However, his work was largely unrecognised until after his death in 1865, which coincided with Pasteur's promotion of the Germ Theory (see p.22).

Dr John Snow (1813–1858), known as the father of (modern) epidemiology, discovered that the cause of cholera was not in fact miasmic, but due to drinking water contaminated with sewage. Initially, his theories were ignored but in 1854 there was a terrible outbreak in Soho that caused hundreds of deaths in a few days. Snow managed to isolate the source of the cholera as a single water pump in Broad Street, thus proving his theory. On microscopic examination of the pump water, Dr Snow saw 'white, flocculent particles', the probable source of the cholera. He eventually managed to get the handle removed from the pump, thereby preventing further deaths. The original source was thought to be a leaking cesspit, not three feet from the pump. However, as Snow's theory was still not taken up by the Board of Health, subsequent recommendations for the removal of the cesspits went unheeded (Summers 1989).

Dr Snow was also a pioneer in the use of ether in anaesthesia, something that probably contributed to his early demise as his kidneys were ruined (found on autopsy) by his self-experimentation. Interestingly, he was a lactovegetarian for most of his life, and was teetotal until his physician advised him to take moderate amounts of red wine, following a bout of renal disease in 1845, which actually improved his health (Frerichs 2009).

1.2.3 THE RISE OF THE GERM THEORY

Louis Pasteur (1822–1895) discovered that contact with air was required to cause bacterial or fungal growth in fermented products such as wine, beer and vinegar and he developed special glass retorts that would keep the air (and contaminants) at bay. In 1858 he published his observations on microbes growing in a test ferment of beer yeast, which he named 'lactic-yeast' because they caused lactic acid fermentation. However, belonging to the school of Sponteparists, he offered no explanation for the phenomenon, believing, instead, that germs appeared by spontaneous generation. This was despite the fact that a contemporary of his, Antoine Béchamp (see p.24) had shown, in experiments between 1855 and 1857, that sugar water did not ferment unless it was in contact with air and thus exposed to moulds, and that the moulds were therefore the causative organism of the fermentation.

Pasteur continued with his own experiments, taking on board some aspects of Béchamp's work, and he eventually moved towards the airborne organism theory.

Box 1.2 The first vaccine

Edward Jenner (1749–1823) was an English country doctor who observed that milkmaids were generally unaffected by the smallpox that ravaged most other people in the area. He deduced that this was due to their exposure to cowpox, although he may have been helped in this deduction by the work of Benjamin Jesty (among others), who, in 1774, inoculated his wife and children with cowpox as a preventative for smallpox. In 1796, Jenner inoculated an eight-year-old boy with pus from the cowpox blisters of a milkmaid and then later challenged him with smallpox – with no infection resulting. This proved that humans could be protected from the smallpox. Thus was born the first ever 'vaccine' (named from the Latin for 'of the cow', *vaccinus*). Jenner is sometimes referred to as the 'father of immunology' for his work in this arena; not just for the vaccine idea but for showing that it worked.

In 1862 Pasteur was seeking a remedy for the spoiling of ferments of beer, wine and vinegar, and also the souring of milk. Together with Claude Bernard (see p.25) he developed a heating protocol that helped to prolong the life of the ferments by destroying any vegetative organisms within. This process came to be known as pasteurisation.

In 1864 he succeeded in convincing the scientific community that germs were the cause of illness and the spoilage of foodstuffs. In 1865 he proposed the Germ Theory, developed in conjunction with Robert Koch (see below). The Germ Theory stated that microorganisms invade a healthy body and cause disease; and that each germ produces one disease, thus, eliminating that germ would eliminate the disease. This theory was 'monomorphic' – the germs took only one form and could not change.

Pasteur was also famed for producing vaccines for anthrax (in 1881, for use in cattle) and for rabies (in 1885). However, the efficacy of the latter is debatable as, prior to the vaccine being introduced, the average number of deaths from rabies in France was 30 per year; after the vaccine was introduced, this rose to 45 per year (Douglas-Hume 1923).

Robert Koch (1843–1910) is renowned for isolating *Bacillus anthracis* (anthrax) in 1875, *Mycobacterium tuberculosis* (tuberculosis) in 1882 and *Vibrio cholerae* (cholera) in 1883 (identified by Italian Filippo Pacini in 1854 but ignored because of the then-prevalent miasma theory). Koch worked with Pasteur and was another proponent of the Germ Theory, for which he put together four postulates. He said that to establish that an organism is the cause of a disease, it must be:

1. found in every case of the disease examined (but must never be found apart from the disease)

2. capable of being isolated from a diseased organism and maintained in a pure culture outside the body

3. capable of producing, by injection, the same disease as that undergone by the body from which the disease germs were taken

4. capable of being re-isolated from the inoculated diseased experimental organism and shown to be the same as the original inoculated causative agent.

Originally the theory included that the germ, on introduction to a healthy body, *must* cause the original disease, but this (and the first postulate) had to be altered on the discovery of healthy 'carriers' of germs.

These postulates were originally developed for tuberculosis and cholera only, although they were extended to other microbes, but there are many microorganisms to which they do not apply, including several viruses.

Koch and Pasteur together are often regarded as the 'fathers of bacteriology and the Germ Theory'.

Joseph Lister, 1st Baron Lister (1827–1912) started trying to eliminate germs from the surgical arena in order to reduce post-operative infections, mostly gangrene. In 1867 he began using a spray of carbolic acid (phenol) to disinfect the instruments, the gloves and the wounds. However, there were problems with this:

In the earlier antiseptic operations of Lister the patients died in great numbers, so that it came to be a gruesome sort of medical joke to say that 'the operation was successful, but the patient died'. But Lister was a surgeon of great skill and observation, and he gradually reduced his employment of antiseptic material to the necessary and not too large dose, when his 'operations were successful and his patients lived'. (Leverson, Introduction, Béchamp 1912)

Paul Ehrlich (1854–1915) was a great histologist, haematologist and immunologist. He is renowned for his concept of 'the magic bullet' – a target-specific cure for disease-causing organisms – and for coining the term 'chemotherapy'. His other work included:

- early tissue and microbe staining techniques, including the forerunner of the Gram stain

- discovery of atoxyl, useful against sleeping sickness

- development of Salvarsan (asphenamine) for treating syphilis

- illumination of the blood brain barrier.

1.2.4 ALTERNATIVES TO THE GERM THEORY

Pleomorphism

Pierre Jacques Antoine Béchamp (1816–1908) was contemporaneously and quietly working on similar subjects to Pasteur. Despite his Beacon experiments of 1855–1857 showing that moulds were the cause of fermentation in sugar water (as mentioned above), and that creosote, if presented prior to any fungal activity, could prevent its growth, these discoveries were discounted at the time, largely because Pasteur, then in the ascendant, chose to deny them and the Germ Theory had not yet been proposed.

Béchamp also observed the digestive life processes of yeast: 'I became assured that that which is called fermentation is, in reality, the phenomenon of nutrition, assimilation, disassimilation and excretion of the products disassimilated' (Béchamp 1912, p.17).

While studying the products of these ferments under the microscope, Béchamp discovered the existence of units smaller than a cell. He went on to show that they were present in all things, living and dead and called them 'microzyma' (small fermenters). He suggested that they were pleomorphic, that is, able to change their form according to their surroundings. He saw under the microscope these tiny 'scintillating corpuscles' of chemical activity and believed that, by coalescing, they could grow into microbes. He reported seeing some microzyma expanding into coccal bacteria (Douglas-Hume 1923). Thus he believed that disease came from within, that the microzyma were behaving in a pathological way, leading them to generate potentially harmful microbes, because certain circumstances were causing them to do so.

He wrote:

In a state of health the microzymas of an organism act harmoniously... In a state of disease, the microzymas do not act harmoniously and the fermentation is disturbed; the microzymas have either changed their function or are placed in an abnormal situation by some modification of the medium. (Béchamp 1912, p.397)

In other words, harmful microzymas arise *because* the body is out of balance, they do not *cause* the imbalance, as the Germ Theory suggests. Once the body is out of balance, it becomes vulnerable to external attack – germs become symptoms that then stimulate the occurrence of more symptoms. So our bodies are in effect mini-ecosystems, or biological terrains, in which nutritional status, levels of toxicity and metabolic balance play key roles.

Because of this, Béchamp was vehemently against the use of vaccines. He said that 'the most serious disorders may be provoked by the injection of living organisms into the blood' (Douglas-Hume 1923, p.276) as this would cause a disruption to the balance of the system and the microzymas would start to develop into pathogens.

Milieu interieur

Claude Bernard (1813–1878), another contemporary of Pasteur, worked with him to develop the process called pasteurisation. Although he shared several of Pasteur's beliefs, he differed in one major aspect – he believed in the supremacy of the 'milieu interieur', the internal terrain. Thus, in a departure from the Germ Theory, he believed that the state of the body, rather than any invading organism, was the most important factor in disease. If the body were healthy, the organism would not take hold and no disease would result.

He wrote:

The fixity of the milieu supposes a perfection of the organism such that the external variations are at each instant compensated for and equilibrated... All of the vital mechanisms, however varied they may be, have always one goal, to maintain the uniformity of the conditions of life in the internal environment... The constancy of the internal environment is the condition for a free and independent life. (Bernard 1974)

This last idea is the first principle of homeostasis. However, these beliefs were largely ignored until the early part of the twentieth century, when Walter Cannon (see p.30) laid down his principles of homeostasis.

Bernard was also a great student of scientific methodology and wrote *An Introduction to the Study of Experimental Medicine* in 1865. His points about what makes a good scientist include this very important note: 'Authority versus Observation – "When we meet a fact which contradicts a prevailing theory, we must accept the fact and abandon the theory, even when the theory is supported by great names and generally accepted"' (Bernard 1974).

Louis Pasteur, on his deathbed, finally acknowledged that 'the germ is nothing, the terrain is everything', in other words, that his old partner, Claude Bernard, had the right idea and that he, Pasteur, had been wrong.

The Cellular Theory

This is a composite of the principles of pleomorphism and milieu interieur.

1.3 The twentieth century

1.3.1 ANTIBIOTICS

Antibiotics were in development during the early part of the twentieth century and some of the earliest were called the sulpha drugs. Sulphonamide, which saved Winston Churchill's life in Carthage during the Second World War, was developed in Germany and produced in Britain.

Alexander Fleming (1881–1955) is famed for the discovery of the first truly effective antibiotic, penicillin, in 1928. Having served in the army in the First World War, he saw the deaths of many soldiers through septicaemia, and acknowledged that many of these were due to the antiseptics used at the time. He proposed that the antiseptics were depressing the patients' immune systems more effectively than any microbes, because the antiseptics killed aerobic microbes, including ones beneficial to the body, thus allowing the dangerous anaerobes deep within the tissues to proliferate unchecked. Penicillin comes from the fungus, *Penicillium* species. It was effective against many disease-causing agents, including those responsible for scarlet fever, meningitis, pneumonia, diphtheria and gonorrhoea.

Fleming also noticed that antibiotic resistance could arise if the wrong dose was used or if treatment was stopped too early. He therefore advised that it should only be used in appropriately diagnosed cases and that patients should take the full course prescribed for the full length of time.

Scientists working in a British team, Florey, Chain and Heatley, cultivated, stabilised and tested penicillin around 1940 and American pharmaceutical interests collaborated to produce vast amounts of the antibiotic by 1944.

Since then, many more antibiotics have been developed in an attempt to counter antibiotic resistance, which, as predicted, has become increasingly prevalent. Among certain strains of bacteria it can occur rapidly, creating life-threatening situations. To combat these resistant bacteria, more toxic antibiotics are created, with concomitant health risks.

OTHER IMPORTANT ADVANCES IN MEDICINE

Marie Sklodowska Curie (1867–1934) was a physicist who gained two joint Nobel Prizes (for Physics and Chemistry). She and her husband Pierre Curie coined the term 'radioactivity' and they spent many years working together on the isolation of radioactive isotopes and the use of radiation therapy in the treatment of cancers. After Pierre's accidental death in 1906, his Chair at the Sorbonne passed to Mme Curie, allowing her to become the first female Professor there. Ironically, Mme Curie died of aplastic anaemia, almost certainly as a result of her longterm exposure to radiation.

Linus Pauling (1901–1994), another holder of two Nobel Prizes (for Chemistry and Peace), had a great interest in the chemical bond and x-ray crystallography. He created Pauling's Rules and was a renowned scientist but his place in this book is due to his creation of the concept of orthomolecular medicine: the use of the 'right molecules in the right amount'. Pauling believed that diseases could be treated and prevented by providing the body with optimal amounts of substances that are natural to the body.

Pauling published an article on psychiatry in *Science* in 1968, in which he coined the term orthomolecular medicine. In this article he discussed the need for optimal amounts of nutrients in restoring health in mental disease. He proposed that optimal amounts may be different from that provided by the diet and endogenous synthesis; and different from the 'recommended' (average) daily amounts suggested to avoid symptoms of deficiency. He was also aware that individuals have different requirements based on their genetics. He wrote: 'I believe that mental disease is for the most part caused by abnormal reaction rates, as determined by genetic constitution and diet and by abnormal molecular concentrations of essential substances' (Pauling 1968). Thus he recommended 'the use, where effective, of supplemental vitamins C, B3 (niacin), B12 (cyanocobalamin), B6; and of "vitamin P" (bioflavonoids) and L-glutamic acid'. He also strongly recommended further research in this area (Pauling 1968).

Pauling had first been introduced to the idea of food supplements in 1941 by Dr Thomas Addis, who treated Pauling for Bright's disease with a low salt, low protein diet, and who prescribed vitamin and mineral supplements for all his patients. Pauling gave a lecture on molecular medicine in the early 1950s and by the late 1950s was working on enzymes in brain function. However, it was reading Abram Hoffer's *Niacin Therapy in Psychiatry* in 1965 that prompted him to think about vitamin deficiencies in terms of more than just their associated deficiency disease states. In 1966 Irwin Stone brought the concept of high-dose vitamin C to his notice and from then on Pauling took 3g/day to prevent colds. In 1971 he started to collaborate with Ewan Cameron, a British cancer surgeon, on the use of vitamin C, orally and intravenously, as a therapy for terminal cancer patients. However, the medical establishment dismissed Pauling's claims for vitamin C as 'quackery' after two studies failed to substantiate Pauling's work. He in turn denounced these studies as they did not follow the same protocol as he had, but he was effectively discredited and became isolated from funding sources and academic support. Intravenous vitamin C has recently been proposed again as a therapy for cancer, appearing to be selectively toxic against cancer cells (Chen *et al.* 2007).

In 1973, in conjunction with two colleagues, Pauling founded the Institute of Orthomolecular Medicine, since renamed the Linus Pauling Institute, now a part of Oregon State University. Today it continues to research micronutrients, phytochemicals and other dietary components as treatments and preventives for disease. Francis Crick dubbed Linus Pauling the 'father of molecular biology'. He and Einstein were the only two scientists of the twentieth century listed in *New Science*'s 'Twenty Greatest Scientists of All Time'.

Ancel Keys (1904–2004) started out studying chemistry but later transferred to biological sciences. He set up the Laboratory of Physical Hygiene at Minneapolis University, which later led to him working with the US army in 1941 to develop rations for combat troops – these were called K rations.

Towards the end of the Second World War, Keys started the 'starvation experiment' to discover how best to combat starvation in war-torn countries. Using consenting conscientious objectors, he put them on half the normal calories for adult males for five months, with regular exercise. In that time the average weight loss was 25 per cent, strength reduction was limited but endurance dropped to half. More importantly he found that it took more than three months of above-normal calorie intake to reverse the responses, and higher protein intake was essential. In 1950 he published his results in what was considered the definitive work on human starvation, *Biology of Human Starvation*.

Statistics from the postwar period showed that heart disease had dropped markedly when food supplies were restricted. This led Keys to the conclusion for which he is most famous – and gave him his nickname of 'Monsieur Cholesterol' – that diets high in fat, and particularly saturated fat, cause excessive blood cholesterol and lead to heart disease. He was more interested in finding dietary factors to help prevent heart disease than he was in finding a cure, and from the 1950s onwards he travelled the world with his biochemist wife, collecting data on heart disease in different populations. He found that heart disease correlated with blood cholesterol levels and dietary saturated fat intake. Keys advocated a proper diet, exercise, emotional stability and the avoidance of smoking and fad dieting (he was also no fan of jogging) (Hoffman 1979).

Both the US Dietary Association's (USDA) specific dietary guidelines of the 1980s and the Food Guide Pyramid of 1992 were based partly on Keys' work (Davis and Saltos 1999). These promoted a low fat, high carbohydrate diet, and the replacement of animal fats with vegetable oils. However, this supposedly healthy way of eating is now being challenged as there is a growing body of scientific opinion that saturated fats and cholesterol pose less of a risk to health than do *trans* fats, polyunsaturated fatty acid (PUFA) imbalances and/or excessive dietary sugars and starches (Ottoboni and Ottoboni 2004).

Keys himself was a great proponent of the Mediterranean Diet and wrote his third book, *Eat Well, Stay Well the Mediterranean Way*, in 1975. Around this time, he moved to Italy and remained there until the year before he died, aged 100.

Elucidation of the double helix structure of DNA in 1953 came about by the combined efforts of **Francis Crick** and **James D. Watson** in Cambridge, helped enormously by the excellent x-ray crystallography of **Rosalind Franklin** at King's College, London. **Maurice Wilkins**, a co-worker of hers, showed the Cambridge scientists an unpublished x-ray diffraction picture of deoxyribonucleic acid (DNA) and it was this picture that allowed them to finally put all the pieces of the jigsaw together and model the double helix structure of DNA. Sadly Rosalind Franklin died in 1958, aged 37, of ovarian cancer – if she had lived, she might have also been a recipient of the Nobel Prize that went to Crick, Watson and Wilkins (Wright 1999).

The elucidation of the structure of DNA has allowed immense leaps forward in biological and medical science. Since the mapping of the human genome in 2003 it has become possible to identify an individual's particular pattern of gene variants that may predispose him or her to specific diseases. As more is learnt about the involvement of specific genes and genetic polymorphisms in particular diseases, we will become increasingly adept at predicting an individual's risk and devising personally tailored nutrition and lifestyle prevention programmes (Nicolle 2007) and personalised drug treatments with individually tailored dosing. (This approach, being predictive and individualised, shares some of the principles of FM – see section 3 of this chapter.)

However, one should not overlook the ethical issues involved, nor the fact that the aetiologies of most human diseases involve more than simply a genetic predisposition. For example, genetic diagnostic tools do not generally identify epigenetic changes, that is, the transfer of genetic information without the use of the genetic code. Such changes are increasingly considered important in the risk for diseases such as cancer (World Cancer Research Fund 1997). Also see Chapter 8 for a discussion of the importance to human health of the millions of genes contained in the microbiome.

1.3.3 MODERN SUPPORT FOR BÉCHAMP'S THEORY

Returning to Béchamp's theory of pleomorphism (see 1.2.4), there is some debate as to the real identity of the microzymas. It has been suggested that he was seeing some kind of ribonucleic acid (RNA), or perhaps that they were microsomes (James 1995).

Dr E.C. Rosenow (1875–1966) first demonstrated pleomorphic bacteria around 1910, when he observed that different strains of streptococcal bacteria could transform into other strains when placed in different culture media (Rosenow 1914). He also established that the streptococcal bacteria found in pus-filled wounds would change over time to staphylococci, due to the breakdown of blood (the bacterial medium). However, his work was not accepted at the time.

Microbiologists at this stage in medical history were split into the Filtrationists and the non-Filtrationists. The former believed that bacteria were able to change (pleomorphic) and pass through fine filters, while the latter believed that bacteria were monomorphic and were therefore too large to do so, and that only viruses could pass through filters.

Royal Raymond Rife (1888–1971) developed microscopes that had unprecedented magnification of up to x50,000. His use of refracting quartz prisms that allowed variable light frequencies to be employed allowed him to see objects far smaller than any other contemporary laboratory. In 1925 he saw tiny sub-cellular units (cellules), refracting in different colours, that had come from preparations of various tumours, so he called them cancer viruses. Naming them BX (from bacillus X), he demonstrated that the cancer virus could morph into various forms, including viral and fungal, depending on the medium in which it was grown, finally reverting back to the non-pathogenic 'bacillus coli'. Using Koch's postulates, he inoculated the BX virus into mice and re-created the initial tumour from which the virus had been isolated (Rife 1953). The electron microscope (developed during the 1930s and 1940s) is the only other type to achieve such magnification, but the electron microscope alters, even kills, what is being viewed. Rife's microscope allowed living organisms to be seen in their natural state.

Rosenow, along with Dr Arthur Kendall and Rife, viewed the tuberculosis bacteria under the Rife microscope and saw it in different stages – as the almost colourless bacillus, as a small independent turquoise cellule and at an in-between stage. What they saw showed that the tubercule bacillus was pleomorphic – it could disintegrate its larger structure, leaving only the tiny turquoise cellule that could pass through the filters (like a virus) and, when placed in an appropriate medium, it could expand back into a tubercle bacillus (Bird 1976). These cellules are possibly the microzymas that Béchamp saw, decades earlier.

These findings all indicate that it is the *medium*, or environment, in which the organism grows that determines its state, thus supporting the Cellular Theory (see p.26) and questioning the Germ Theory.

Pleomorphic bacteria have since been found in the blood of healthy individuals, an environment that had been thought to be microbially sterile (McLaughlin *et al.* 2002); this follows on from the discovery of similar bacteria living parasitically inside erythrocytes, where they were discovered to be taking up thymidine, uracil and glycine – not a function normally associated with red blood cell (RBC) metabolism (Tedeshi, Amici and Paparelli 1969). *Candida albicans* is a well-known example of a pleomorphic fungus.

The discussion above is by no means exhaustive; there are many other figures who have played significant roles in shaping modern medicine as we know it.

2. Homeostasis and allostasis

2.1 Homeostasis

Walter Cannon (1871–1945) defined the first principles of homeostasis in the first half of the twentieth century, shortly after the discovery of penicillin, and following on from Bernard's proposals in the previous century:

- 'Constancy in an open system, such as our bodies represent, requires mechanisms that act to maintain this constancy.' (Cannon based this proposition on insights into the ways by which steady states such as glucose concentrations, body temperature and acid-base balance were regulated.)

- Steady-state conditions require that any tendency toward change automatically meets with factors that resist change. An increase in blood sugar results in thirst, as the body attempts to dilute the concentration of sugar in the extracellular fluid.

- The regulating system that determines the homeostatic state consists of a number of co-operating mechanisms acting simultaneously or successively. Blood sugar is regulated by insulin, glucagon and other hormones that control its release from the liver or its uptake by the tissues.

- Homeostasis does not occur by chance, but is the result of organised self-government.

(Cannon 1932, pp.299–300)

The word homeostasis comes from the Greek for 'same' (*homo*) and 'stable' (*stasis*). Homeostasis thus means 'remaining stable by staying the same' and was the perceived 'health' goal – everything in the body working to maintain a static position. Many pharmaceutical interventions work towards this goal of maintaining a static 'norm' by suppressing extreme responses.

Nowadays, this model seems somewhat restrictive and cannot explain many of the common complaints of modern life, such as hypertension and metabolic syndrome. Thus a new paradigm was suggested – that of allostasis.

2.2 Allostasis

Peter Sterling and **Joseph Eyer** (1988) proposed the theory of allostasis: *allo* from the Greek for other, different, varied or the opposite of normal, depending on the context. Thus allostasis can be defined as 'remaining stable by changing'. According to Sterling, allostasis should replace homeostasis as the model of physiological regulation; it should not be considered as merely a modulator of homeostasis (Sterling 2003). The allostasis model is better able to explain chronic conditions like hypertension, obesity and diabetes, as well as problems like drug addiction.

In his 2003 essay **John C. Wingfield** states: 'The concept of allostasis, maintaining stability through change, is a fundamental process through which organisms actively adjust to both predictable and unpredictable events' (pp.807–816). Wingfield defines 'allostatic load' as the cumulative cost to the body of allostasis. In other words, the amount of work that has to be done to re-establish homeostasis can be detrimental. When 'load' becomes 'overload', this can result in illness or disease. With **Bruce S. McEwen**, he goes on to propose two types of allostatic overload, which have different responses and outcomes:

Type I – energy demand exceeds supply. This activates 'survival mode' in extreme circumstances, decreasing allostatic load in order to regain a positive energy balance. When the challenge has passed, normal service can resume. This could be allied with the 'fight or flight' mechanism, wherein all energies are channelled to the rapid responses required to save immediate life, leaving all non-essential processes devoid of energy until the crisis has passed.

Type II – there is sufficient or even excessive energy intake, but there are other stressors in terms of social interactions – conflict, repression, fear, loneliness and other dysfunctional scenarios.

(McEwen and Wingfield 2003)

In 2003 Sterling put forward six underlying principles that drive allostasis:

1. Organisms are designed to be efficient.

2. Efficiency requires reciprocal trade-offs.

3. Efficiency also requires being able to predict future needs.

4. Such prediction requires each sensor to adapt to the expected range of input.

5. Prediction also demands that each effector adapt its output to the expected range of demand.

6. Predictive regulation depends on behaviour, while neural mechanisms also adapt.

In allostasis, the body has a relatively high level of flexibility in response to challenges but after a while the maintenance of allostatic changes where the body fails to revert to 'normal status', leading to overload, begins to have consequences. These are likely to be pathological in nature, for example hypertension, obesity, type 2 diabetes, addictive behaviours and psychological problems.

Hypertension is a good example: during the day, our blood pressure will fluctuate around the 'norm' of approximately 110/70, where this value is the most frequently required. It can reach 170/90 in times of extreme physical activity and drop to 55/40 during deep sleep. None of this is pathological – the need meets the demand. However, if the demand is frequently or even constantly set at a higher level, due to stress for example, then the 'norm' will be reset higher. This is 'adaptation of response' and, although it may result in pathology, it is not necessarily inappropriate, nor is it due to any level of dysregulation. Environmental factors have been responded to in a 'normal' fashion – it is the environmental factors (or, more accurately, the individual's interpretation of these) that are dysregulated and inappropriate, not the response.

As the physiological response is normal, not dysfunctional, where should therapeutics intervene? Current interventions aim at the body's reactions, rather than the instigators of the reactions, but this has three main problems:

1. Every signal has multiple cascading effects; affecting one signal will affect many cascades, some inappropriately and detrimentally (iatrogenic effects).

2. The brain is driving the response – altering the response by drug intervention causes the brain to compensate by driving other mechanisms harder.

3. 'Clamping' responses to a set level reduces the ability of the body to respond to changing need, thus blocking physiological regulation.

Drugs can force the response back to the 'norm' but this reduces the range of responsiveness.

In allostasis, therapy should aim to shift the demand range back to its 'normal' level. In many cases this can be achieved by altering lifestyle and diet. The allostasis model also implies that better health could be achieved by restoring small satisfactions in life, in work and in leisure.

3. Functional medicine (FM)

The model of allostasis is the bedrock upon which are firmly planted the roots of FM. While allostatic load refers to the cumulative negative effects of stress (such as poor diet, exposure to environmental toxins and destructive relationships) over an individual's lifetime, FM aims to identify the individual's (current and previous) problematic challenges and environments, understand how they have affected him or her and provide interventions to help redress the consequent biochemical changes.

The Functional model draws on the knowledge areas of nutrition science and molecular biology and is defined as a science-based 'patient-centred healthcare approach to assessing, preventing and treating complex chronic disease' (Institute for Functional Medicine 2007). Created in the 1980s by the nutritional biochemist Dr Jeff Bland, it has become a fast-growing movement amongst North American doctors who believe that allopathic medicine is limiting because it does not treat 'the whole person'. Instead of asking, 'what disease does the patient have?' and then prescribing agents that suppress the symptoms (the allopathic model), FM asks, 'what sort of individual has the disease?' It then sets about identifying and modifying the unique set of biochemical imbalances that are present in that individual. This, in turn, is claimed by the model's creators to ultimately halt or slow the disease process and thus attain better patient outcomes than the conventional allopathic approach of controlling signs and symptoms (Jones, Bland and Quinn 2005, pp.5–10). (Note that FM's departure from the allopathic model is specific to chronic care, not acute care.)

This principle of 'biochemical individuality', together with the significance of 'inputs' during the individual's whole life history, are embedded within the FM model, as they are in the model of allostatic load. As mentioned above, the FM model is at the heart of this book. A full list of the principles of FM can be seen at the Institute for Functional Medicine's website: www.functionalmedicine.org/about/whatis.asp.

As well as its holistic approach and its grounding in the biochemical sciences, another advantage claimed by FM's advocates is that the model includes therapies like diet, food supplements and exercise, which (although there are exceptions) tend to have fewer side-effects than prescription medications.

3.1 The adoption and usage of the FM model among UK nutritional therapists

According to a recent literature search, as yet there appear to be no published statistics regarding the current usage of the model, nor any recorded objections to the use of FM, by any type of healthcare practitioner worldwide. This lack of information is not altogether surprising, given that FM is still a minority healthcare paradigm compared to allopathic medicine, partly due to lack of awareness, but also because it does not adhere to the principles of reductionism and specialisation that underlie most conventional medical training.

However, a qualitative survey of UK nutritional therapists (NTs) (Nicolle 2008)[1] found that FM is increasingly becoming adopted as their model of choice. (For more information on the training, qualifications and quality standards of NTs see the Nutritional THerapy Council (NTC) Professional Standards Council at www.nutritionaltherapycouncil.org.uk and the regulatory body at www.cnhc.org.uk. The regulatory body also holds a register of competent practitioners.) The survey found that FM users who also had experience of using other models believe that they benefit from:

- improved patient outcomes

- improved patient understanding of his/her health issues

- enhanced practitioner understanding of the individual patient's case

- enhanced practitioner knowledge of human physiology and biochemistry.

Logically, this could lead to more constructive communications with conventional medical practitioners and a greater ability to provide a multi-disciplinary healthcare service to patients.

The only real drawback of FM that came out of the qualitative data was its perceived relative expense to the patient, due to the significant investment of practitioner time and the use of functional tests. Despite this, the survey found that FM was still seen as being overall better value for money than other models, due to its improved precision of diagnosis and treatment.

4. The chapters

We have brought together the information in the following chapters because we firmly believe that the FM approach to patient care may be the most logical, useful and enlightening *modus operandi* for our healthcare system in the twenty-first century.

Of the ten chapters that follow, the first nine each focus on a particular type of biochemical imbalance. Many of the book's contributors are clinicians and are therefore acutely aware of the difficulties of interpreting incomplete and sometimes seemingly contradictory scientific data for use in the real world. Thus the concluding chapter comprises a detailed case example, which is designed to walk the reader through the FM approach as it may be applied in practice. It can be read before, after or in conjunction with the technical information of Chapters 2–10.

Chapter 2, 'Gastro-Intestinal Imbalances' – A two-part review of the digestive system in health and imbalance and the usage of probiotics and other natural interventions to help with re-establishing correct function.

---

1   This is qualitative study and, as such, is limited in its sample size and type. The findings must therefore be taken as indicative, rather than as truly representative, of the UK NT population. Furthermore, the study was conducted by an 'insider' to the profession, and thus the researcher's own preconceptions, as a positive supporter of the model, need to be taken into account.

Chapter 3, 'Compromised Detoxification' – A chapter comprising information on tests for detoxification capacity and a range of interventions to reduce the patient's toxic load and improve detoxification function.

Chapter 4, 'Polyunsaturated Fatty Acid (PUFA) Imbalances' – A discussion of the role of PUFAs in health and disease, followed by a focus on PUFAs in neurological health.

Chapter 5, 'Metabolic Syndrome: Insulin Resistance, Dysglycaemia and Dyslipidaemia' – An involved look at imbalances in the control of blood sugar and lipid levels; the metabolic syndrome and some nutritional and lifestyle interventions to consider.

Chapter 6, 'Compromised Thyroid and Adrenal Function' – A detailed discourse on the thyroid and adrenal glands, what can happen when they are not functioning optimally and the nutritional interventions that may help to manage the resulting hormonal imbalances.

Chapter 7, 'Sex Hormone Imbalances' – A range of insights into the effects of environmental inputs on sex hormone balance in the body and the resulting (ill-) health conditions.

Chapter 8, 'Dysregulation of the Immune System: A Gastro-Centric Perspective' – A review of the immune system and how imbalances can contribute to systemic inflammation and other conditions of ill health.

Chapter 9, 'Poor Energy Production and Increased Oxidative Stress' – A discussion of oxidative stress, especially with regard to its effects on the mitochondria; and the importance of antioxidants.

Chapter 10, 'Dysregulated Neurotransmitter Function' – A look at a range of functional neurological imbalances and some natural interventions to consider.

Chapter 11, 'Putting Knowledge into Practice: A Case Study' – An in-depth case example of how the functional model can be applied nutritionally to a patient with multiple presenting symptoms, in this case, rheumatoid arthritis, fatigue, slow cognition and irritable bowel syndrome.

We have found this an exciting book to put together – we hope you will find it a stimulating read.

AN IMPORTANT NOTE

We must stress that the nutritional guidelines and cautions for nutritional supplementation given in these chapters are not exhaustive, nor are they prescriptive. Patients of nutrition practitioners should also consult an appropriate medical professional if they have a medical condition and/or undiagnosed symptoms.

Nutritional supplements should only be used where dietary intake is inadequate for the patient's needs, and in conjunction with dietary modification, taking into account any drug/nutrient interactions. Supplementation should be managed and reviewed in line with regular medical monitoring and laboratory testing. Individuals should not discontinue, or alter the dosage of, any medication without the knowledge of their medical practitioner.

References

Béchamp, A. (1912) *The Blood and Its Third Anatomical Element: Application of the Microzymian Theory*, translated by M.R. Leverson. London: John Ouseley.

Bernard, C. (1974) *Lectures on the Phenomena Common to Animals and Plants*, translated by H.E. Hoff, R. Guillemin and L. Guillemin. Springfield, IL: Charles C. Thomas.

Bird, C. (1976) 'What has become of the Rife microscope?' *New Age Journal* (March 1976), 41–47.

Bryan, C.S. and Podolsky, S.H. (2009) 'Dr. Holmes at 200 – the spirit of skepticism.' *New England Journal of Medicine 361*, 9, 846–847.

Cannon, W. (1932) *The Wisdom of the Body*. New York: W.W. Norton and Company.

Chen, Q., Espey, M.G., Sun, A.Y., Lee, J.H. *et al.* (2007) 'Ascorbate in pharmacologic concentrations selectively generates ascorbate radical and hydrogen peroxide in extracellular fluid in vivo.' *Proceedings of the National Academy of Sciences 104*, 21, 8749.

Davis, C. and Saltos, E. (1999) 'Dietary recommendations and how they have changed over time.' In E. Frazao (ed.) *America's Eating Habits: Changes and Consequences*. Washington, DC: US Department of Agriculture.

Douglas-Hume, E. (1923) *Béchamp or Pasteur?* London: C.W. Daniel.

Frerichs, R. (2009) 'John Snow's final rest.' Available at www.ph.ucla.edu/epi/snow/death.html, accessed on 28 October 2009.

Hoffman, W. (1979) 'Meet Monsieur Cholesterol.' University of Minnesota *Update* (winter). Available at www.mbbnet.umn.edu/hoff/hoff_ak.html, accessed on 28 October 2009.

Hyman, M. and Jones, D. (2009) *Healthcare Watch*. Available by email via suesabol@fxmed.com.

Institute for Functional Medicine (2007) *What is Functional Medicine?* Gig Harbour, WA: Institute for Functional Medicine. Available at www.functionalmedicine.org, accessed on 28 October 2009.

James, W. (1995) *Immunization: The Reality Behind the Myth*, 2nd edn. Santa Barbara, CA: Greenwood Publishing Group.

Jones, D. and Quinn, S. (2005) 'Why Functional Medicine?' In D. Jones (ed.) (2005) *The Textbook of Functional Medicine*. Gig Harbour, WA: Institute for Functional Medicine.

Jones, D.S., Bland, J.S. and Quinn, S. (2005) *Introduction to Functional Medicine*. In D.S. Jones (2005) *The Textbook of Functional Medicine*. Gig Harbour, WA: IFM.

Louis, P.C.A. (1844) *Researches on Phthisis, Anatomical, Pathological and Therapeutical*, 2nd edn, translated by W.H. Walshe. London: Sydenham Society.

McEwen, B.S. and Wingfield, J.C. (2003) 'The concept of allostasis in biology and biomedicine.' *Hormones and Behaviour 43*, 1, 2–15.

McLaughlin, R.W., Vali, H., Lau, P.C.K., Palfree, R.G.E. *et al.* (2002) 'Are there naturally occurring pleomorphic bacteria in the blood of healthy humans?' *Journal Of Clinical Microbiology 40*, 12, 4771–4775.

National Association of Naturopathic Physicians (1970) *Outline for Study of Services of Practitioners Performing Health Services in Independent Practice – Part II – The Discipline*, report presented to US Congress.

Neeb, K. (2001) *Fundamentals of Mental Health Nursing*, 2nd edn. Philadelphia: F.A. Davis.

Nicolle, L. (2007) 'Nutrigenomics in practice: The use of genetic and allied screening tools on a client with known genetic risks for developing a chronic disease.' *Nutrition Practitioner 8*, 3, 4–12.

Nicolle, L. (2008) 'A critical exploration of nutritional therapists' perceptions of the use and value of the Functional Medicine model in nutritional therapy practice and education.' Unpublished paper.

Ottoboni, A. and Ottoboni, F. (2004) 'The Food Guide Pyramid: Will the defects be corrected?' *Journal of American Physicians and Surgeons 9*, 4, 109–113.

Pauling, L. (1968) 'Orthomolecular psychiatry.' *Science n.s. 160*, 3825, 265–271.

Rife, R.R. (1953) *History of the Development of a Successful Treatment for Cancer and other Virus, Bacteria and Fungi.* San Diego, CA: Research Laboratory Data, Allied Industries.

Rosenow, E.C. (1914) 'Transmutations within the streptococcus-pneumococcus group.' *Journal of Infectious Diseases 14.*

Smallwood, C. (2005) *The Role of Complementary and Alternative Medicine in the NHS.* London: Freshminds.

Sterling, P. (2003) 'Principles of Allostasis: Optimal Design, Predictive Regulation, Pathophysiology, and Rational Therapeutics.' In J. Schulkin (ed.) *Allostasis, Homeostasis, and the Costs of Physiological Adaptation.* Cambridge, MA: MIT Press.

Sterling, P. and Eyer, J. (1988) 'Allostasis: A New Paradigm to Explain Arousal Pathology.' In S. Fisher and J. Reason (eds) *Handbook of Life Stress, Cognition and Health.* New York: John Wiley & Sons.

Summers, J. (1989) *Soho – A History of London's Most Colourful Neighbourhood.* London: Bloomsbury. Available at www.ph.ucla.edu/epi/snow/broadstreetpump.html, accessed on 28 October 2009.

Tedeshi, G.G., Amici, D. and Paparelli, M. (1969) 'Incorporation of nucleosides and amino-acids in human erythrocyte suspensions: possible relation with a diffuse infection of mycoplasmas or bacteria in the L form.' *Nature 222*, 1285–1286.

Wingfield, J.C. (2003) 'Anniversary essay: Control of behavioural strategies for capricious environments.' *Animal Behaviour 66.*

World Cancer Research Fund (1997) *Food, Nutrition and the Prevention of Cancer: A Global Perspective.* Washington, DC: American Institute for Cancer Research.

Wright, R. (1999) 'The Time 100 – James Watson & Francis Crick.' *Time Magazine* (29 Mar).

Chapter 2

GASTRO-INTESTINAL IMBALANCES

Part 1 The gastro-intestinal tract – Use and abuse

Laurence Trueman and Justine Bold

1. Gastro-intestinal imbalances and disease

Imbalances in the gastro-intestinal (GI) tract are now widely believed to be contributory factors to the development of many chronic diseases, including inflammatory bowel disease (IBD) (O'Hara and Shanahan 2006) and rheumatic disease (Chong and Wang 2008). This chapter will investigate the ways in which GI imbalances can lead to a wide range of symptoms.

Gastro-intestinal disease itself frequently exists with other disease, as there are many well-documented co-morbidities. For instance, coeliac disease, Crohn's disease and ulcerative colitis are all associated with an overall increased risk of cancer (Goldacre *et al.* 2008), whilst Seaman *et al.* (2008) report that women with endometriosis are more likely to have irritable bowel syndrome (IBS). Further, Hillilä *et al.* (2008) suggest that not only are depressed patients more likely to have IBS but that there is a positive correlation between depression and GI problems in the general population. The frequent occurrence of such co-morbidities supports the view of The Institute for Functional Medicine, which has pioneered the functional medicine (FM) philosophy, in which underlying imbalances are addressed in order to both prevent and treat chronic disease (Jones 2005).

Gastro-intestinal diseases are often extremely distressing for patients, and studies on the health-related quality of life report a significant reduction with conditions such as Crohn's disease (Cohen 2002) and IBS (Rey *et al.* 2008). One study reports the reduction in health-related quality of life among IBS sufferers as of a similar magnitude to that experienced by patients with congestive heart failure (Whitehead *et al.* 1996).

There is much the practitioner can do to relieve the symptoms associated with digestive imbalances, and some management strategies are detailed later. However, many such problems start with simple disturbances in the functioning of the digestive system due to modern day living, and it is thus worth considering how such imbalances arise.

2. Physiological imbalances of the human digestive system

This section seeks to give a brief understanding of how to maximise the digestive function using an evidence-based exploration of physiology. Whenever possible, references detailing attributes of the human digestive system have been used, but with ethical considerations rightly restricting experimentation in live subjects, some references detail work on human cadavers, *in vitro* cell lines or other mammals. Many of these will accurately predict the response of the living human digestive system, but caution must be exercised when constructing therapeutic plans based on this data.

2.1 Oral cavity and oesophagus

Digestion starts with chewing, which has three main functions: to reduce particle size, expel air and to mix the food thoroughly with saliva in order to form a bolus. The reduction in particle size increases the surface area of the food allowing the digestive enzymes to function more efficiently, thus poor or painful dentition can impact on the thoroughness of chewing and impair digestion. Perhaps a more serious consequence is the avoidance of tough and fibrous foods such as fruits and vegetables in favour of processed foods, with an associated decrease in the intake of fibre and micronutrients, such as zinc and vitamins A and E (Krall, Hayes and Garcia 1998).

Poor chewing also results in the improper mixing of sufficient volumes of saliva with the food and is often experienced as an uncomfortable slow moving bolus through the oesophagus due to a lack of mucins and statherins that act as lubricants. Mucin secretion occurs throughout the digestive system, aiding lubrication and protecting the mucosa against chemical (e.g. the stomach) and bacterial (e.g. the small intestine) attack. Saliva also has many other functional components, with the presence of the enzymes salivary α-amylase and lipase being well known. The action of the former releases maltose via the digestion of starch.

Saliva has its own pH buffer system in the form of secreted bicarbonate and the enzyme carbonic anhydrase. This enzyme not only adjusts the pH of the bolus to optimise starch and lipid digestion, but is also believed to have a role in protecting taste buds from premature apoptosis (Leinonen *et al.* 2001). Carbonic anhydrase function can be disrupted by zinc insufficiency, and in both humans and rats this has been shown to affect taste acuity. Zinc-deficient rats had an increased preference for salt in their food (Komai *et al.* 2000).

Saliva production can slow or cease (xerostomia) as one gets older (Lopez-Jornet and Bermejo-Fenoll 1994), or in interventions such as chemotherapy, and the risk of dental caries is seen to increase (Garg and Malo 1997). Artificial saliva exists in several forms; gel, spray, pastille or tablet and is taken before/with a meal and sometimes at night to stop a dry palate disturbing sleep. Many forms however, only lubricate the bolus (Preetha and Banerjee 2005) and do not contain α-amylase or lipase, which can have an effect on food flavour and texture (Wijk *et al.* 2004).

Saliva also initiates sterilisation of the food, having antibacterial, antiviral and antifungal activity, including candidacidal action (Xu *et al.* 1991). Inflammation of the gums (periodontal disease and gingivitis) due to the indigenous oral bacteria is extremely common in the UK, with 72 per cent of adults with their own teeth showing evidence of plaque and 54 per cent showing periodontal pocketing (Office for National Statistics 2000).

Natural ways to encourage saliva production (which assumes functional epithelia) is by appreciating the sight and smell of food before consumption, although, as Pavlov famously showed with his dogs, other recurrent stimuli could be used, emphasising the power of expectation and routine. Sufficient chewing will also encourage saliva production, due to a direct synaptic link between the taste buds and salivary glands.

On formation of a bolus, the food, pushed by the tongue, exits the oral cavity and is swallowed, travelling down the oesophagus and into the stomach. One major problem encountered by practitioners is gastric reflux. This is when acid seeps past the lower oesophageal sphincter (LOS) back into the oesophagus. The nutritional strategy to alleviate gastric reflux relies on the reduction of meal size to minimise stomach distension, proper bolus formation to reduce the ingestion of air, avoiding constriction of the upper abdomen by tight clothes or bad posture and avoiding foods that reduce muscular tone of the LOS. Such foods include chocolate, coffee, tea, alcohol, mint or meals high in fat (Castell 1975). Other foods such as citric juices, spicy food and tomato juice do not appear to lower oesophageal sphincter pressure significantly in healthy individuals, but may irritate an already inflamed sphincter due to their pH-lowering activity (Castell 1975). This scenario can also be applied to the consumption of protein-rich food prior to sleep or lying down, as this allows the gastric acid, which is usually confined to the lower part of the stomach, to come into contact with the LOS.

2.2 The stomach

The stomach is a 'J-shaped' sac with four main functions: acting as a reservoir for food; continuing the digestive process; preparing the food to enter the small intestine and as an endocrine gland signalling future digestive status.

Preparation for digestive functions occurs before food enters the stomach due to cephalic reflexes that initiate the secretion of acid and the hormone gastrin. This latter response is further enforced when food enters the stomach, stretching the mucosa as well as stimulating the secretion of digestive enzymes. Finally, the low pH inhibits further gastric secretions. The pH achieved depends on the composition and volume of the food present. In the absence of food the pH is about 1.5, but rises to between 3 and 5 during feeding (Hill 2002). Peptides are found to strongly stimulate acid secretion, while carbohydrates, lipids (Low 1990) and dietary fibre (Tadesse 1986) have only weak effects.

The pH of the lumen (the biological name given to the space inside an anatomical structure that is tubular in form) is an important factor in the ability of the stomach to sterilise the food, with a pH below 2.5 being optimal to kill *Escherichia coli* and *Helicobacter pylori*, but a pH of 3.5 showing little effect (Zhu *et al.* 2006). The amount of acid produced is thus important for health.

2.2.1 HYPOCHLORHYDRIA AND ACHLORHYDRIA

Hydrochloric acid production decreases with age, leading to low (hypochlorhydria) or no (achlorhydria) acid secretion. This used to be attributed to gastric mucosa atrophy (Nilsson-Ehle 1998), due to an autoimmune response, but there is increasing evidence that *H. pylori* infection frequently initiates the condition via gastritis (Lo *et al.* 2005). *H. pylori* infection can be determined by blood or stool tests and can be treated allopathically (90% effective), using a combination of antimicrobial agents for two weeks and a gastric antisecretory drug (Timbury *et al.* 2002). A range of foods and food extracts have also been suggested to aid removal of the bacterium. A recent systematic review of randomised controlled studies on humans demonstrated that fermented milk probiotic preparations improve *H. pylori* eradication rates by 5–15 per cent (Sachdeva and Nagpal 2009) and cranberry juice (2x250mL per day) has also been found to suppress infection (Zhang *et al.* 2005). A laboratory study of manuka honey has suggested that it has antimicrobial activity against *H. pylori* isolated from gastric ulcer biopsy samples, at concentrations consistent with an oral dose (Al Somal *et al.* 1994). The UK government recommends that honey should not be given to babies under 12 months of age owing to the risk of infant botulism (Advisory Committee on the Microbiological Safety of Food 2006, p.3). Other natural substances and common culinary herbs or spices have an inhibitory effect on *H. pylori* bacteria *in vitro*. For instance, allicin, the active component in garlic, inhibited *H. pylori* growth *in vitro* at 20–30μg/mL (Ohta *et al.* 1999), although there is a loss of potency when the garlic is cooked.

There are several clinical consequences of achlorhydria:

- In mice it is associated with bacterial overgrowth and intestinal metaplasia, eventually leading to cancer (Friis-Hansen 2006); bacterial overgrowth has also been recorded in humans (Theisen *et al.* 2000). This can lead to food fermenting in the stomach, increasing burping, acid reflux into the oesophagus and bloating, the main symptoms of low gastric acid, as well as competition for essential nutrients.

- Vitamin B12 (the cobalamins), which is unstable in the alkali conditions that exist in the small intestine, is stabilised by its conjugation to intrinsic factor (IF) secreted by the gastric mucosa. Gastric atrophy leads not only to a reduction in IF, but impaired release of bound B12 from the food, due to insufficient acidification of the lumen. Furthermore, bacterial overgrowth competes for this nutrient. Vitamin B12 malabsorption may also be a side-effect of acid-reducing drugs (Andrès, Noel and Abdelghani 2003). Cobalamins are effectively recycled by the body. Thus deficiency symptoms, such as pernicious anaemia, may take several years to appear. Achlorhydric individuals may require B12 injections, although high dose (1000µg/day) supplementation has also been demonstrated to be effective (Lane and Rojas-Fernandez 2002; Lederle 1991).

- The uptake of some minerals and vitamins may be affected, such as iron (Skikne, Lynch and Cook 1981), calcium (Recker 1985), and folate (Krasinski *et al.* 1986).

Some of the consequences of hypochlorhydria and achlorhydria can be supported by taking hydrochloric acid (HCl) supplements, normally in the form of betaine-HCl capsules – but these are contraindicated in gastritis and if ulcers are present. They normally do not contain proteases, nor IF, but may help to control gastric flora and the regulation of GI pH. A simple test to help assess acid production can be done using a bicarbonate solution (see Box 2.1).

Box 2.1 The bicarbonate test for the assessment of gastric acid secretion

The stomach must be empty of food. Take a glass of water and stir in one teaspoon of bicarbonate of soda. Induce acid secretion by cephalic reflex (thinking, smelling or observing desired food for several minutes). Drink the entire contents and wait 10–15 minutes. If acid is present it will react with the bicarbonate producing carbon dioxide, resulting in eructation (burping). If there is no effect then acid levels may be low.

2.2.2 HYPERCHLORHYDRIA

The ability to stimulate natural secretion of gastric acid will depend on the functionality of the gastric mucosa. Cephalic-vagal-mediated reflex due to the anticipation, sight and smell of food, preparation and routine meal times, has been estimated to account for a third of gastric acid secretion (Richardson *et al.* 1977).

Hyperchlorhydria is the production of excess gastric acid; this is related to the volume, not the pH. The most common cause is due to delayed gastric evacuation and has very similar symptoms to hypochlorhydria (burping, oesophageal reflux and bloating). In general the rate of gastric emptying is controlled by the small intestine and depends on meal composition with macronutrients exiting in the order of carbohydrates, proteins and fats.

Gastric emptying is also controlled by diurnal rhythms, with faster emptying occurring in the morning than the afternoon. Knowledge of this may aid in the treatment of one of the most common oesophageal complaints, gastroesophageal reflux. It is well documented (although not scientifically) that some forms of food combining can reduce the incidence of this condition by, in its most basic form, partitioning bulk protein and carbohydrate (starch) ingestion to separate meals in the day. This limits those combinations of foods that result in a low acid environment and the potential for microbial fermentation which can lead to gastric bloating, burping and an increased risk of reflux. Eating the protein-based meal earlier in the day when gastric emptying is faster may lead to a reduced risk of reflux during this period of low gastric pH and the longer retention time required to process protein. This is further aided by the increased probability that an upright posture will be maintained and that the greater feeling of satiation that protein induces may translate into a smaller meal, thus reducing the volume of the gastric lumen and the proximity of gastric acid to the lower oesophageal sphincter. Later in the day, carbohydrate-based meals will result in a higher pH of the lumen and thus reduce the severity of burning of the oesophagus if reflux occurs, particularly because sleeping or 'lounging' places the stomach in a more lateral orientation, thus increasing the proximity of gastric acid to the sphincter. Care must be taken as to the processing of this latter meal in order to reduce the microbial load present, thus reducing the potential for fermentation, and also to its composition in order to avoid problems with glycaemic control.

2.3 The small intestine

The small intestine is the longest of all the sections of the GI tract and is formed from three histologically distinct regions: the duodenum, the jejunum and the ileum.

As the chyme (partially-digested food) passes through the pyloric sphincter it enters the duodenum, which has a high density of Brunner's glands that secrete protective alkali mucus. The pancreas has already responded to cephalic and hormonal influences by initiating secretion of small but concentrated amounts of pancreatic juice, including bicarbonate, however, the majority of secretion (60–70%) occurs when chyme enters the duodenum (Barrett 2006).

The jejunum is the major site of digestion and water, ion and nutrient uptake. Up to this point, between 7 and 10L of fluid has been secreted into the digestive system of a typical adult in a 24-hour period. The water stress a large meal can impose on a person who is not hydrated must be appreciated. Most of this water is reabsorbed in the small intestine.

The small intestinal mucosa is coated with a matrix of enzymes, including peptidases, oligosaccharidases and disaccharidases such as sucrase, maltase and lactase. This last enzyme is often missing from non-Caucasian adults, resulting in lactose intolerance. The result of digestion is the simple monomers that make up the complex macromolecules (amino acids, fatty acids, monosaccharides and nucleotides).

There is currently a lot of interest in jejunal flora, particularly concerning the possible link between the presence of bacterial overgrowth and IBS. In Western countries, jejunal microflora of healthy individuals mainly consists of Gram-positive, facultative bacteria such as *Lactobacillus* species (spp.); while the Gram-negative *Enterobacteriaceae* are absent or few in numbers (Cain *et al.* 1976). Generally, the jejunum naturally maintains low bacterial numbers by a rapid transit rate.

Jejunum bacterial overgrowth appears to be associated with protein-energy malnutrition (PEM) and has been reported in many populations where kwashiorkor[1] is common (Cain *et al.* 1976), apparently due to raised gastric pH reducing the ability of the stomach to sterilise the chyme and promoting gastric mucosa atrophy (Winick 1979). Another consequence of PEM is reduced expression of enzymes by the enterocytes (Römer *et al.* 1983), leading to decreased nutrient availability.

Jejunum floral overgrowth leads to deconjugation of bile acids even by genera considered to be beneficial (Klaver and van der Meer 1993), which leads to malabsorption of the bile acids by the distal ileum, leading to steatorrhoea in mild cases and diarrhoea if more severe. It is suggested that up to 50 per cent of cases of watery diarrhoea is due to bile malabsorption (Galatola and the Italian 75 SeHCAT Multicenter Study Group 1992).

Alcohol abuse is also associated with jejunum bacterial overgrowth, with greater numbers of both anaerobic and aerobic bacteria; the bacterial load correlates with raised gastric pH (Bode *et al.* 1984).

The proximal ileum continues to absorb nutrients, but about halfway along the length of the ileum the *plicae circulares* (large valvular flaps that project into the lumen) disappear in humans, suggesting a change in function. In this distal region, bile salts are reabsorbed (Craddock *et al.* 1998); in the rat there has been found a reduced capacity for ion secretion and uptake (Young and Levin 1989) and this is supported in humans (Silk *et al.* 1975).

Transition from the small to the large intestine is demarcated by the ileocaecal junction, which regulates the flow of material out of the ileum and into the caecum. Relaxation of the valve is stimulated in response to food entering the stomach and also by the presence of short chain fatty acids (SCFAs) (Malbert 2005). This latter stimulus could be regarded as a response to bacterial overgrowth, but may also be a response to caecal reflux.

Caecal pressure causes an increase in muscular tone of the sphincter (Dinning *et al.* 1999) and a structure that naturally causes the valve to close. Despite this, it is estimated that in 10–20 per cent of people the valve is incompetent, with colonic pressure resulting in reflux back into the ileum (Chang, Shelton and Welton 2005). There are many reports of symptoms of caecal reflux, including low back pain, headaches, shoulder pain, nausea, neck stiffness, sinusitis, dizziness, fatigue, pallor, dark circles under the eyes and so on (Pollard, Bablis and Bonello 2006).

A pattern of behaviour that reduces colonic pressure should be adopted to minimise caecal reflux:

1. Regular defecation to reduce colon pressure is important and steps should be taken to increase the transit time of people with constipation.

2. The size and timing of meals is also important. Overeating should be avoided, with the body being allowed to become hungry in between.

---

1 This is a commonly-used synonym for protein-energy malnutrition among organisations such as the World Health Organisation.

3. Another consideration should be the minimal inclusion of food constituents that stimulate the smooth muscle to relax; these include alcohol, caffeine, 'hot' spices, castor oil and magnesium supplements. In this latter case the tolerable upper limit (UL) for adults has been estimated to be 350mg/day (Institute of Medicine 1997), which is based on a lowest observable adverse effect level (LOAEL) of 360mg/day, although they go on to state that 'many other individuals have not encountered such effects even when receiving substantially more than this UL of supplementary magnesium' (p.246). (Note that therapeutic doses may need to be higher when working to correct an identified dietary deficiency of magnesium, especially in certain fatigue-related conditions.)

2.4 The colon

The colon can be divided into six regions: the caecum, the ascending colon, the transverse colon, the descending colon, the sigmoid colon, and the rectum and anus. The main function of the proximal colon is one of absorption of water and sodium ions (Sandle et al. 1986), while the presence of *plicae semilunares* (permanent folds in the mucosa) increases the surface area of the colon by 10–15 times, giving it a high absorptive capacity capable of reducing the 2L of soft faecal material that enters per day into less than 200mL. The colonic mucosa atrophies with advanced age and is associated with changes in water and electrolyte absorption (Yamagata 1965).

Many chronic diseases of the colon are associated with a change in colon pH and some have been related to changes in SCFA composition, as well as potentially increasing the risk of colon cancer (Hong, Ying Qiang and Shan Jun 2004).

The three main SCFA salts found in the colon are acetate, propionate and butyrate. They are formed as the result of fermentation of undigested carbohydrate, particularly cellulose, fructo-oligosaccharides and resistant starches. This last group appears to reduce the risk of colon cancer, with a significant negative association between resistant starch consumption and malignancy; but no such correlation is found with non-starch polysaccharides (NSP) alone (Cassidy, Bingham and Cummings 1994). This may be largely due to the protective effects of butyrate (Hamer et al. 2007). It is estimated that, in a typical Western diet, 10 per cent of ingested starch reaches the colon (Wilson 2005); although this proportion can increase with inefficient chewing and/or with a greater proportion of the starch being unprocessed (Englyst, Kingman and Cummings 1992).

SCFA salts, particularly butyrate, are a source of energy for the mucosa, supplying an estimated 9 per cent of its energy requirement (Wilson 2005). Acetate, the main SCFA salt synthesised, is metabolised by peripheral tissues and can also stimulate cholesterol synthesis; while propionate is metabolised by the liver and can inhibit cholesterol synthesis (Wong et al. 2006).

Many vitamins are also synthesised by the colon microflora, including Vitamin K and the B vitamins thiamine (B1), riboflavin (B2), nicotinic acid (B3), pyridoxine (B6), biotin, folate and cobalamins (B12). *Bifidobacterium* spp. are the most important in terms of vitamin synthesis, but *E. coli*, *Enterococcus* spp. and other enterobacteria also contribute.

2.4.1 DIARRHOEA

As the faecal material reaches the distal colon, absorption of sodium, potassium, chloride and water continues. Disruption of this process can lead to diarrhoea. Generally there are two factors that need to be taken into account when considering the cause of diarrhoea: whether the basis of the condition is osmotic or secretory and/or related to osmolyte malabsorption or whether it is due to increased motility (Field 2003; Sellin 2001). This leads to three main classifications:

- **Secretory diarrhoea** results from irritation of the lumen by bacterial endotoxins, deconjugated bile acids or mediators of inflammation. The faeces contain levels of chloride, potassium and sodium and are iso-osmotic with the plasma. It is important that these ions and water are replaced quickly in people with this form of diarrhoea to prevent vascular collapse.

- **Osmotic diarrhoea** is due to high levels of osmolytes in the lumen drawing more water than usual in an attempt to produce iso-osmotic chyme. There are three main causes:

    1. The high concentration of a nutrient that has saturated the normal uptake mechanism; this commonly occurs with high dose nutrient supplements such as high-strength vitamin C preparations.

    2. The presence of non-absorbable, osmotically active compounds such as sorbitol and lactulose – the *modus operandi* of osmotic laxatives.

    3. The presence of compounds that would normally be digested and absorbed except that there is malabsorption of the nutrient, as found in coeliac and Crohn's disease.

- The mechanism behind **motility-related diarrhoea** depends on whether peristalsis is:

    1. too rapid: due to conditions such as hyperthyroidism or opiate withdrawal, leading to insufficient time for water absorption

    2. impaired/slow transit: this is due to bacterial overgrowth causing irritation, inflammation and malabsorption which can result in both secretory and/ or osmotic diarrhoea. Causes of reduced motility include large diverticula, autonomic neuropathy such as that associated with diabetes, and smooth muscle damage due to muscular dystrophy or inflammatory conditions.

2.4.2 CONSTIPATION

Constipation is defined as infrequent bowel movements, typically less than three times a week; difficulty during defecation with straining during more than 25 per cent of bowel movements, or a subjective sensation of hard stools and/or the sensation of incomplete bowel evacuation. Constipation is associated with several physical causes including: a poor diet lacking fibre that results in low stool volume; anatomical defects, frequently due to surgery, polyps or tumours; or a lack of GI tract motility due to a sedentary lifestyle, hypothyroidism or abnormality. Psychological problems can also impact on the regularity of defecation.

Major control of motility in the colon is inherent in the smooth muscle function; although other influences such as cephalic stimulation and signals from further up the GI tract can influence peristalsis, particularly the gastrocolic reflex. This is the rapid increase in colon motility after eating, the severity of which is associated with calorie content, with fat being the most potent stimulator. Hormones such as progesterone can inhibit contractions, causing variation in bowel movement throughout the menstrual cycle.

Please see Part 2 of this chapter for further discussion of treatment options for constipation.

3. Microflora supplementation and the human gut

There is much public and medical interest in the role of bacteria in the gastro-intestinal tract. Indeed, the market for functional food products containing the so-called 'friendly bacteria' is valuable and growing across most countries in Europe. Sales of probiotic yoghurts and milks are estimated to account for 25 per cent of the UK functional foods market (Mintel Reports 2006) and are estimated to be worth £164 million per annum (Lawrence 2009).

Marteau *et al.* (2001) state that 'friendly bacteria' are 'non-pathogenic micro-organisms that, when ingested, exert a positive influence on the health of the host'. Probiotic bacteria could therefore be viewed as human symbionts, naturally inhabiting the gut and conferring a range of health benefits. Rolfe (2000) expresses similarly positive views in concluding 'probiotics represent a potentially significant therapeutic advance' (p.396S) and that, in addition, 'probiotics offer dietary means to support balance of the intestinal flora. They may be used to counteract local immunological dysfunction, to stabilise the intestinal mucosal barrier function, to prevent infectious succession of pathogenic microorganisms and to influence intestinal metabolism' (p.400S). However, he goes on to say that 'any postulated benefit from the consumption of probiotics and prebiotics should be accepted as fact only after extensive, multicenter testing in human clinical trials' (p.400S).

The British Nutrition Foundation has raised concerns about trials undertaken up to 2007, citing that many studies have been conducted on animals or *in vitro* or without adequate controls or adequately defined study end points (Miles 2007). However, more positive findings were published in a review paper in the *American Journal of Clinical Nutrition*, which assessed human intervention studies and analysed 49 papers produced between 1988 and 1998 on the health effects of probiotic bacteria (de Roos and Katan

2000). They reviewed 26 studies on the role of probiotic bacteria in the prevention and treatment of diarrhoea and concluded that *Lactobacillus rhamnosus* GG is effective against rotavirus, a common cause of gastroenteritis and diarrhoea, with it shortening the diarrhoeal phase by a day.

A more recent systematic review of probiotics in the therapy of IBS concludes that overall 'probiotics appear efficacious in IBS but the magnitude of benefit and the most effective species and strains are uncertain' (Moayyedi *et al.* 2008).

Other studies demonstrate the benefits of probiotics, as in the treatment of travellers' diarrhoea (Sazawal *et al.* 2006). Positive effects on the duration and severity of diarrhoea due to other viruses and bacteria are less conclusive, with perhaps the main advocacy of probiotic use being for nosocomial diarrhoea (acquired in hospital) and antibiotic-associated diarrhoea (de Vresem and Marteau 2007).

The main cause of nosocomial diarrhoea is *Clostridium difficile* (McFarland 2006), which is associated with the use of broad-spectrum antibiotics and is an increasingly common problem, particularly amongst elderly patients (O'Connor *et al.* 2004). The most promising microbial candidates, as part of treatment and reducing recurrent infection, are *Lactobacillus rhamnosus* and the yeast *Saccharomyces boulardii* (Bartlett 2009). The proposed mechanism for the latter is the production of a protease that cleaves *C. difficile* toxins A and B, thus preventing binding to the mucosal receptor (Castagliuolo *et al.* 1999).

Other studies show *L. rhamnosus* GG reduces the three-week recurrence rate of *C. difficile* infection (Pochapin 2000). In this study patients also reported less abdominal cramping and the earlier disappearance of diarrhoea. Prebiotic supplementation has also been reported to lessen the associated diarrhoea (Lewis, Burmeister and Brazier 2005).

There are also nine preliminary studies on the role of probiotics in reducing the risk of cancer or the formation of carcinogens, which demonstrate a 'smaller recurrence' of some tumours (de Roos and Katan 2000). In other studies human volunteers receiving *Lactobacillus casei* (Hayatsu and Hayatsu 1993) or *Lactobacillus acidophilus* (Lidbeck *et al.* 1992) have been found to have lower levels of mutagens from food.

However, there are now concerns about the use of probiotics in the immuno-compromised and in critically ill patients, such as those in intensive care units. This is because there have been reports of probiotics causing problems such as sepsis in these patients (Singhi and Baranwal 2008).

One possibility for the relative lack of evidence for the effectiveness of probiotics is the concentration on genera associated with dairy products, such as *Lactobacillus* and *Bifidobacter* (Wilson 2005), which are only naturally present in small numbers in the small intestine and colon.

There are many genera of enterobacteria that are also found in the soil, and there are brands of probiotics on the market containing such organisms. However, a lack of evidence pertaining to their benefit, coupled with the suggestion that many of these species have 'virulence' traits that may become pathogenic or cause problems in the immuno-compromised (Kayser 2003) have made this a controversial topic. More research is needed to establish the therapeutic potential and the risks associated with ingestion of soil bacteria-containing supplements. It is perhaps worth remembering that soil organisms can easily be ingested through food, especially via home-grown or organic vegetables that commonly have soil still on the produce.

Survival in the gut is essential for the effectiveness of any probiotic strain that is being supplemented in patients that do not fall into the at-risk, immuno-compromised category. Gibson *et al.* (2005) report on *in vitro* experiments validated to assess survival in the human GI tract. They conclude that that some strains of *Lactobacillus* spp. and *Bifidobacterium* spp. can survive the gastric environment, although the latter show more sensitivity. The researchers also tested selected strains against bile salts and pancreatic enzymes with a view to determining survival in the intestines. *Lactobacillus* spp. showed sensitivity to upper intestinal content (six strains were tested independently), whereas *Bifidobacterium* spp. demonstrated good survival. They also report that the inclusion of oligosaccharides and ingestion at the same time as food can affect the survival of probiotic bacteria.

Functions attributed to probiotics:

- enhance barrier function and prevent enterotoxins, including pathogenic bacteria, from binding to epithelial cells (Elmer 2001)

- produce antimicrobial substances, e.g. organic acids, hydrogen peroxide and bacteriocins (Rolfe 2000)

- modulate secretory immunoglobin A (IgA) production (Elmer 2001)

- stabilise the colon pH of the gut via SCFA synthesis, with the lower pH aiding mineral absorption and the control of pathogens

- synthesise SCFAs, which increases the flow of blood to the colon (Schwiertz *et al.* 2002). SCFAs are also a major energy source for the colonocytes

- produce lactase to aid digestion of lactose (Marteau *et al.* 2001)

- produce B vitamins and vitamin K (Hill 1997)

- stop pathogenic bacteria from attaching to mucosal binding sites (Elmer 2001)

- compete for nutrients with pathogenic and dysbiotic flora and so help to control the population of these. Hence, these effects help prevent production of harmful bacterial enzymes, such as beta-glucuronidase

- lower serum cholesterol (*Lactobacillus acidophilus*) (de Roos and Katan 2000)

- reduce the production of mutagens after a meal (Hayatsu and Hayatsu 1993; Lidbeck *et al.* 1992).

In conclusion, it appears that, in many common conditions affecting the GI tract, supplemental probiotics or functional foods containing probiotics present a valid therapeutic option to complementary and allopathic health professionals alike.

4. Diagnostic testing

The digestive system is physiologically complex, and there is still much research to be done. However, enough is known about the human digestive function for a functional approach to be taken in managing age-related decline, GI imbalance and organic disease. Often the first step is to determine the imbalances that are leading to functional changes and thus symptoms, by undertaking an empirical analysis of the patient's diet with respect to the scientific literature; and engaging in laboratory testing where appropriate.

A description of some of the conventional diagnostic tests for diseases and conditions associated with the digestive system can be found at Lab Tests Online (Lab Tests Online 2009). However, the functional medicine approach is concerned with determining the biochemical and physiological irregularities underlying the patient's symptoms and which, if not challenged, would lead to disease. It is, therefore, concerned with prevention of disease. It might be argued that mainstream testing techniques are similarly preventative tools, but many of these are actually tests for the early detection of disease. This is not to say that these do not have their place, they most certainly do, but the main difference between the FM approach and that of conventional diagnostic testing is one of chronology.

Although it is outside the scope of this chapter to recommend a laboratory, placing the following term 'functional testing laboratory' into an internet search engine should list the major players. Most have detailed descriptions of the tests they offer.

Some symptoms, however, termed 'red flags', require an immediate referral of the patient to their GP or to a hospital emergency department. (Note that patient consent is normally required prior to referral to a GP.) A list of red flags associated with the digestive system is given in Table 2.1.

Table 2.1 Red flags that could relate to the digestive system

Category	Symptom	Notes
Discomfort	Persistent severe pain in the abdomen	
	Absence of pain in ulcers, fissures, etc.	
Appearance	Blood in sputum, vomit or stools (*)	
	Vomit containing coagulated blood (*)	'coffee grounds' appearance
	Black tarry stools (*)	GI bleeding?
Persistent	Vomiting and/or diarrhoea	
	Vomiting and/or diarrhoea in an infant (*)	
	Thirst	
	Unexplained weight loss	500g (1lb) per week or more
Sudden	Swelling of face, lips, tongue or throat (*)	
Difficulty	Swallowing	

Category	Symptom	Notes
Change	In bowel habit (especially in patients over 60)	lasting more than 6 weeks with looser and/or more frequent stools
Others	Unexplained swelling or lumps	
	Anaemia	
	Raised inflammatory markers in blood	could indicate IBD

Symptoms marked with (*) need immediate medical attention

Part 2 Functional disorders of the gastro-intestinal tract

Justine Bold

5. Functional gastro-intestinal tract disorders

The rest of this chapter aims to explore functional disorders, which can affect many areas of the GI tract. According to Drossman *et al.* (1993) functional disorders include functional dysphagia (FD), IBS, functional abdominal pain (FAP) and functional bloating (FB). All functional disorders are characterised by an absence of biological markers for the condition, having normal histopathology. However, research is emerging to support the view that GI imbalances (in terms of, for example, altered digestive secretions and/or microflora imbalances) may be a factor in their development.

5.1 Irritable bowel syndrome (IBS)

The general prevalence of IBS is between 10 and 15 per cent in industrialised countries. IBS is defined by Rome III (classification system for functional gastro-intestinal disorders) as recurrent abdominal pain for at least three days a month for at least the three previous months, with improvement of symptoms upon defecation; onset with a change in stool frequency, form or appearance (Hotoleanu *et al.* 2008). IBS is normally diagnosed after investigations to rule out other organic diseases (e.g. inflammatory bowel disease, diverticulitis and colon cancer).

The National Institute of Clinical Excellence (NICE) in the UK has published a quick guide on the diagnosis of IBS (NICE 2008). NICE recommends the following:

- full blood count (FBC)

- erythrocyte sedimentation rate (ESR) or plasma viscosity

- C-reactive protein (CRP)

- antibody testing for coeliac disease.

NICE recommends thyroid function test, ova and parasite test (faecal), hydrogen breath test (for lactose intolerance and bacterial overgrowth) and tests such as sigmoidoscopy, colonoscopy, barium enema and ultrasound if there is a family history of bowel or ovarian cancer or if red flag symptoms are present (see Table 2.1).

The aetiology of IBS is not clear, but there may be a genetic involvement (Hotoleanu *et al.* 2008) and some studies report an increased prevalence in women (Wilson *et al.* 2004). Other factors implicated in its development include stress and food sensitivities, including lactose intolerance. The role of immune-mediated food sensitivity is still generally viewed with scepticism, but there is evidence that elimination of foods to which raised IgG antibodies exist can reduce symptoms in IBS (Andersson *et al.* 2001; Atkinson *et al.* 2004).

The main risk factor in the development of IBS is gastroenteritis, principally of infectious origin (Bercik, Verdu and Collins 2005). Pathogenic bacterial species, such as those belonging to the genera *Campylobacter, Salmonella* and *Shigella,* are commonly implicated (Spiller 2007). Post-infectious IBS has a prevalence of 4–31 per cent following bacterial gastroenteritis, with 6–17 per cent of IBS patients believing that an infection triggered their condition (Spiller 2007). The underlying mechanism is disruption of the microfloral balance of the GI tract, leading to damage of the gut mucosa, which can cause increased intestinal permeability. A study in 2003 reported a link between the amoeba (of flagellate origin) *Dientamoeba fragilis* (DF), *Blastocystis hominis* (BH) and IBS symptoms, and recommended that patients should be screened for these parasites before a diagnosis of IBS is given (Windsor *et al.* 2003). This view is controversial and not widely accepted. However, a later paper from Australia also concludes that these organisms may play a role in IBS and that patients should undergo routine parasitological screening (Stark *et al.* 2007). Tests for these organisms are not routine in the UK; yet many patients seeking help from complementary practitioners eventually test positive for these organisms and report an easing of symptoms once the infection has been addressed. Many patients, paradoxically, are able to obtain medication from their GP once the infection has been identified.

A small study has suggested that the oil extracted from oregano (*Oreganum vulgare*) contains natural agents effective against these parasites (Force, Sparks and Ronzio 2000). The study of 14 adult patients with enteric parasites identified by stool tests (*Blastocystis hominis, Entamoeba hartmanni* and *Endolimax nana*), received six weeks of supplementation with 600mg emulsified oil of oregano daily. There was total eradication of *E. hartmanni* in four cases, one case of *E. nana,* and eight cases of *B. hominis.* In three other test subjects with *B. hominis* levels were reduced and symptoms improved, hence natural agents may help manage such infections.

5.1.1 LOW-GRADE INFLAMMATION IN IBS

Studies of post-infectious IBS (after *Campylobacter jejuni* infection) demonstrate increased numbers of enterochromaffin cells and inflammation (Spiller 2007), which is consistent with other recent research suggesting that IBS is a condition in which low-grade inflammation is present (De Giorgio and Barbara 2008). Indeed, a paper published in 2005 suggested that IBS and IBD are part of the same continuum, with low-grade inflammation present in IBS and in patients with IBS symptoms where IBD is in remission (Bercik *et al.* 2005). Gasbarini (1987) states that mast cell activation in the gut mucosa is a contributory factor to this low-grade inflammation in IBS. Nutritional management of inflammation should therefore also be considered (see Chapter 4).

5.1.2 SMALL INTESTINAL BACTERIAL OVERGROWTH

Small intestinal bacterial overgrowth (SIBO) is one form of microflora imbalance and is reported to be associated with diarrhoea and weight loss (Rana and Bhardwaj 2008). Carrara *et al.* (2008) report that SIBO is relatively common in IBS patients. SIBO is also associated with increased age, antibiotic use, appendectomy and the use of proton pump inhibitors (PPIs), commonly prescribed for conditions such as gastritis and acid reflux (Lauritano *et al.* 2008). The consequences of achlorhydria in humans in relation to bacterial overgrowth (Theisen *et al.* 2000) have been described in Part 1 of this chapter; this should thus be another area of investigation.

5.1.3 QUICK GUIDE: PREVALENCE AND SYMPTOMS OF IBS (WILSON *ET AL.* 2004)

- Prevalence of IBS = 10.5% adult population (6.6% men, 14% women).
- 25.4% of patients suffer from diarrhoea.
- 24.1% of patients suffer from constipation.
- 46.7% suffer from alternating symptoms.
- 56% of patients have consulted their GP in the last six months.
- 16% of patients have seen a specialist.
- Almost half of patients are on medication.
- The majority of patients are self-treating in some form.

5.1.4 IBS AND SEROTONIN

Neurotransmitters are emerging as a significant factor in functional disorders, including IBS. Spiller (2007) reports that IBS-D (characterised by diarrhoea) and post-infective IBS are associated with higher postprandial release of the neurotransmitter serotonin, which is also commonly seen in inflammatory bowel conditions, such as Crohn's disease, whilst patients with IBS-C (constipation) show a lower release. Significantly, IBS-D has been shown to be associated with the serotonin re-uptake transporter (SERT)

SERT-P deletion (Yeo *et al.* 2004). Serotonin (5HT), produced by enteroendocrine cells in the mucosa of the stomach and in the enteric nervous system in response to the ingestion of food, stimulates peristaltic waves in the GI tract. Transit is regulated by the removal of serotonin from its site of action by SERT. A polymorphism in SERT can therefore reduce serotonin removal, resulting in speedier transit, possibly leading to diarrhoea. Type 3 serotonin antagonists are often used in treating IBS-D as they inhibit the serotonin receptor, making it less sensitive to increased serotonin levels at the site of action. This rationale also explains why selective serotonin re-uptake inhibitors (SSRIs), commonly prescribed for depression, have side-effects that can include nausea, vomiting, abdominal pain and diarrhoea.

5.1.5 QUICK GUIDE: THE NUTRITIONAL MANAGEMENT OF IBS (NICE 2008)

- Have regular meals and take time to eat.
- Avoid missing meals or leaving long gaps between eating.
- Drink at least eight cups of fluid per day, especially water or other non-caffeinated drinks such as herbal teas.
- Restrict tea and coffee to three cups per day.
- Reduce intake of alcohol and fizzy drinks.
- Consider limiting intake of high-fibre food (for example, wholemeal or high-fibre flour and breads, cereals high in bran, and whole grains such as brown rice).
- Reduce intake of resistant starch (starch that resists digestion in the small intestine and reaches the colon intact), often found in processed or re-cooked foods.
- Limit fresh fruit to three portions (of 80g each) per day.
- For diarrhoea, avoid sorbitol, a sugar polyol found in sugar-free sweets (including chewing gum), drinks and in some diabetic and slimming products.
- For wind and bloating consider increasing intake of oats (for example, oat-based breakfast cereal or porridge) and linseeds (up to 1 tablespoon per day).

NICE probably recommend limiting high-fibre foods due to the possible irritant effects of such foods. However, as lack of fibre can cause constipation (which is one of the main symptoms of some types of IBS), the author would recommend that this is considered carefully in IBS-C. Limiting fresh fruit to three 80g portions a day is probably recommended owing to the fructose content, as excess sugar may in itself contribute to bloating. As fruit is nutritious, it is still important to include it in the diet. Clinical experience indicates that, more often than not, a very low fruit and vegetable diet and a low-fibre diet contribute to the development of many functional GI disorders.

Essentially, an individualised assessment of the patient's diet, including the fibre intake, is recommended, along with an assessment of symptoms. This should help to determine more accurately whether or not low fibre might be a contributory factor in the patient's symptoms. As allopathic advice normally includes a reduction of fibre, it is important for any complementary practitioner to understand this and work with the patient and his/her other health professionals to inform them of the results of any dietary assessment, or of other findings, that point to low fibre being significant in the patient's symptoms.

A functional approach to IBS would include the development of an individualised programme, based on the contributory factors and history of the patient (including such factors as infection or stress). The strategy should also assess any potential imbalances in the gut flora, given their role in the maintenance of the gut mucosa, with a view to restoring balance. A systematic review of the efficacy of probiotics in IBS treatment published in the journal *Gut* has concluded there is evidence of benefit, with most trials scoring above placebo (Moayyedi *et al.* 2008) (see Part 1 of this chapter, section 3, for further discussion.)

Other studies suggest benefit in certain subgroups of IBS patients, notably less pain in those with alternating symptoms; and improved stool frequency in those with constipation (Drouault-Holowacz *et al.* 2008). Probiotics may thus be a key therapeutic tool, with some patients potentially benefiting from supplementation with *Lactobacilli*, *Bifidobacterium* spp. and the yeast *Saccharomyces boulardii*.

A comprehensive digestive stool analysis (CDSA) can help assess the balance of the gut flora in patients, whilst also ruling out any potential pathogens that may be aggravating the GI tract. This can be used to determine requirements of supplemental probiotics (that is, the species and/or strain of probiotic and the appropriate dose and length of the initial course of supplementation). This approach is consistent with the strategy outlined by the Institute for Functional Medicine.

5.1.6 QUICK GUIDE: OTHER CONSIDERATIONS IN THE NUTRITIONAL MANAGEMENT OF IBS

- Try to eat when relaxed and chew food thoroughly.

- Avoid possible triggers such as wheat bran.

- Optimise stomach acid production (see Part 1 of this chapter, 2.2.1). For example, investigate and address zinc deficiency, for HCl synthesis.

- Manage flare-ups. For example, increase intake of soups and mashed foods, as these are easier to digest.

- Consume a range of fruits and vegetables (of many different colours) to optimise intake of beneficial phytochemicals, such as allicin in garlic, which has antibacterial activity (Ohta *et al.* 1999) (see Part 1 of this chapter, 2.2.1).

- Identify any food intolerances or sensitivities, as addressing these may reduce symptoms (Atkinson *et al.* 2004).

- Identify any enzyme deficiencies (such as lactase deficiency, which causes lactose intolerance) as these can lead to IBS-like symptoms.

- It may also be necessary to tackle low-grade inflammation with nutrients such as essential fats (especially omega-3) (see Chapter 4 for a discussion on essential fats).

5.2 Functional abdominal pain (FAP)

The aetiology of FAP is not fully defined but, as with the other functional disorders, organic disease is not present and histopathology is normal. It is defined by positive symptoms criteria, which are largely unrelated to food intake and defecation and it has higher co-morbidity with psychiatric disorders than other GI problems (Clouse *et al.* 2006). However, studies show increased visceral perception and the involvement of alterations in the visceral sensory nerve transmission routes (Hasler 2001). Allopathic treatments of FAP include acid-suppressing drugs, antispasmodics and antidepressants. The main consideration is the implications for health-related quality of life, as this can be negatively affected. In a prospective cohort study of 237 children with FAP, Saps *et al.* (2009) report higher rates of anxiety and depression, with 23 per cent of children absent from school during the course of the research. Development of an individualised plan is recommended, using FM philosophy and appropriate functional testing.

5.3 Functional bloating (FB)

The mechanism underpinning FB is not clear; although no one will be surprised that current research suggests colonic fermentation is involved. Di Stefano *et al.* (2006) measured breath hydrogen before and after injection of lactulose and concluded that colonic fermentation may be implicated. Significantly, bloating is often ranked as the most bothersome symptom in IBS, being most prevalent in IBS constipation (Houghton *et al.* 2006). Bloating is, however, a common problem and not always related to a diagnosis of IBS. In some cases it can be caused by food sensitivity or intolerance (Atkinson *et al.* 2004).

5.4 Functional constipation (FC)

Constipation without an organic cause is also considered a functional disorder, as well as being one of the main problems that affects some IBS patients. The anatomical/physiological basis for constipation has already been discussed in Part 1 of this chapter (see 2.4.2). This section will review contributory factors in more detail and treatment options. The prevalence of constipation in children (0–18 years) is estimated to be between 0.7 and 29.6 per cent (Van den Berg, Benninga and Di Lovenzo 2006), and can be persistent, with over a third of UK children still suffering six years after referral to a specialist paediatric gastroenterology clinic (Procter and Loader 2003). Risk factors for constipation in children are varied and include dietary, genetic and psychological factors. Inan *et al.* (2007) identify the following risk factors:

- never having used school toilets
- problems with bowel control after the age of two years
- less regular physical activity
- diets lower in fruits and vegetables
- diets higher in milk-based foods, biscuits and macaroni
- a history of constipation in family members.

5.4.1 PROBIOTICS AND FC IN CHILDREN

Bekkali *et al.* (2007) undertook a small study to determine the value of supplemental probiotics in children aged 4–16 years with constipation (as defined by the Rome III criteria). After treatment to remove any rectal impaction, the children received a daily probiotic supplement (*Bifidobacteria bifidum, B. infantis, B. longum, Lactobacillus casei, L. plantarum* and *L. rhamnosus*) over a four-week period. The results were positive, showing an increase in bowel movements from an average of 2.0 to 4.2 in week two of the study, and 3.8 (2.1–7.0) movements in week four. In the 12 children presenting with fewer than three bowel movements per week, movements increased significantly from an average of 1.0 to 3.0 in week two, and 3.0 in week four, both of which are statistically significant (p=0.05). Less abdominal pain was reported, as was an absence of adverse effects. Hence, in children a CDSA may be useful to determine if probiotics could also be considered as part of a treatment strategy for constipation.

5.4.2 FIBRE AND FC

There are several studies that suggest that dietary fibre can be useful in treating constipation in adults and children (BMJ 2007). It increases the bulk of stool, affecting stool form and consistency (usually making stools softer and easier to pass), caused in part by the swelling of insoluble fibres and the fermentative action of gut microflora. It is thus a main nutritional consideration in dealing with functional constipation and the associated bloating. Most adults in the UK do not eat the recommended amount of fibre, that is, 18g a day, with older children requiring proportionally less. Pre-school children should have fibre introduced slowly into the diet, as too much may lead to the child becoming prematurely full thus affecting total nutrient intake. However, it is important to remember than many clinicians are cautious when recommending high-fibre diets to young children and patients with GI conditions, owing to the poor digestibility of high-fibre diets (Tan and Seow-Choen 2007) and the fact that an excess of fibre (particularly insoluble fibre) can aggravate many conditions. Patients should be encouraged to eat the correct amount of fruits and vegetables, as this alone may help to improve the situation. Soluble fibre food sources can also be introduced gradually to help increase overall fibre intake.

5.4.3 QUICK GUIDE: NUTRITIONAL MANAGEMENT OF CONSTIPATION

- Drink plenty of fluids (6–8 glasses a day), as dehydration may be a factor (Arnaud 2003).

- If the diet is low in fibre, increase intake to the recommended 18g a day for an adult (Department of Health 1991).

- Increase whole foods rich in soluble fibre such as oats and legumes. Avoid an excess of insoluble fibre, such as wheat bran, as this may aggravate the problem in some people.

- Consume five 80g portions of fruits and vegetables a day.

- Include foods such as prunes, psyllium husks and/or soaked linseeds.

If there are no improvements from these general dietary modifications, an individualised programme should be developed. This should be based on contributory factors and should assess possible imbalances in gut flora (via the use of a CDSA), consider the supplemental use of probiotics and oligosaccharides and correct any nutrient deficiencies. Magnesium sulphate (Epsom salts) has long been used as a treatment for constipation, and some researchers report that mineral water with higher levels of magnesium sulphate improves constipation (Arnaud 2003).

In conclusion, whilst functional disorders show no abnormal histopathology, they do cause significant problems and reductions in quality of life. Whilst the aetiologies of functional disorders and inter-relationships to GI disease are not fully understood, it is evident that an imbalance of microflora is, in many cases, a contributory factor to their development, and that other factors, such as fibre intake, enzyme deficiencies, food sensitivities and psychological issues are also likely to be involved.

References

Advisory Committee on the Microbiological Safety of Food (2006) *Ad Hoc Group on Infant Botulism: Report on Minimally Processed Infant Weaning Foods and the Risk of Infant Botulism.* London: Food Standards Agency.

Al Somal, N., Coley, K.E., Molan, P.C. and Hancock, B.M. (1994) 'Susceptibility of Helicobacter pylori to the antibacterial activity of manuka honey.' *Journal of the Royal Society of Medicine 87,* 1, 9–12.

Andersson, R., Olaison, G., Tysk, C. and Ekbom, A. (2001) 'Appendectomy and protection against ulcerative colitis.' *New England Journal of Medicine 344,* 11, 808–814.

Andrès, E., Noel, E. and Abdelghani, M.B. (2003) 'Vitamin B12 deficiency associated with chronic acid suppression therapy.' *Annals of Pharmacotherapy 37,* 11, 1730.

Arnaud, M. (2003) 'Mild dehydration: a risk factor of constipation?' *European Journal of Clinical Nutrition 57,* 2, S88–S95.

Atkinson, W., Sheldon, T., Shaath, N. and Whorwell, P.J. (2004) 'Food elimination based on IgG antibodies in irritable bowel syndrome: A randomised controlled trial.' *Gut 53,* 1459–1464.

Barrett, K.E. (2006) *Gastrointestinal Physiology.* New York: McGraw-Hill.

Bartlett, J. (2009) 'New antimicrobial agents for patients with Clostridium difficile infections.' *Current Infectious Disease Reports 11*, 1, 21–28.

Bekkali, N., Bongers, M., Van den Berg, M., Liem, O. and Benninga, M. (2007) 'The role of a probiotics mixture in the treatment of childhood constipation: A pilot study.' *Nutrition Journal 5*, 6, 17.

Bercik, P., Verdu, E. and Collins, S. (2005) 'Is irritable bowel syndrome a low-grade inflammatory bowel disease?' *Gastroenterology Clinics of North America 34*, 2, 235–245.

BMJ (2007) 'Clinical evidence: Constipation in adults.' Available at http://clinicalevidence.bmj.com/ceweb/conditions/dsd/0413/0413_I17.jsp, accessed on 30 October 2009.

Bode, J.C., Bode, C., Heidelbach, R., Dürr, H.K. and Martini, G.A. (1984) 'Jejunal microflora in patients with chronic alcohol abuse.' *Hepatogastroenterology 31*, 1, 30–34.

Cain, J.R., Mayoral, L., Hertlan Lotero, M.S., Bolaños, O. and Duque, E. (1976) 'Enterobacteriaceae in the jejunal microflora: Prevalence and relationship to biochemical and histological evaluations in healthy Colombian men.' *American Journal of Clinical Nutrition 29*, 1397–1403.

Carrara, M., Desideri, S., Azzurro, M., Bulighin, G.M. *et al.* (2008) 'Small intestine bacterial overgrowth in patients with irritable bowel syndrome.' *European Review for Medical and Pharmacological Sciences 12*, 3, 197–202.

Cassidy, A., Bingham, S.A. and Cummings, J.H. (1994) 'Starch intake and colorectal.' *British Journal of Cancer 69*, 937–942.

Castagliuolo, I., Riegler, M.F., Valenick, L., LaMont, J.T. and Pothoulaki, C. (1999) '*Saccharomyces boulardii* protease inhibits the effects of *Clostridium difficile* toxins A and B in human colonic mucosa.' *Infection and Immunity 67*, 1, 302–307.

Castell, D. (1975) 'Diet and the lower oesophageal sphincter.' *American Journal of Clinical Nutrition 28*, 1296–1298.

Chang, J.G., Shelton, A. and Welton, M. (2005) 'Large Intestine.' In G. Doherty and L. Way (eds) *Current Surgical Diagnosis and Treatment*, 12th edn. New York: McGraw-Hill/Appleton and Lange.

Chong, V.H. and Wang, C.L. (2008) 'Higher prevalence of gastrointestinal symptoms among patients with rheumatic disorders.' *Singapore Medical Journal 49*, 5, 419–424.

Clouse, R.E., Mayer, E.A., Aziz, Q., Drossman, D.A. *et al.* (2006) 'Functional abdominal pain syndrome.' *Gastroenterology 130*, 5, 1492–1497.

Cohen, R.D. (2002) 'The quality of life in patients with Crohn's disease.' *Alimentary Pharmacology and Therapeutics 16*, 9, 1603–1609.

Craddock, A.L., Love, M.W., Daniel, R.W., Lyndon, C.K. *et al.* (1998) 'Expression and transport properties of the human ileal and renal sodium-dependent bile acid transporter.' *American Journal of Physiology 274*, 157–169.

De Giorgio, R. and Barbara, G. (2008) 'Is irritable syndrome an inflammatory disorder?' *Current Gastroenterology Reports 10*, 4, 385–390.

de Roos, N.M. and Katan, M.B. (2000) 'Effects of probiotic bacteria on diarrhea, lipid metabolism, and carcinogenesis: A review of papers published between 1988 and 1998.' *American Journal of Clinical Nutrition 71*, 2, 405–411.

de Vresem, M. and Marteau, P.R. (2007) 'Probiotics and prebiotics: Effects on diarrhea.' *Journal of Nutrition 137*, 3, 803S–811S.

Department of Health (1991) *Dietary Reference Values for Food Energy and Nutrients for the United Kingdom. Report of the Panel on Dietary Reference Values of the Committee on Medical Aspects of Food Policy.* London: HMSO.

Di Stefano, M., Miceli, E., Missanelli, A., Mazzocchi, S., Tana, P. and Corazza, G. (2006) 'Role of colonic fermentation in the perception of colonic distension in irritable bowel syndrome and functional bloating.' *Clinical Gastroenterology and Hepatology 4*, 10, 1242–1247.

Dinning, P.G., Bampton, P.A., Kennedy, M.L., Kajimoto, T. *et al.* (1999) 'Basal pressure patterns and reflexive motor responses in the human ileocolonic junction.' *American Journal of Physiology – Gastrointestinal and Liver Physiology 276*, 331–340.

Drossman, D., Li, Z., Andruzzi, E., Temple, R. *et al.* (1993) 'US householder survey of functional gastrointestinal disorders. Prevalence, sociodemography, and health impact.' *Digestive Diseases and Sciences 38*, 9, 1569–1580.

Drouault-Holowacz, S., Bieuvelet, S., Burckel, A., Cazaubiel, M., Dray, X. and Marteau, P. (2008) 'A double blind randomized controlled trial of a probiotic combination in 100 patients with irritable bowel syndrome.' *Gastroenterologie Clinique et Biologique 32*, 2, 147–152.

Elmer, G.W. (2001) 'Probiotics: Living drugs.' *American Journal of Health-System Pharmacy 58*, 12, 1101–1109.

Englyst, H., Kingman, S. and Cummings, J. (1992) 'Classification and measurement.' *European Journal of Clinical Nutrition 46*, suppl. 2, S33–S50.

Field, M. (2003) 'Intestinal ion transport and the pathophysiology of diarrhea.' *Journal of Clinical Investigation 111*, 7, 931–943.

Force, M., Sparks, W. and Ronzio, R. (2000) 'Inhibition of eneteric parasites by emulsified oil of oregano in vivo.' *Phytotherapy Research 14*, 3, 213–214.

Friis-Hansen, L. (2006) 'Achlorhydria is associated with gastric microbial overgrowth and development of cancer: Lessons learned from the gastrin knockout mouse.' *Scandinavian Journal of Clinical and Laboratory Investigation 66*, 7, 607–622.

Galatola, G. and the Italian 75 SeHCAT Multicenter Study Group (1992) 'The prevalence of bile acid malabsorption in irritable bowel syndrome and the effect of cholestyramine: An uncontrolled open multicenter study.' *European Journal of Gastroenterology and Hepatology 4*, 533–537.

Garg, A. and Malo, M. (1997) 'Manifestations and treatment of xerostomia and associated oral effects secondary to head and neck radiation therapy.' *Americal Dental Association 128*, 1128–1133.

Gasbarini, G. (1987) 'Fasting breath hydrogen in coeliac disease.' *Gasterenterology 93*, 53–58.

Gibson, G., Rouzaud, G., Brostoff, J. and Rayment, N. (2005) 'An evaluation of probiotic effects in the human gut: Microbial aspects.' Available at www.food.gov.uk/news/newsarchive/2005/mar/probiotics, accessed on 30 October 2009.

Goldacre, M., Wotton, C., Yeates, D., Seagroatt, V. and Jewell, D. (2008) 'Cancer in patients with ulcerative colitis, Crohn's disease and Coeliac disease: Record linkage study.' *European Journal of Gastroenterology and Hepatology 20*, 4, 297–304.

Hamer, H.M., Jonkers, D., Venema, K., Vanhoutvin, S., Troost, F.J. and Brummer, R.J. (2007) 'Review article: The role of butyrate on colonic function.' *Alimentary Pharmacology and Therapeutics 27*, 2, 104–119.

Hasler, W. (2001) 'Augmented visceral perception.' *Current Treatment Options in Gastroenterology 4*, 4, 339–349.

Hayatsu, H. and Hayatsu, T. (1993) 'Suppressing effects of Lactobacillus casei administration on the urinary mutagenicity arising fom the ingestion of ground beef in the human.' *Cancer Letters 73*, 173–179.

Hill, M. (1997) 'Intestinal flora and endogenous vitamin synthesis.' *Cancer Prevention 6*, 1, S43–S45.

Hill, M.J. (2002) 'Factors Controlling the Microflora of the Healthy Upper Gastrointestinal Tract.' In M. Hill and P. Marsh (eds) *Human Microbial Ecology*. Boca Raton, FL: CRC Press.

Hillilä, M., Hämäläinen, J., Heikkinen, M. and Färkkilä, M. (2008) 'Gastrointestinal complaints among subjects with depressive symptoms in the general population.' *Alimentary Pharmacology and Therapeutics 28*, 5, 648–654.

Hong, F.U., Ying Qiang, S.H.I. and Shan Jin, M.O. (2004) 'Effect of short-chain fatty acids on the proliferation and differentiation of the human colonic adenocarcinoma cell line Caco-2.' *Chinese Journal of Digestive Diseases 5*, 3, 115–117.

Hotoleanu, C., Popp, R., Trifa, A., Nedelcu, L. and Dumistrascu, D. (2008) 'Genetic determination of irritable bowel syndrome.' *World Journal of Gastroenterology 14*, 43, 6636–6640.

Houghton, L., Lea, R., Agrawal, A., Reilly, B. and Whorwell, P. (2006) 'Relationship of abdominal bloating to distension in irritable bowel syndrome and effect of bowel habit.' *Gastroenterology 131*, 4, 1003–1010.

Inan, M., Aydiner, C.Y., Tokuc, B., Aksu, B. *et al.* (2007) 'Factors associated with childhood constipation.' *Journal of Paediatrics and Child Health 43*, 10, 700–706.

Institute of Medicine (1997) *Dietary Reference Intakes for Calcium, Phosphorus, Magnesium, Vitamin D, and Fluoride.* Washington, DC: National Academy Press.

Jones, D.S. (ed.) (2005) *Textbook of Functional Medicine.* Gig Harbor, WA: Institute for Functional Medicine.

Kayser, F. (2003) 'Safety aspects of enterococci from the medical point of view.' *International Journal of Food Microbiology 88*, 2–3, 255–262.

Klaver, F.A.M. and van der Meer, R. (1993) 'The assumed assimilation of cholesterol by Lactobacilli and Bifidobacterium bifidum is due to their bile salt-deconjugating activity.' *Applied and Environmental Microbiology 59*, 4, 1120–1124.

Komai, M., Goto, T., Suzuki, S., Takeda, T. and Furukawa, Y. (2000) 'Zinc deficiency and taste dysfunction: Contribution of carbonic anhydrase, a zinc-metalloenzyme, to normal taste sensation.' *Biofactors 12*, 1–4, 65.

Krall, E., Hayes, C. and Garcia, R. (1998) 'How dentition status and masticatory function affect nutrient intake.' *Journal of the American Dental Association 129*, 9, 1261–1269.

Krasinski, S.D., Russell, R.M., Samloff, I.M., Jacob, R.A. *et al.* (1986) 'Fundic atrophic gastritis in an elderly population: Effect on hemoglobin and several serum nutritional indicators.' *Journal of the American Geriatrics Society 34*, S00–S06.

Lab Tests Online (2009) Available at www.labtestsonline.org.uk/, accessed on 30 October 2009.

Lane, L.A. and Rojas-Fernandez, C. (2002) 'Treatment of vitamin b(12)-deficiency anemia: oral versus parenteral therapy.' *Annals of Pharmacotherapy 36*, 7, 1268–1272.

Lauritano, E., Gabrielli, M., Scarpellini, E., Lupascu, A. *et al.* (2008) 'Small intestinal bacterial overgrowth recurrence after antibiotic therapy.' *American Journal of Gastroenterology 103*, 8, 2031–2035.

Lawrence, F. (2009) 'Are probiotics really that good for your health?' *Guardian* (25 July). Available at www.guardian.co.uk/theguardian/2009/jul/25/probiotic-health-benefits, accessed on 1 November 2009.

Lederle, F.A. (1991) 'Oral cobalamin for pernicious anemia. Medicine's best kept secret.' Journal of the American Medical Association *265*, 94–95.

Leinonen, J., Parkkila, S., Kaunisto, K., Koivunen, P. and Rajaniemi, H. (2001) 'Secretion of carbonic anhydrase isoenzyme VI (CA VI) from human and rat lingual serous von Ebner's glands.' *Journal of Histochemistry and Cytochemistry 49*, 5, 657–662.

Lewis, S., Burmeister, S. and Brazier, J. (2005) 'Effect of the prebiotic oligofructose on relapse of Clostridium difficile-associated diarrhea: A randomised, controlled study.' *Clinical Gastroenterology and Hepatology 3*, 5, 442–448.

Lidbeck, A., Nord, C., Gustafsson, J.A. and Rafter, J. (1992) 'Lactobacillus anticarcinogenic activities and the human intestinal microflora.' *European Journal of Cancer Prevention 1*, 341–353.

Lo, C.-C., Hsu, P.-I., Lo, G.-H., Lai, K.-H. *et al.* (2005) 'Implications of anti-parietal cell antibodies and anti-Helicobacter pylori.' *World Journal of Gastroenterology 11*, 30, 4715–4720.

Lopez-Jornet, M. and Bermejo-Fenoll, A. (1994) 'Is there an age-dependent decrease in resting secretion of saliva of healthy persons? A study of 1493 subjects.' *Brazilian Dental Journal 5*, 2, 93–98.

Low, A.G. (1990) 'Nutritional regulation of gastric secretion, digestion and emptying.' *Nutrition Research Reviews 3*, 229–252.

Malbert, C.H. (2005) 'The ileocolonic sphincter.' *Neurogastroenterology and Motility 17*, S1, 41–49.

Marteau, P.R., De Vresse, M., Cellier, C. and Schrezenmeir, J. (2001) 'Protection from gastrointestinal diseases with the use of probiotics.' *American Journal of Clinical Nutrition 73*, 2, 430S–436S.

McFarland, L. (2006) 'Meta-analysis of probiotics for the prevention of antibiotic associated diarrhea and the treatment of Clostridium difficile disease.' *American Journal of Gastroenterology 101*, 4, 812–822.

Miles, L. (2007) 'Are probiotics beneficial for health?' *Nutrition Bulletin 32* (British Nutrition Foundation), 2–5.

Mintel Reports (2006) *Functional Foods –UK*. London: Mintel International Group.

Moayyedi, P., Ford, A., Talley, N., Cremonini, F. *et al.* (2008) 'The efficacy of probiotics in the therapy of irritable bowel syndrome: A systematic review.' *Gut* epub ahead of pages: http://gut.bmj.com/cgi/content/abstract/gut.2008.167270v1.

NICE (2008) 'Irritable bowel syndrome in adults.' London: NICE. Available at www.nice.org.uk/nicemedia/pdf/CG61IBSQRG.pdf, accessed on 1 November 2009.

Nilsson-Ehle, H. (1998) 'Age-related changes in cobalamin (vitamin B) handling: Implications for therapy.' *Drugs and Aging 12*, 4, 277–292.

O'Connor, K.A., Kingston, M., O'Donovan, M., Cryan, B., Twomey, C. and O'Mahony, D. (2004) 'Antibiotic prescribing policy and Clostridium difficile diarrhoea.' *QJM 97*, 7, 423–429.

Office for National Statistics (2000) 'Adult dental health survey: Oral health in the United Kingdon 1998.' Available at www.statistics.gov.uk/downloads/theme_health/DHBulletinNew.pdf, accessed on 22 February 2009.

O'Hara, A.M. and Shanahan, F. (2006) 'The gut flora as a forgotten organ.' *EMBO Reports 7*, 7, 688–693.

Ohta, R., Yamada, N., Kaneko, H., Ishikawa, K. *et al.* (1999) 'In vitro inhibition of the growth of Helicobacter pylori by oil-macerated garlic constituents.' *Antimicrobial Agents and Chemotherapy 43*, 7, 1811–1812.

Pochapin, M. (2000) 'The effect of probiotics on Clostridium difficile diarrhea.' *American Journal of Gasteroenterology 95*, 1, S11–13.

Pollard, H., Bablis, P. and Bonello, R. (2006) 'Commentary: The ileocecal valve point and muscle testing: A possible mechanism of action.' *Chiropractic Journal of Australia 36*, 4, 122–126.

Preetha, A. and Banerjee, R. (2005) 'Comparison of artificial saliva substitutes.' *Trends in Biomaterials and Artificial Organs 18*, 2, 178–186.

Procter, E. and Loader, P. (2003) 'A 6-year follow-up study of chronic constipation and soiling in a specialist paediatric service.' *Child Care, Health and Development 29*, 2, 103–109.

Rana, S. and Bhardwaj, S.B. (2008) 'Small intestinal bacterial overgrowth.' *Scandinavian Journal of Gastroenterology 43*, 9, 1030 –1037.

Recker, R.R. (1985) 'Calcium absorption and achlorhydria.' *New England Journal of Medicine 313*, 2, 70–73.

Rey, E., García-Alonso, M.O., Moreno-Ortega, M., Alvarez-Sanchez, A. and Diaz-Rubio, M. (2008) 'Determinants of quality of life in irritable bowel syndrome.' *Journal of Clinical Gastroenterology 42*, 9, 1003–1009.

Richardson, C.T., Walsh, J.H., Cooper, K.A., Feldman, M. and Fordtran, J.S. (1977) 'Studies on the role of cephalic-vagal stimulation in the acid secretory response to eating in normal human subjects.' *Journal of Clinical Investigation 60*, 2, 435–441.

Rolfe, R. (2000) 'The role of probiotic cultures in the control of gastro-intestinal health.' *Journal of Nutrition 130*, 396S–402S.

Römer, H., Urbach, R., Gomez, M.A., Lopez, A., Perozo-Ruggeri, G. and Vegas, M.E. (1983) 'Moderate and severe protein energy malnutrition in childhood: Effects on jejunal mucosal morphology and disaccharidase activities.' *Journal of Pediatric Gastroenterology and Nutrition 2*, 3, 459–464.

Sachdeva, A. and Nagpal, J. (2009) 'Effect of fermented milk-based probiotic preparations on Helicobacter pylori eradication: A systematic review and meta-analysis of randomized-controlled trials.' *European Journal of Gastroenterology and Hepatology 21*, 1, 45–53.

Sandle, G.I., Wills, N.K., Alles, W. and Binder, H.J. (1986) 'Electrophysiology of the human colon: Evidence of segmental heterogeneity.' *Gut 27*, 999–1005.

Saps, M., Seshadri, R., Sztainberg, M., Schaffer, G., Marshall, B. and Di Lorenzo, C. (2009) 'A prospective school-based study of abdominal pain and other common somatic complaints in children.' *Journal of Pediatrics 154*, 3, 322–326.

Sazawal, S., Hiremath, G., Dhingra, U., Malik, P., Deb, S. and Black, R. (2006) 'Efficacy of probiotics in prevention of acute diarrhoea: A meta-analysis of masked, randomised, placebo-controlled trials.' *Lancet Infectious Diseases 6*, 6, 374–382.

Schwiertz, A., Lehmann, U., Jacobasch, G. and Blaut, M. (2002) 'Influence of resistant starch on the SCFA production and cell counts of butyrate-producing Eubacterium spp. in the human intestine.' *Journal of Applied Microbiology 93*, 1, 157–162.

Seaman, H., Ballard, K., Wright, J. and de Vries, C. (2008) 'Endometriosis and its coexistence with irritable bowel syndrome and pelvic inflammatory disease: Findings from a national case-control study – Part 2.' *BJOG 115*, 11, 1392–1396.

Sellin, J.H. (2001) 'The pathophysiology of diarrhea.' *Clinical Transplantation 15*, 4, 2–10.

Silk, D., Kumar, P.J., Webb, J.P., Lane, A.E., Clark, M.L. and Dawson, A.M. (1975) 'Oleal function in patients with untreated adult coeliac disease.' *Gut 16*, 261–267.

Singhi, S.C. and Baranwal, A. (2008) 'Probiotic use in the critically ill.' *Indian Journal of Pediatrics 75*, 6, 621–627.

Skikne, B.S., Lynch, S.R. and Cook, J.D. (1981) 'Role of gastric acid in food iron absorption.' *Gastroenterology 81*, 1068–1070.

Spiller, R. (2007) 'Serotonin, inflammation, and IBS: Fitting the jigsaw together?' *Journal of Pediatric Gastroenterology and Nutrition 45*, 2, 115–119.

Stark, D., van Hal, S., Marriott, D., Ellis, J. and Harkness, J. (2007) 'Irritable bowel syndrome: A review on the role of intestinal protozoa and the importance of their detection and diagnosis.' *International Journal of Parasitology 37*, 1, 11–20.

Tadesse, K. (1986) 'The effect of dietary fibre isolates on gastric secretion: Acidity and emptying.' *British Journal of Nutrition 55*, 507–551.

Tan, K. and Seow-Choen, F. (2007) 'Fiber and colorectal diseases: Separating fact from fiction.' *World Journal of Gastroenterology 13*, 31, 4161–4167.

Theisen, J., Nehra, D., Citron, D., Johansson, J. *et al.* (2000) 'Suppression of gastric acid secretion in patients with gastroesophageal reflux disease results in gastric bacterial overgrowth and deconjugation of bile acids.' *Journal of Gastrointestinal Surgery 4*, 1, 50–54.

Timbury, M.C., Sleigh, J.D., McCartney, A.C., Thakker, B. and Ward, K.N. (2002) *Notes on Medical Microbiology.* London: Churchill Livingstone.

Van den Berg, M.M., Benninga, M.A. and Di Lorenzo, C. (2006) 'Epidemiology of childhood constipation: A systemic review.' *American Journal of Gastroenterology 101*, 10, 2401–2409.

Whitehead, W.E., Burnett, C.K., Cook, E.W. and Taub, E. (1996) 'Impact of irritable bowel syndrome on quality of life.' *Digestive Diseases and Sciences 41*, 11, 2248–2253.

Wijk, R., Prinz, J., Engelen, L. and Weenen, H. (2004) 'The role of α-amylase in the perception of oral texture and flavour in custards.' *Physiology and Behaviour 83*, 1, 81–91.

Wilson, M. (2005) *Microbial Inhabitants of Humans.* Cambridge: Cambridge University Press.

Wilson, S., Roberts, L., Roalfe, A., Bridge, P. and Singh, S. (2004) 'Prevalence of irritable bowel syndrome: A community survey.' *British Journal of General Practice 54*, 504, 495–502.

Windsor, J., Macfarlane, L., Hughes-Thapa, G., Jones, S. and Whiteside, T. (2003) 'Detection of Dentamoeba fragilis by culture.' *British Journal of Biomedical Science 60*, 2, 79–83.

Winick, M. (ed.) (1979) *Hunger Disease. Studies by the Jewish Physicians in the Warsaw Ghetto.* New York: John Wiley and Sons.

Wong, J.M., de Souza, R., Kendall, C.W., Emam, A. and Jenkins, D.J. (2006) 'Colonic health: Fermentation and short chain fatty acids.' *Journal of Clinical Gastroenterology 40*, 3, 235–243.

Xu, T., Levitz, S.M., Diamond, R.D. and Oppenheim, F.G. (1991) 'Anticandidal activity of major human salivary histatins.' *Infection and Immunity 59*, 8, 2549–2554.

Yamagata, A. (1965) 'Histopathological studies of the colon in relation to age.' *Japanese Journal of Gastroenterology 62*, 229–235.

Yeo, A., Boyd, P., Lumsden, S., Saunders, T. *et al.* (2004) 'Association between a functional polymorphism in the serotonin transporter gene and diarrhoea predominant irritable bowel syndrome in women.' *Gut 53*, 10, 1452–1458.

Young, A. and Levin, R.J. (1989) 'The rat distal ileum has a reduced absorptive and secretory capacity compared with proximal ileum – is it to facilitate its chemosensing function?' *Quarterly Journal of Experimental Physiology 74*, 4, 561–563.

Zhang, L., Ma, J., Pan, K., Go, V.L., Chen, J. and You, W.-C. (2005) 'Efficacy of cranberry juice on Hellcobacter pylori infection: A double-blind, randomized placebo-controlled trial.' *Helicobacter 10*, 2, 139–145.

Zhu, H., Hart, C.A., Sales, D. and Roberts, N.B. (2006) 'Bacterial killing in gastric juice – effect of pH on Escherichia coli and Helicobacter pylori.' *Journal of Medical Microbiology 55*, 1265–1270.

Chapter 3

COMPROMISED DETOXIFICATION

Angelette Müller and Christabelle Yeoh

1. Introduction

Detoxification is a process that involves all organ systems in the body. Understanding detoxification chemistry, and its effects on neuro-immuno-endocrinology, allows the healthcare practitioner to integrate skills for addressing problems at any level of complexity. Detoxification is a key part of undertaking a functional medicine health programme. It is important not only because we live in an increasingly toxic world but also because detoxification processes put a greater metabolic demand on the body than any other biochemical process, using a large proportion of mitochondrial adenosine triphosphate (ATP).

Toxins are molecules that are capable of inducing disease when inside the human body. Detoxification processes not only handle waste from the environment, but also molecules in the body that have served their purpose and need to be removed. These include: ammonia left over from protein metabolism; hormones no longer needed by the endocrine system; neurotransmitters from the nervous system; and by-products of the immune system. All these molecules undergo biotransformation processes, being changed before being excreted safely from the body.

In this chapter the focus will be on biochemical pathways involved in detoxification of xenobiotics and the factors that govern these. Xenobiotics are molecules that are foreign, do not exist in nature and thus need to be transformed and removed from the circulation. Nutritional therapy is essential in enhancing these pathways and an individualised programme of detoxification often forms a key part of a functional medicine approach towards improving a patient's health.

2. Sources and routes of entry of toxins

Toxins are mainly sourced from our air, food and water. Pollution is present in both indoor and outdoor environments. Outdoor pollution represents combustion and synthetic products from industrial and traffic pollution. The levels vary daily and seasonally and are influenced by the weather. Indoor pollution comprises that which has been generated outside and inside buildings and thus can potentially be worse for a chemically sensitive patient. Indoor pollution arises from, for example, cleaning materials, scents, building materials and cigarette smoke.

The respiratory system is the largest surface area in the body and is a major route of entry for toxins. From the mucosal surfaces of the nasal passages down to the lining of the alveoli in the lungs the body has at its disposal various forms of protection, including mucus, cilia, macrophages, commensals (microflora) and detoxification enzymes, to deal with toxins and foreign bodies.

Oral ingestion of toxins is another major route of entry. The mucosal lining, acidity of gut, tight junctions, digestive enzymes, gut-associated lymphoid tissue (GALT) immunity, detoxification enzymes and peristalsis all work together to help to reduce entry of pathogens or toxins into the body from the gut. The gut has the capacity to reduce the absorption of chemicals, thus we see a wide variety of responses to medication between individuals. The portal blood supply to the liver is the next major step in dealing with absorbed substances in the blood. Blood travels through hepatocyte-lined passages known as sinusoids, where Kupffer cell macrophages help to filter out microorganisms such as bacteria and other potential pathogens.

Food is a major source of toxins entering the body. The portal vein delivers the toxins that have been absorbed through the gut directly to the liver to be metabolised and detoxified, although fat-soluble toxins will first enter the lymphatic system. Some estimates suggest that we process approximately 60 tonnes of food in a lifetime, with a possible combination of residues of agricultural pesticides, fertilizers, additives, aluminium (mostly through cooking utensils) and other toxic metals. In addition, natural plant substances, such as phytonutrients and substances produced during cooking, have to enter detoxification pathways (Furst 2002).

Alcohol consumption clearly impacts on detoxification capacity and also alters the protective barriers, such as tight junctions (in the gut) and the blood brain barrier (Reeves *et al.* 2007).

Residues and liquids, including personal care products and household cleaning agents, as well as paints and adhesives, are other sources of toxic exposure through the skin and respiratory system. Lipid-soluble toxins which are absorbed through the skin transfer directly to adipose tissue, where they accumulate and are only slowly modified by detoxification enzymes. There is much debate over the toxic effects of mercury (Hg) exposure from amalgam fillings, with differing opinions on the potential health impacts of amalgams. However, concerns related to dental amalgam continue, due to multiple links between amalgam Hg and various pathologies (Lorscheidf, Vimy and Summers 1995).

Endogenous sources of toxins from metabolic processes, including hormones and inflammatory mediators, also impact on the use of the detoxification pathways.

As a practitioner, the study of each group of substances that impact the detoxification systems should involve an understanding of:

- what they are
- where they are found
- how they may effect signs and symptoms.

This comprehension is important for each individual's case analysis.

3. Biochemical pathways of detoxification

The body has an incredible potential for recognising, breaking down and eliminating toxins. It achieves this through a specialised system of enzymes, transporters, eliminatory pathways and physical expulsion. Up to 95 per cent of the enzymes are hepatic (present in the liver) but they are also present throughout the body.

3.1 Phase I (biotransformation)

Phase I enzymes largely belong to the Cytochrome P450 enzyme family. These enzymes are proteins with an active iron centre. They are often written as 'CYP' enzymes – for example, CYP1A1, CYP1A2, etc. The CYP enzymes perform oxidation, reduction and hydrolysis to increase water solubility of many xenobiotics, steroids, bile acids and fatty acids. These reactions are dependent on nutrient co-factors. Vitamins A, C, E, thiamine (B1), niacin (B3) and riboflavin (B2) all alter phase I P450 activity (Hodgson 2004). Toxic metals can also interfere with P450 metabolism (Moore 2003). A summary of phase I biotransformation is below:

- P450 activity occurs in the inner mitochondrial membrane or endoplasmic reticulum.
- Activated niacin is required (as reduced nicotinamide adenine dinucleotide, NAD^+), which complexes with CYP450 enzymes to perform oxidation, reduction or hydrolysis. It involves the addition of electrons, or of functional groups, such as hydroxy (-OH) or carboxyl (-COOH).
- Oxidation and hydrolysis allows the compound to enter phase II conjugation and increases its water solubility.

By adding a polar group and increasing the water solubility, phase I metabolites may either be rendered nontoxic, and thus be excreted, or, alternatively, may have increased reactivity and therefore become more toxic. Reactive oxygen species (ROS) are produced as part of the phase I detoxification process. The liver is therefore more susceptible to damage, due to the concentration of phase I activity and its high oxidant generation.

Oxidation promotes damage to phospholipids, thus increasing the rigidity of the cell membrane and affecting the transport of nutrients in and out of the cell. Excessive oxidative damage to DNA can promote and initiate carcinogenesis (Cejas *et al.* 2004).

Local and hepatic tissue protection is present through an antioxidant defence system, including antioxidant enzymes such as superoxide dismutase (SOD) and catalase. These work together with dietary-derived antioxidants, playing a protective role against cellular damage. Depletion of dietary antioxidants or endogenous antioxidant enzymes can reduce this cellular protection, resulting in tissue damage. This damage over time can reduce the effective function of the organ. The key antioxidant enzymes are listed below:

- superoxide dismutase (SOD)
- glutathione peroxidase (GSH-Px)
- glutathione reductase (GR)
- glutathione-S-transferase (GST)
- methionine sulphoxide reductase (MSRA).

See Chapter 9 for a fuller discussion of antioxidants.

3.2 Phase II (conjugation)

The fate of phase I toxic metabolites is phase II detoxification or conjugation, which means to 'join together'. The conjugating enzymes add an organic donor molecule (see Table 3.1) that generally reduces the reactivity of the metabolite, although it can also increase its reactivity. Some water-soluble metabolites bypass phase I and enter straight into phase II detoxification (McCarver and Hines 2002).

3.3 Phase III (transporters)

Transporters are present in the cell membranes of liver, intestine, kidney, brain and other tissues. Phase III transporters are also known as ATP-binding cassette transporters (ABC). They transport substances across the membrane, including amino acids, ions and lipids, as well as xenobiotics, medications and conjugated substances.

The intestines contain phase III transporters in the enterocytes. These work with phase I enzymes to reduce the absorption of toxins from the lumen of the gut. If a substance is not processed using brush border phase I enzymes, it can pass into the enterocyte, where the phase III transporter pumps it back into the gut lumen for a second chance for detoxification. This is also known as the anti-porter system. Toxins that manage to evade this system travel via the hepatic portal vein to the liver to be processed (Dietrich, Geier and Oude Elferink 2003).

Table 3.1 Major conjugating processes and enzymes

Conjugation	Conjugating Enzyme	Processes
Sulphate	Sulphotransferase	• Conjugation of bile acids, neurotransmitters, hormones and many other endogenous and exogenous compounds • Occurs in all tissues and involves a sulphation reaction followed by hydrolysis of the sulphate ester hence using significant amounts of ATP
Glutathione	Glutathione S-transferase	• Occurs in almost all tissues with the highest concentration in the brain, liver and kidney • Glutathione conjugation dramatically increases the water solubility of metabolites • Glutathione also independently scavenges free radicals
Acetyl	N-acetyltransferase	• Requires acetyl Co-A as the donor, which activates phase II acetyltransferase, transferring its acetyl group to reduce hydrophilic properties • Foreign exogenous amines are removed this way • Fast and slow acetylators exist, with slow acetylators being susceptible to the toxic effects of compounds detoxified by acetylation
Amino acid	Amino acid-transferases	• Takes place in inner mitochondrial membrane • Requires specific amino acids such as glycine, taurine and cysteine • Many aromatic compounds are removed this way
Methyl	N-and O-methyl-transferases	• Involves the addition of a methyl group and is involved in the detoxification of a large number of exogenous (such as toxic metals) and endogenous (including neurotransmitters and hydrogen sulphide) compounds
Glucuronide	UDP-glucuronosyl-transferase	• Glucuronidation is one of the most common phase II conjugation reactions in humans, being the major pathway for the elimination of many lipophilic xenobiotics • It involves the addition of uridine 5-diphosphoglucoronic acid to functional groups • It occurs in liver microsomal cells, the kidney, intestine and other tissues

3.4 Metallothioneins

Metallothioneins perform multiple functions, including detoxification. These cysteine-rich proteins function as storage units for zinc and copper within the cell. They have a high affinity for zinc and copper, but an even greater affinity for the toxic metals cadmium and mercury. The metallothioneins can preferentially bind cadmium and mercury, displacing zinc and copper. This cleaving and transfer of toxic metals across the cell membrane has a protective effect, as accumulation of such metals within the cell would promote oxidative damage.

Metallothioneins are synthesised in the presence of free zinc (Borghesi and Lynes 1996). From a clinical perspective, low or deficient levels of zinc could reduce metallothionein synthesis, as observed in animal studies (Szczurek *et al.* 2009).

4. Factors affecting detoxification processes

Table 3.2 Factors affecting detoxification processes

Age	• Infants express phase I and II within 2 weeks of birth
	• Levels in infants and children differ from adults; hence the need for age-dependent doses of medication, vitamins and minerals
	• The degree and efficiency of detoxification lowers with age, exacerbated by decreased absorption from the gut, resulting in lower nutrient/amino acid uptake
Gender	• Men and women have varying levels of phase I detoxification enzymes The oestrogen and progesterone ratio influences the expression of specific enzymes, such as CYP3A4
	• Pre-menopausal women have 30–40 times the availability of enzymes than post-menopausal women
	• Pregnancy up-regulates many of the enzymes
Genetics	• Genetic polymorphisms exist in human population in both P450 and conjugating enzymes. Genetic variations in CYP1A1, CYP1A2 and CYP1A3 result in enormous inter-individual variation in detoxification capacity. Individuals can be categorised as either a 'poor' or an 'efficient' metaboliser, depending on their detoxification ability
	• An example of a poor metaboliser exists in the expression of CYP2D6 in 5–10% of the Caucasian population. Lowered CYP2D6 activity affects the ability to detoxify a wide variety of xenobiotics and can result in an increased risk of side-effects from medications
	• Efficient metabolisers have a greater ability to detoxify medication and environmental toxins. This may have consequences when medication is prescribed, as they may require higher doses for a treatment effect

Sources: Liska, Lyon and Jones 2006; Piñeiro-Carrero and Piñeiro 2004; Williams *et al.* 2004

5. The impact of toxins on nutrients

Detoxification capacity is determined by both the environmental exposure to toxins and the endogenous production and removal of toxins. Clinical expressions of ill health depend on the combination of the toxic load and the individual's capacity to detoxify. Understanding this dynamic requires some knowledge of the ways in which common toxins interact with nutrients, in terms of inhibiting both nutrient function and biochemical pathways.

The practitioner should also remember that detoxification pathways are metabolically demanding. Energy and nutrients are consumed in all toxin-modifying pathways. Box 3.1 gives some examples of the impact of various toxins on nutrients.

Box 3.1 Examples of how toxins impact on nutrients

- **Toxins can affect food quality**
  The glycoalkaloid solanine, an anticholinesterase, accumulates in potatoes, turning green when exposed to light. Solanine poisoning can cause GI upset, which can lead to malabsorption of nutrients.

- **Toxins can inhibit energy pathways**
  Uncoupling of oxidative phosphorylation in glucose metabolism, by a large number of drugs and chemicals, such as fluoride and cyanide.

- **Toxins can inhibit nutrient catabolism**
  For example, the inhibition of methionine synthase (a B12-dependent enzyme which catalyses the methylation of homocysteine to methionine) by lead, aluminium and mercury.

- **Toxins can inhibit nutrient function**
  Cadmium prevents the release of copper from mucosal cells, reducing the levels of copper in plasma.
  Fluoride acts as a cellular poison because it interferes with calcium metabolism, causing raised intracellular calcium and thus disrupting membrane action potential functions (Xu *et al.* 2007). Due to its pervasive disruptive nature in biological systems, the wide use of water fluoridation is a controversial issue, with strong opposition. For further information, see the recommended reading list at the end of this chapter.

- **Toxins can deplete nutrient pools required for detoxification**
  Paracetamol depletes glutathione levels, which can affect phases I and II. Toxicity occurs when sulphation and glucuronide conjugation pathways become saturated, causing paracetamol metabolites from cytochrome P450 metabolism to accumulate. These metabolites are neutralised by binding to the sulphydryl group of glutathione. Further acute toxicity and hepatic cellular necrosis, as seen in paracetamol overdose, occurs when glutathione is no longer available and excess peroxynitrite (from the oxidative stress generated by fever or infection) causes widespread lipid peroxidation (James, Mayeux and Hinson 2003).

- **Toxins can damage DNA repair mechanisms**
  DNA adducts to a large range of widely distributed environmental chemicals, such as diamine dyes, phthalates from plastic and nitrosamines from cured or burnt foods. Chemicals may be adducted to a particular nucleotide on a gene thus inhibiting DNA replication, RNA synthesis and DNA repair mechanisms. If a gene coding for enzymes involved in nutrient metabolism is inhibited by a chemical adduct, this can have multiple consequences for a cascade of nutrients involved.

- **Toxins can impair renal function, causing poor elimination or retention of nutrients**
  Cadmium significantly reduces renal tubular and glomerular function.

- **Toxins can competitively inhibit nutrient absorption**
  Lead is absorbed by competitively binding with calcium-binding proteins.

The common scenario observed clinically is of multiple nutrient deficiencies in a person, despite having what might be considered a reasonable diet. The negative impacts of toxins on biochemical pathways underlie this, combined with the overall toxic load. The logical approach is therefore to increase nutrients for optimising detoxification pathways, in order to reduce toxic loads. The source of toxin should also be sought and then avoided or significantly reduced.

6. Clinical assessment of detoxification capacity and the body burden of toxins

6.1 Tests to consider

Assessment of the patient with compromised detoxification requires an in-depth environmental and medical history, examination of physical signs and laboratory investigations to guide further management. The clinical history is likely to lead the practitioner to consider detoxification therapy, but investigations help to develop an individualised approach and help motivate the patient to undertake therapy.

Investigations should be considered for:

- assessing the patient's detoxification capacity (Table 3.3)
- assessing the patient's toxic load (Table 3.4).

The practitioner should also understand that the clinical scenarios of toxic overload and chemical sensitivity are closely linked. Therapeutic detoxification of the chemically sensitive patient is detailed in this chapter but direct treatment of a sensitivity state is beyond its scope. The patient with compromised detoxification may present in many ways but a patient with chemical sensitivity always has compromised detoxification.

Table 3.3 Tests to investigate detoxification capacity

Assessment of nutrients	Functional tests	Genetic tests: polymorphisms in genes coding for
Plasma cysteine	B vitamins	Cytochrome P450 activity
Plasma sulphate	Urinary methylmalonic acid	Methylation
Plasma glutathione	Urinary pyroglutamic acid	Acetylation
Red blood cell glutathione	24-hour urinary amino acids	Glutathione conjugation
Plasma methionine	Urinary caffeine challenge	Superoxide dismutase activity
Plasma taurine	Urinary salicylate challenge	
Plasma and red cell minerals	Urinary paracetamol challenge	
Plasma antioxidants		

Table 3.4 Tests to investigate toxic load

Biochemical markers of toxic exposure
Urinary organic acids: *D Glucaric*   *Mercapturic acid*   *Orotate*   *Benzoate*
24-hour urinary amino acids: *ammonia metabolism*
Stool, urine (baseline and challenged), hair and sweat tests for toxic metals
Blood samples for DNA adducts to xenobiotics in cells
Fat biopsies
Blood levels of metals, pesticides, solvents and cholinesterase activity

1. **Routine blood chemistry** to measure renal and liver function must be the initial screen to ensure there is no gross renal or liver pathology. This should be undertaken by the patient's GP. Elevated levels of alanine transferase (ALT) and aspartate transaminase (AST) indicate liver pathology. Serious liver diseases, such as viral hepatitis and hepatocellular carcinoma, must be excluded, after which the practitioner may consider whether liver derangements could be due to inefficient detoxification pathways and a toxic patient.

2. **Elevated blood urea nitrogen** (or urea) indicates renal clearance failure. If this is significantly elevated, further tests, such as creatinine clearance and urine protein assessment, should be performed. A slightly high urea and normal creatinine is most commonly due to dehydration.

3. **The level of bilirubin** should be considered a functional liver marker as it can be improved by enhancing other phase II pathways. An elevated bilirubin with normal liver enzymes indicates impaired glucuronidation (Gilbert's syndrome).

6.2 Functional tests

Functional testing looks at the way nutrients are being used or how toxins are challenging an individual's biochemical pathways. Such tests include urinary tests of amino acids and organic acids and detoxification pathway challenges (see below and Table 3.3). Commonly used challenges involve ingesting paracetamol, salicylate and/or caffeine to assess hepatic capacity for detoxification. B vitamins are measured by enzyme stimulation assays. Amino acids and methylmalonic acid collected over 24-hour samples reflect the total requirement and excretion over a day.

The challenge tests work on the basis that different drugs use different hepatic detoxification pathways. Not all of these pathways can be tested but:

- Caffeine clearance can indicate the rate of phase I enzymatic function.

- A paracetamol challenge can indicate the activity of glutathione, glucuronide and sulphate conjugation.

- A salicylate challenge can indicate whether or not glycine and glucuronide conjugation (see Table 3.1) may be compromised.

Abnormal ratios of phase I and II detoxification reactions indicate potential adverse toxicological or pharmacological effects of toxins in the body. A low phase I:II ratio, that is, slow phase I oxidation with cytochrome P450 systems, tends to cause higher tissue accumulation of xenobiotics, as the duration of toxic or pharmacological effects will be prolonged. A high phase I:II ratio, that is, slow phase II reactions, will lead to increased circulation of toxic intermediate metabolites, causing oxidative damage and increasing the risk for carcinogenesis.

In Table 3.5 some commonly prescribed medicines and factors that affect phase I are listed. It is useful to be aware of these when assessing your patient with polypharmacy or with abnormal liver function.

Table 3.5 Examples of inhibitors and substrates of cytochrome P450 enzymes

Inhibitors		
Drugs	*Diet*	*Environmental chemicals*
Azole anti-fungals	Grapefruit juice	Nitric dioxide
Metronidazole	Iron deficiency	Toxic metals
Macrolide antibiotics (erythromycin)		
Quinolone antibiotics (ciprofloxacin)		
Selective serotonin re-uptake inhibitor (SSRI) antidepressants		
Substrates		
Drugs/chemicals	*Diet*	*Endogenous*
Oral contraceptive pill	Caffeine	Oestrogen
Paracetamol	Ethanol	Testosterone
Warfarin	PAHs (chargrilled or roasted meats, cigarette smoke, exhaust smoke)	
Zolmitriptan		
NSAIDs		
Beta blockers		
Polyaromatic hydrocarbons (PAHs)		

Source: Johns Cupp and Tracy 1998

For further details on such functional tests of hepatic pathways, as well as on the assessment of nutrients, please refer to Bralley and Lord (2005), Chapters 3, 4 and 8.

6.3 Genetic tests of detoxification capacity

These tests are useful for understanding a person's genetic susceptibility to the adverse effects of toxins. They explain the huge variation in people's ability to tolerate different degrees of exposure to environmental toxins. A genetic test helps to further individualise detoxification regimes and provides the experienced practitioner and the motivated patient with invaluable insights into his/her genetic susceptibilities, thus providing a platform for preventive medicine, whereby the diet and environment are considered together in order to optimise health. It must be understood, however, that measuring a patient's genotype cannot fully inform one of the phenotype; and functional tests are still necessary to understand the current state of a person's detoxification pathways.

Single nucleotide polymorphisms (SNPs) may be present in one or both alleles coding for an enzyme. SNPs in the genes coding for a particular enzyme usually decrease the activity of the enzyme, but less commonly may increase it. Susceptibility to both increased and decreased activity may be harmful. For example, an increased phase I clearance without increasing phase II activity can lead to increases in circulating toxic metabolites. Table 3.6 gives examples of genes that can be tested for SNPs that may affect the associated detoxification enzyme activity.

Table 3.6 Commercially available genetic tests of detoxification capacity

Cytochrome P450	Methylation	Acetylation	Glutathione conjugation	Oxidative protection
CYP 1A1	Catechol-O-	N-Acetyl-	Glutathione-S-	Super oxide
CYP 1A2	Methyl-	transferase:	transferase:	dismutase:
CYP 1B1	transferase	NAT1	GST M1	SOD1
CYP 2A6	(COMT)	NAT1	GST P1	SOD2
CYP 2CP				
CYP 2C19				
CYP 2D6				
CYP 2E1				
CYP 34A				
PON 1				

Detecting abnormalities in these important enzymes should give the practitioner clues for appropriate treatments. For example, the tolerance of supplemented methyl groups will vary, according to COMT status. With reduced COMT activity, supplementation with methyl donors and methyl groups (such as methylcobalamin, methionine, choline, folinic acid and trimethylglycine) can cause imbalances of dopamine, causing hyperactivity and mood swings (Yasko 2005).

Further genetic testing of the methylation process can be carried out to guide clinical treatment (Lampe 2007) but is beyond the scope of this text. For details on genetic testing refer to Trent (2005), pp.119–140.

6.4 Assessment of toxic exposure or load

Accurately assessing a patient's toxic load requires information from several sources. It involves understanding the mechanisms of uptake of the toxins into the body, the toxin's half life, tissue distribution and elimination, and being aware of any synergistic activity of toxins. Currently available tests do not provide a complete picture of metal and/or chemical toxicity but they can show a snapshot of the load of chemicals or metals currently being eliminated by the body at the time of testing. These tests should therefore be performed and interpreted with care, ensuring the patient does not get a falsely negative picture, nor get unduly concerned about a toxin that appears to be abnormally high, when it may reflect a normal process.

Chemical industries provide data on acute poisoning of the chemical but there is limited knowledge on the chronic low-level exposure that people are undergoing. There is insufficient human data to document long-term carcinogenic effects. Furthermore, there is minimal data on the effects of chemical combinations acting synergistically within biological systems. Current toxicological research can provide fixed concepts but each individual will have varying responses, due to huge genetic variations of enzyme systems.

It is also necessary for the practitioner to be aware that the speed and response to detoxification can vary widely, according to the individual mix of accumulated toxic loads.

6.4.1 RED BLOOD CELL CHOLINESTERASE ACTIVITY

Cholinesterase enzymes are inhibited by two classes of organic chemicals: organophosphates and carbamates. Both are present in pesticides, herbicides and fungicides used in agriculture and gardens. The test is useful only for acute exposures within two weeks.

6.4.2 BLOOD LEVELS OF CHLORINATED PESTICIDES, ORGANOPHOSPHATES AND THEIR METABOLITES

Once again, this is only useful following acute exposure. However, in patients with chemical sensitivity and compromised detoxification, the half-life in serum may be much longer, due to its persistence, and it may therefore be detectable over longer periods of time.

6.4.3 ASSESSMENT OF TOXIC METALS

Serum

Tests for lead and mercury are usually unhelpful as metals are rapidly removed from the blood stream into tissues. In blood the half-life of mercury is 3 days but in tissues it is 69 days. These are helpful in an acute medical setting only.

Whole blood

This is a more sensitive measure, as it includes the total concentration of the elements in serum and intracellular compartments. Excess levels of toxic metals such as cadmium, nickel, mercury, lead and uranium can be assessed. It also determines deficiency of essential minerals and should be done after an overnight fast. Once again, it is limited by not reflecting the toxic loads in other tissue compartments.

Hair

Levels of toxic metals such as lead, mercury, cadmium and arsenic in the hair are highly correlated with exposure (Marlow and Vukelja 1988). However, this test cannot directly imply clinical toxicity. The hair, functioning as an excretory tissue, absorbs these toxic metals so that they do not circulate in the blood. The absence of toxic metals is as important as their presence and must be considered in conjunction with the presence or absence of essential minerals, such as sulphate. In patients with well-functioning detoxification systems, hair levels of sulphate should be well within range. If the hair analysis shows abnormally low levels of sulphate and other minerals (hair mineral analysis has been validated for testing essential minerals: Druyan 1998), the practitioner should be aware that:

- further investigation of detoxification systems is warranted
- the absence of toxic metals in the hair in such a scenario cannot be used to indicate an absence of exposure or metal toxicity (Holmes, Blaxill and Haley 2003).

With treatment to improve detoxification pathways, hair levels of toxic metals should increase, reflecting their circulation in the body and improved excretory function. With continued detoxification treatment and chelation therapy, the hair level of toxic metals should reduce again, with a maintained presence of essential minerals.

Stool

Bile comprises bile pigments (from porphyrin degradation), bile acids (from cholesterol and phospholipids) and bile salts (containing a cocktail of minerals such as lead, iron, copper, tin and manganese). Stool tests can therefore reflect gastro-intestinal elimination of toxic metals. The largest burdens of ingested toxic metals are from fish, seafood and mercuric vapours from dental amalgams. Ninety per cent of mercury ingested is excreted via the biliary faecal route. Stool testing does not measure the retained body burden of metals and cannot be used to imply clinical toxicity. It is helpful for showing toxic exposures.

Urine baseline and challenge tests

Excretion of toxic metals is performed mostly by the liver and excreted through bile. Therefore urinary measurement of toxic metals does not yield information on the body burden of metals. Provocation with a chelating agent is necessary for yielding a range of metals in urine, their excretion depending upon the pharmacokinetics of the chelation agent used. (Note that blood tests for renal function must be checked beforehand.)

Provoking chelating agents used are dimercapto succinic acid (DMSA), ethylene diamine tetraacetic acid (EDTA) and 2,3-dimercapto-1-propanesulphonic acid (DMPS). Six-hour urine collection post provocation recovers 90 per cent of the mobilised metals. The mobilised metals reflect a total body burden of the metal excreted (Hibberd, Howard and Hunnisett 1998). (Note that fish and shellfish should be avoided for a week prior to the test and mineral supplements stopped 24 hours beforehand.)

This is currently the best available method for indicating excessive body burdens of metals. A common mistake, however, is to assume that the level excreted directly indicates how much toxic metal remains in the body. No clinical toxicology tests can directly measure the distribution and load remaining in the body. Urinary excretion tests should be used in succession to determine ongoing toxic metal excretion and thus guide treatment, such as chelation therapy. It is also a mistake to conclude, from one single test, that a patient does not have significant toxic metal excretion if the test does not show increased urinary metal excretion. This depends on the combination of toxins, the tissue distribution of metals and the type and dosage of the chelating agent given. If a practitioner suspects a significant toxic metal load in a patient, this test should be repeated after taking steps to improve liver detoxification pathways (Lee *et al.* 1995).

Sweat

Certain labs offer sweat measurements of toxic and essential minerals. In the clinical context, this test is not needed to guide detoxification therapy, but may be helpful for research purposes.

6.4.4 FAT BIOPSY

This is a sensitive way of detecting a large range of fat-soluble chemicals or their metabolites that have been stored with chronic exposure. These include solvents, pesticides and plastics. The levels of chemicals are reported, with normal ranges indicating the expected background exposure in the general population. Elevated levels of specific chemicals should prompt the practitioner to seek a relevant source, which may have come from previous exposure and/or be in the current environment.

6.4.5 DNA ADDUCTS

Serum levels of DNA adducts indicate the presence of pro-mutagenic markers. Thus treatment to remove them is important for the prevention of cancer initiation. Numerous DNA adducts have been found in people with environmental illnesses and improving zinc status has a protective effect (McLaren Howard 2002). Zinc plays important roles in the cross-bridging and repair mechanisms of DNA. Zinc supplementation has been shown to reduce lipid peroxidation and DNA adducts (Prasad *et al.* 2004).

A large range of chemicals and metals are tested for their presence as DNA adducts. At times, the source of the chemical present as a DNA adduct may not be obvious, but an abnormal test result should prompt the need for detoxification treatment and encourage a chemical-free lifestyle and eating habits. For example, phthalates may be found adducted to DNA if a person prepares food with, or eats and drinks from, plastic products, particularly when heated. This may reflect excessive use of soft plastic products, but may also represent 'normal' exposure with underlying compromised detoxification and DNA repair mechanisms.

7. The detoxification programme

The dietary management of detoxification is a complex issue. The client's current signs and symptoms, medical conditions, digestive health, lifestyle and motivation all play a role in the design of the programme. Inter-individual variation means that manipulation of the diet is personalised. It is important as a practitioner to have evidence and informed understanding of detoxification, as detoxification diets are associated with a degree of controversy. As diets have to be individualised, a set protocol has not been given. Instead, various considerations are given to support the practitioner in making recommendations.

7.1 New and/or exacerbated symptoms during detoxification

The client should understand that new symptoms may be experienced when elimination or addition of specific foods takes place. For example, cutting out caffeine can be associated with headaches. A sudden significant increase in fibre intake can promote symptoms of constipation or bloating, especially where there is insufficient fluid intake. Some individuals may experience rashes and spots. The literature does not support a link between detoxification and skin eruptions and the exact mechanisms are unknown. However, the authors believe that a link may exist, as the skin is a major organ of detoxification.

It is important to explain to the patient that symptoms of pain, bleeding, excessive thirst and vomiting (in addition to other red flag symptoms) can have multiple causes and should not be ignored or thought to be a consequence of dietary intervention. The practitioner should advise the client to visit their general practitioner (GP) if new symptoms arise and are concerning to the patient. Working with a GP is also necessary when designing a detoxification programme for patients with medically diagnosed conditions and prescribed medication.

7.2 Considerations for the detoxification programme

When designing a detoxification programme it is necessary to begin by considering the following:

- The weight of the client. Rapid weight loss can promote the release of toxins. If the client is overweight, gradual weight loss should be promoted (about 2lbs or 1kg a week – although higher amounts may be lost in the initial weeks).

- Digestive and eliminative functions. Consider the type and frequency of stools, the estimated gut transit time and urinary frequency (water intake). If the client is constipated, it is important to address this first as entero-hepatic recirculation of toxins can occur with slow passage and constipation. Evaluate the likelihood of microflora imbalance and/or gastro-intestinal permeability, where appropriate. (See Chapters 2 and 11 for a fuller discussion of digestive function.)

- Promoting an antioxidant-rich diet and supporting antioxidant enzyme systems. Generation of ROS is a natural consequence of the detoxification process. (See Chapter 9 for more information on antioxidants.)

- Supporting the reduction or avoidance of alcohol, smoking, caffeinated products and/or recreational drugs.

In addition, where clients can afford to use natural cosmetic and hygiene products, household cleaning products and water filters, this should be encouraged in order to reduce accumulative exposure to toxins.

8. The dietary management of detoxification

8.1 Aims of a dietary detoxification programme

- Increase foods that promote and support the detoxification process.
- Increase antioxidant-rich foods.
- Modify intake of foods or beverages that significantly promote imbalance between the induction of phase I P450 enzymes and phase II conjugation processes.
- Choose foods that are organic or wild, wherever possible.
- Ensure adequate macronutrient intake, with particular attention to protein, and low glycaemic index foods.

8.2 Protein

A low-protein diet is associated with a lower detoxification capacity. Protein deficiency can cause impaired hepatic function, leading to decreased levels of hepatic proteins, DNA and P450 enzymes. It can also lead to reduced plasma binding of xenobiotics. Animals fed a low-protein diet have increased mortality from exposure to pesticides, chlorinated hydrocarbons and organophosphates (Yu 2005). Conversely, excessive intake of protein, as observed in high-protein weight loss diets, may place a burden on detoxification systems. The by-products of elevated amino acids – ammonia, homocysteine and asymmetric dimethylarginine – have been associated with pathological processes, such as oxidative stress (Wu 2009). The recommended dietary reference values for protein levels vary according to gender, age and lifestyle, and can be found in good nutritional textbooks (Gropper, Smith and Groff 2009).

There is some debate over the type of protein that is recommended for a detoxification diet. Animal proteins are rich in sulphur amino acids, necessary for some of the phase II conjugation reactions. They have higher levels of methionine, for example, compared to plant proteins, such as beans. Methionine is synthesised to cysteine and then to taurine (in the presence of B6), although dietary taurine is the more common source in humans.

Despite the importance of the sulphur amino acids in detoxification, direct evidence of animal protein consumption increasing conjugation has not been found by the authors. In fact, some studies indicate that a lower level of methionine may play a protective role in detoxification, through the preservation of glycine (Meakins, Persaud and Jackson 1998), which is crucial for the amino acid phase II pathway. (Meakins found that high-methionine diets can deplete glycine.) Lower levels of methionine (achieved by consuming a plant-based diet) also appear to reduce mitochondrial oxidative stress (Fontana 2009; McCarty, Barroso-Aranda and Contreras 2009).

In practice, patients are advised to have a diet abundant in all essential amino acids and antioxidants. In the author's clinical experience, vegetarian patients with compromised detoxification pathways are often deficient in sulphur amino acids. Thus patients who are limiting or avoiding animal protein should be encouraged to consume plant foods higher in methionine, such as corn, sunflower seeds, oats, cashews and almonds (Parcell 2002).

As methionine is the chief source of sulphur in the body, supplementation of methionine may be necessary in certain circumstances. This has been observed in specific conditions, such as fatty liver disease and HIV infection; and may also be advisable in some vegans with signs of compromised detoxification systems. Also consider supplementing vitamin B12 and folate and monitor homocysteine levels in patients at increased risk of high homocysteine (Parcell 2002).

An additional benefit of plant-based protein is the rich phytonutrient content. Ellagic acid present in nuts has been shown to have protective effects on indices of liver damage, lipid peroxidation and conservation of antioxidant enzymes (Devipriya et al. 2007). Plant protein foods also contain fermentable fibre, associated with greater excretion of specific toxins, such as polychlorinated biphenyls (PCBs) via the urine (Kimura, Nagata amd Buddington 2004). Plant proteins have a lower potential renal acid load (PRAL) value than animal proteins and may therefore have a greater alkalinising effect, which is associated with increased renal clearance of toxins (Minich and Bland 2007). These benefits offer particular support for detoxification processes.

When eating animal protein, lean meat is preferable, as fat is a storage site for toxins. Organically reared animals are farmed without the unnecessary use of antibiotics and have been found to have fewer xenobiotics as a result (Food and Agriculture Organisation 2000). Wild fish is considered preferable to farmed fish for its lower levels of fat and microbial contamination, such as sea lice (Boxshall and Defaye 1994) and significantly lower levels of pollutants (Hites *et al.* 2004).

8.3 Carbohydrates

8.3.1 STARCHY CARBOHYDRATES

Starchy carbohydrates that are high in fibre and phytonutrients, with a lower glycaemic index, favourably support detoxification: for example, grains contain phenolic acid in their bran layer, which has been found to induce phase II detoxification pathways (Slavin *et al.* 1999).

Gluten

Total exclusion of gluten as part of the detoxification diet may be recommended. In certain individuals, gliadin, a component of gluten, promotes the disassembly of intestinal tight junctions that precedes the onset of gliadin-induced hypersensitivity (Lammers *et al.* 2008). Intestinal permeability is associated with increased susceptibility to toxins and partially-digested substrates, which pass through the gut's tight junctions. Gluten's impact on detoxification in susceptible individuals like Coeliac patients is partly due to its negative association with small intestine mucosal glutathione-S-transferase; this may be linked to increased susceptibility to carcinogenesis (Wahab *et al.* 2005) and gluten-stimulated liver dysfunction (Davison 2002).

Rice may be used as a substitute, with additional starchy carbohydrates, such as millet and quinoa (Lyon, Bland and Jones 2006).

8.3.2 NON-STARCHY CARBOHYDRATES: FRUIT AND VEGETABLES

Fibre

Fruit and vegetables offer a great deal of detoxification support because they are high in fibre (particularly gums, fructans, lignins, cellulose and hemicellulose) and phytonutrients (including plant sterols). There are many benefits of a gradual increase to a high-fruit (where tolerated) and vegetable diet to support detoxification.

For example, increased fermentable fibres, such as fructo-oligosaccharides and inulin, improve stool consistency and transit time, thus potentially reducing constipation (Kelly 2009). Pectin increases the secretion of glycine-conjugated bile acids (Ide *et al.* 1989). High-fibre diets were associated with reduced enterohepatic recirculation of oestrogen when compared to low-fibre diets in women taking oral contraceptives (Sher and Rahman 1994).

Green leafy vegetables

In addition to fibre, fruit and vegetables contain phytonutrients. Cruciferous vegetables, such as broccoli, Brussels sprouts and cabbage, support detoxification through the action of glucosinolates, activated and released through chewing (Fahey, Zhang and Talalay 1997). An example of this is the activity of indole-3-carbinol or its active metabolite di-indolylmethane. These induce the enzyme CYP1A1, which converts oestrone to 2-hydroxyoestrone rather than 16-alpha-hydroxyoestrone (which increases cell proliferation) and may thus have protective effects against oestrogen-dependent cancers (Auborn *et al.* 2003). (See Chapter 7 for a more detailed discussion.) Younger sprouts of broccoli or cauliflower have significantly higher concentrations of a powerful phase II inducer called glucoraphanin (Fahey *et al.* 1997). Cooking reduces the levels of these inducers. It is preferable to steam them lightly. Alternatively, watercress or rocket can be eaten raw in salads or added to food in sauces or pesto. Many other foods have been associated with liver support, such as onions, garlic and bitter foods like chicory, bitter greens, and beetroot (Craig 1999; Osawa 2007).

Organically grown food is preferable, due to lower levels of agricultural pesticides, environmental pollutants, plant toxins, biological pesticides, nitrates and pathogenic organisms (Baker *et al.* 2002; Magkos *et al.* 2006). All fruit and vegetables should be thoroughly washed before use.

8.4 Fats

Fats both modulate and regulate detoxification, through their structure and ability to store toxins. Excessive dietary fat may lead to increased exposure to chemicals from, for example, pesticides and solvents, because once they are ingested and absorbed, they are stored in adipose tissue. High-fat diets, saturated fat and cholesterol are known to induce P450 enzymes (Yang, Brady and Hong 1992).

8.4.1 POLYUNSATURATED FATTY ACIDS (PUFAS)

Essential fatty acid composition in the cell membrane alters its fluidity (Vognild *et al.* 1998), which affects its function, and may alter cells' detoxification potential. Hydrogenated and oxidised fats decrease membrane fluidity. They are also directly toxic to the cell, causing irreversible cellular damage (Chow 1979).

PUFAs, including docosahexaenoic acid (DHA) and eicosapentaenoic acid (EPA), have multiple double bonds (see Chapter 4), which may make them more prone to oxidation. Takahashi *et al.* (2002) demonstrated that increased lipid peroxidation, secondary to intake of fish oil, promotes increased genetic expression of antioxidant enzymes in the liver. Animals fed fish oil were shown to have increased activities of glutathione peroxidase, superoxide dismutase and catalase. Ruiz-Gutiérrez *et al.* (1999) suggest that this effect of fish oil inducing hepatic antioxidant enzyme systems could arise due to increased free radical presence and lipid peroxidation, in response to higher concentration of PUFAs. Other studies suggest that specific antioxidants, such as alpha-tocopherol, are depleted in response to elevated DHA from fish oil intake (Song, Fujimoto and Miyazawa 2000).

In the authors' opinion, compromised detoxification capacity, certain metabolic disorders and/or inter-individual variability may mean that some individuals are more susceptible than others to the effects of lipid peroxidation. The practitioner should therefore consider enhancing dietary antioxidant support as a preliminary step to following a detoxification programme and increasing PUFAs, especially if supplementing fish oil. This antioxidant support should primarily be supplied through the use of use of wholefoods. Increasing dietary sources of antioxidants has been found to have a protective effect in reducing lipid peroxidation (Venkatraman *et al.* 1998).

Evaluation of the quality of any oil, including fish oil, is necessary. How has it been stored? Might there already be oxidised lipids in the product before consumption? Wander *et al.* (1996) reported on the plasma and urinary lipid peroxidation that arose from supplement consumption, rather than arising *in vivo*.

The clinical experience of the authors suggests that a combination of plant oils and fish oil should be consumed, in a ratio of approximately 4:1, omega-6:omega 3, as this has been found to be optimum for membrane fluidity and function (Yehuda and Carrasso 1993; Yehuda, Rabinovitz and Mostofsky 1997). However, this may vary slightly depending on the individual's circumstances. (See Chapter 4 for a fuller discussion of PUFAs.)

8.4.2 MONOUNSATURATED FATS

Monounsaturated fats, such as olive oil, stimulate bile acid production and lead to a reduction in hepatic cholesterol levels, whereas cholesterol and saturated fat diets reduce bile production (Li *et al.* 2005).

8.5 Dairy

Milk may contain significant levels of persistent organic pollutants. Dairy products, such as milk, can also contain mould aflatoxins from contaminated feeds (Fink-Gremmels 2008). As toxins are stored in fat, higher fat dairy products are more likely to contain greater toxin levels than lower fat products. In the authors' opinion it would follow that lower fat dairy products should be used to replace higher fat versions, where appropriate.

For example hard cheese and butter (typically higher in fat) could be replaced by softer, lower fat creams, yoghurts or cheeses, such as feta and ricotta.

8.6 Herbs and spices

Herbs and spices contain active constituents that offer antioxidant activity (thus conserving antioxidant enzyme systems) (see Table 3.7). They may also induce helpful enzymes, such as glutathione transferases, which are major phase II detoxification enzymes in the cytosol, catalysing electrophilic substrates to glutathione.

Table 3.7 Herbs and their active constituents

Herb	Active constituent	Activity
Turmeric	Curcumin	Induce glutathione transferase activity
		Protective of liver cells (Osawa 2007)
Anise, caraway, celery seed, cilantro, coriander, cumin, dill, fennel, parsley and mint	Coumarins, phthalides, polyacetylenes, and terpenoids	Induce glutathione transferase activity (Craig 1999)
Garlic and onions	Sulphides	
Ginger	Gingerols and diarylheptanoids	Promote antioxidant activity (Craig 1999)
Paprika, saffron	Carotenoid pigments	

8.7 Fasting and dietary restriction

Fasting involves partial or total restriction of food for a limited period and usually allows normal intake of water or clear fluid. It has been traditionally associated with detoxification and liver rejuvenation. The benefits of fasting may include: a reduction in total oxidative stress from the cellular mitochondria; greater processing of metabolic by-products, such as chemical messengers like adrenaline and cortisol, and a reduction of the total burden of toxins. There is some evidence that fasting reduces the processes linked with autoimmunity, such as through the reduction of leptin, which alters T cell function (Kuchroo and Nicholson 2003). A period of fasting was found to promote natural killer cell activity and bactericidal capacity (Martí, Marcos and Martínez 2001).

There are different opinions on the safety and efficacy of fasting. Protein, nutrient and fibre restriction can limit the capacity of detoxification and elimination if the fasting process is prolonged. It can also lead to fasting-induced lipolysis (Kather et al. 1985) and the release of toxins into the circulation, with possibly insufficient capacity to biotransform and eliminate them. Evidence to support the use of fasting for detoxification remains undefined and inconclusive. However, water fasts and fruit and/or vegetable fasts have often been used, with anecdotal evidence suggesting temporary and sometimes lasting benefit. The clinical experience of the authors is that total fasting for several days may lead to temporary symptom relief in the patient, particularly where multiple food intolerances are involved. However, this should only ever take place within a hospital setting, where the patient is under constant supervision by experienced healthcare practitioners. Such fasts are also contraindicated in many medical conditions, especially those involving blood sugar control, such as diabetes. Patients who are toxic can reduce their environmental loads temporarily by fasting but are also likely to feel more unwell, which may be due to withdrawal of certain food dependencies but could be due to metabolic derangements, such as hypoglycaemia or hyponatraemia. Fasting for prolonged periods also leads to depletion of essential amino acids, vitamins and minerals needed for detoxification. Thus, without supervision, intensive fasting may not be suitable for many patients with chronic environmental illness. Partial fasts, however, can often be safely used, even outside the hospital setting. These involve restricting processed foods, additives, caffeine, alcohol, sugar, other non-essential nutrients and chemicals, while ensuring adequate intake of protein, slow-releasing carbohydrates and essential fats, vitamins and minerals.

8.8 Food preparation

Food preparation and cooking can alter the nutrient content and generate toxic metabolites. Frying at high temperatures and repeated use of the same oil alters fatty acids, giving rise to toxic polymer compounds and peroxides. These are associated with increased levels of glutathione peroxide and depletion of the glutathione redox system (Saka, Aouacheri and Abdennour 2002), which is an important antioxidant system. In addition, the process promotes the production of heterocyclic aromatic amines, which induce hepatic P450 enzymes (Hümmerich, Zohm and Pfau 2004).

The authors recommend that food should be prepared simply, by cooking methods such as pressure cooking, steaming, steam frying and/or slow cooking on a low heat. Pre-prepared and packaged foods should be kept to a minimum. A significant proportion of the diet, for example a third of the daily food intake by weight, should also be eaten raw, where this can be tolerated.

9. Lifestyle interventions

9.1 Exercise

- Sweating increases body temperature and can promote toxin elimination through the skin, lungs, kidney and intestinal tract, through increased blood flow.

- Exercise stimulates the mobilisation of fats. The breakdown of fat is associated with the release of toxins. As seen above, caution is therefore required with patients who carry significant excess fat, as they may be at greater risk of detoxification side-effects.

- Exercise promotes blood circulation and filters plasma through the lymphatic organs.

9.2 Sauna

Conventional and far infrared saunas elevate body temperatures to induce sweating. Saunas used as an adjunct method of detoxification may include 2–3 sauna sessions of 10–20 minutes each. The heat generated by a sauna also promotes circulation, carrying toxins in the blood to the liver and kidneys for detoxification and elimination. Sweating can promote the excretion of toxic metals such as lead, cadmium and aluminium (Omokhodion and Howard 1994). Note that essential minerals are also excreted in this way, therefore care should be taken to replace them.

9.3 Hydrotherapy

Hydrotherapy includes a variety of water-based therapies, such as alternate hot and cold treatments, to enhance detoxification processes. Hydrotherapy should be performed by an experienced, qualified practitioner, under medical supervision, where necessary. Hydrotherapy has been found to:

- be effective in the treatment of lead poisoning, with a 250 per cent increase in lead excretion (Bennet 2006)
- increase reduced glutathione in the red blood cells of winter swimmers (cold water application) (Siems *et al.* 1999)
- stimulate sympathetic tone in the extracellular matrix, promoting the circulation of blood and lymph (alternate hot–cold water application) (Bennet 2006).

10. Supplement treatment regimes

Nutritional supplements may be needed in cases of:

- nutritional deficiencies
- imbalances in specific detoxification pathways
- genetic polymorphisms.

Table 3.8 Key nutrients used to enhance detoxification pathways

Nutrient	Daily dose range	Indication and reason for use
Nutrients to aid phase I detoxification processes		
Indicated by:		
• certain P450 polymorphisms being present on genetic test results		
• poor caffeine clearance		
• regular use of P450 inhibitors and substrates (see Table 3.5)		
• an additional detoxification burden of chemicals or metals		
Vitamin C	1–3g	Providing phase I pathways with
Vitamin E (mixed tocopherols)	400–800iu	necessary antioxidants. Deficiencies have also been associated with reduced P450
Beta carotene	25,000–50,000iu	function[r]
Silymarin[a]	250–750mg	Increases glutathione and antioxidant enzymes
Iron citrate or	7–14mg	Iron deficiency reduces P450 activity[q]
Ferrous sulphate	200mg	
Riboflavin	5–10mg	Riboflavin deficiency reduces P450 activity[r]
Nutrients to aid phase II detoxification pathways		
Indicated by:		
• certain conjugation enzyme polymorphisms being present on genetic tests		
• the results of a salicylate and acetaminophen challenge test		
• Gilbert's syndrome		
• allergies		
• autoimmune disorders		
• neurodegenerative disorders		
• an additional detoxification burden of chemicals or metals		
Curcumin	250mg–1.5g	Inhibits phase I whilst stimulating phase II reactions[b]. Use when high phase I/II ratio seen on challenge testing
N-acetyl cysteine	600–1800mg	Use when reduced cysteine levels are seen. Increases cysteine and glutathione levels[c]
Methylsulphonylmethane (MSM)[s]	1–7g	Use when reduced sulphur levels are seen and/or sulphation pathway is slow
Magnesium sulphate (Epsom salts)[d]	500–600g in each bath	This, and other supplements with sulphate, can also provide additional sulphate groups for increasing sulphation[p]

Nutrient	Daily dose range	Indication and reason for use
Reduced glutathione[e]	5–10mg/kg	Use when low glutathione levels are seen. It can also be used for chelation, toxic metal detoxification and systemic inflammation.[o] An alternative would be to take the amino acids that make up this tripeptide (L-glutamic acid, L-cysteine and glycine)*
Selenium	200–400mcg	These nutrients are needed to synthesise glutathione
Alpha lipoic acid	100–600mg	Increases glutathione peroxidase activity[f] Increases glutathione activity[g]
Glycine Dimethylglycine Trimethylglycine	500mg–3g 250–750mg 500–6000mg	For glycine conjugation and metal detoxification, particularly of aluminium and nickel[h, i]
Taurine	1–6g	Supports sulphur amino acid pathway (methionine, cysteine and glutathione)[k]

Additional nutrients for methylation should also be considered, as this cycle and the transsulphuration pathway are interdependent.

L-methionine[m] S-adenosyl-methionine[l] Betaine[j] Choline Lecithin	500–1500mg 200–800mg 3g 2g 2g	Consider using any of these nutrients when low methionine levels are seen All increase plasma methionine levels but, as supplementing methionine alone can increase plasma homocysteine levels, consider other nutrients involved with methionine metabolism and methylation[n]
Methylcobalamin Methylfolate/folinic acid Pyridoxine	1mg 0.8–1mg 50mg	Use when low functional levels of these nutrients are seen and/or to support the methyl cycle

a. Kiruthiga *et al.* 2007; b. Osawa 2007; c. Dodd *et al.* 2008; d. Waring 2004; e. Biswas and Rahman 2009; f. Schnabel *et al.* 2008; g. Exner *et al.* 2000; h. Roth *et al.* 2003; i. Graber *et al.* 1981; j. Olthof and Verhoef 2005; k. Lourenço and Camilo 2002; l. Fetrow and Avila 2001; m. Ditscheid *et al.* 2005; n. Naurath *et al.* 2001; o. Angstwurm *et al.* 2007; p. Coughtrie 2002; q. Kaminksy and Fasco 1992; r. Hodgson 2004; s. Monograph 2003
*Note that L-cysteine should not be given as a supplement in that state but as NAC, due to rare reports of cysteine renal stones where L-cysteine is used

In Table 3.8 the recommended doses are stated in ranges, in order to allow for the individual requirements of each patient, and are for use on a daily basis, in divided doses. The dosage of nutrients should be tailored according to the practitioner's experience and the patient's response to treatment. The nutrients listed are used specifically to enhance and support detoxification pathways and should be used in addition to a comprehensive dietary and lifestyle programme.

A good multi-mineral to provide a broad base of minerals is important. Trace minerals can reduce the absorption of xenobiotics, as divalent cations compete for chelation sites in intestinal contents, as well as for binding sites on transport proteins. Selenium is antagonistic to the absorption of cadmium and mercury and participates at the active site of the antioxidant enzyme glutathione peroxidase. Zinc protects against lead and cadmium toxicities. Iron deficiency leads to a reduction in cytochrome P450 function, which requires iron for its biosynthesis. Lithium increases catalase and superoxide dismutase levels and reduces products of lipid peroxidation (Song, Killeen and Leonard 1994).

Probiotic supplements and fermented foods help to keep unwanted intestinal fermentation to a minimum. Problematic bacteria can cause conjugated toxins to de-conjugate, enabling them to be reabsorbed into the blood stream (Hayes 2007).

11. Chelation therapy

Chelating drugs (including DMSA, EDTA, DMPS) are prescription medicines and must be used with care by the experienced healthcare practitioner. Detailed protocols of chelation therapy are beyond the scope of this text. Chelation therapy, incorporated with a comprehensive detoxification regime, is used to remove specific burdens of toxic metals, such as lead, mercury, aluminium, nickel and arsenic (Anderson and Aaseth 2002).

11.1 Contraindications of chelating drugs

DMSA and DMPS are contraindicated in renal insufficiency. Renal function must be checked prior to administration. EDTA may be given at a reduced dose with renal insufficiency. Pregnancy and lactation are also contraindications to chelation therapy.

12. Other considerations for successful detoxification

The focus of this text has been on the function of the liver's detoxification pathways. However, the successful practitioner will also investigate and address any imbalances in related functions, such as digestion (see Chapter 2), circulation (for example, tissue oxygenation, cell respiration and nutrient supply, blood flow and lymphatic flow), renal function (especially with regard to whether there is sufficient hydration for renal clearance) and adrenal and thyroid function (see Chapter 6).

13. Compromised detoxification and chronic disease

A basic appreciation of the possible links between compromised detoxification and illness is important, as such a scenario applies to many patients seeking medical help and nutritional therapy.

Box 3.2 A clinical case of chemical sensitivity

A 55-year-old woman presented with increasing sensitivities. She had a history of food allergy since her 20s. Numerous foods caused brain fog but she managed this by restricting her diet. In her 40s she had more problems, with mould exposure causing fatigue and generalised pain. She had increasing sensitivities to many chemical agents, including perfume, paint, cars, cleaning products, new furnishings and certain buildings and environments. She felt debilitated, with facial flushing, swollen glands and headaches.

Investigations brought to light the following:

- positive autoimmune antibodies: anti nuclear antibodies

- abnormal liver enzymes: lactate dehydrogenase, aspartate transferase and alanine transferase

- elevated serum levels of DDE (dichlorodiphenyldichloroethylene, a breakdown product of DDT, a banned pesticide)

- low glutathione, cysteine and sulphate levels

- the presence of lindane (a pesticide) and PCP (pentachlorophenol, a wood preservative and fungicide) in fat cells

- lindane and PCP DNA adducts

- genomic profile: four abnormal polymorphisms in phase I enzymes, one in oxidative protection (SOD) and six in the phase II pathways glutathione, acetylation and methylation

- excessively raised aluminium and lead excretion in an EDTA urine challenge. Significantly raised mercury, lead and nickel excretion in a DMPS challenge.

Her treatment included a rotation diet, with an emphasis on supplying protein and essential fatty acids and eating organic whole foods. She also had far infrared hyperthermia, massage and nutritional supplements, including silymarin, NAC, taurine, alpha lipoic acid, pyridoxine, folinic acid, methylcobalamin, B complex, vitamin E, vitamin C, multi-minerals, selenium, zinc, omega 3 and 6 fatty acids and reduced glutathione. Given her genetic profile, supplementing glutathione is likely to always be needed.

13.1 Examples of common conditions and compromised detoxification

Table 3.9 Examples of common conditions and compromised detoxification

Alactasia (Swagerty, Walling and Klein 2002)	One third of the world's population (about 15% of northern Europeans, 80% of people of African and Latin origin, and up to 100% of American Indians and Asians) do not maintain the brush border enzyme lactase after the first five years of life. Without lactase, lactose can be considered a toxin because it cannot be digested by humans, but the gut bacteria can utilise it. This causes fermentation, producing additional toxins. Thus lactose intolerance can increase the burden on detoxification pathways and this may ultimately compromise the function of these pathways.
Gilbert's syndrome (Bosma *et al.* 1995)	Gilbert's syndrome is present in 10% of the population, being much more common in people with chronic fatigue and toxic overloads. Gilbert's syndrome is caused by approximately 75% reduced glucuronidation activity of the phase II enzyme UGT1A1.
Autoimmune diseases (Hess 2002)	1 in 31 people in America suffer from autoimmune disorders. Industrial chemicals, pesticides, drugs and toxic metals are all known contributory factors in autoimmune disease. Cumulative occupational exposures to chemicals can lead to autoimmune disease in those with genetic susceptibilities. According to Hess (2002), impaired detoxification underlies this, with genetic deficits in detoxification pathways giving rise to altered cell membrane permeability and immune processes that cause autoimmunity.
Motor neurone disease (MND) (Steventon *et al.* 1988)	There are significantly fewer sulphur-oxidising and sulphur-conjugating activities in patients with MND. The ability to cope safely with neurotoxins is crucial in the pathogenesis of neuro-degenerative diseases.
Alzheimer's disease (AD) (Steventon *et al.* 1990)	There is reduced sulphoxidation in AD patients, as seen from their reduced ability to form sulphate conjugates with paracetamol. Compromised capacity for xenobiotic metabolism of compounds containing sulphur is a major risk factor for developing Alzheimer's disease.
Food sensitivity (Scadding *et al.* 1988)	Patients with food allergy and sensitivity have significantly lower ability to perform sulphoxidation of xenobiotics.
Rheumatoid arthritis (RA) (Emery *et al.* 1992)	There is a significant reduction in sulphoxidation capacity in patients with RA. Patients with persistent inflammation had a higher prevalence of poor sulphoxidation.

13.2 Some possible mechanisms

There are many other examples of the ways in which a heavy toxic load and/or compromised detoxification systems can contribute to ill health. Some of the mechanisms that may be involved are described below.

Box 3.3 Mechanisms of disease due to toxin exposure

Disruption of immune barriers

The four major barriers in the human body are the skin, lung, intestinal and blood–brain barriers. Disruption to cell membranes can be caused by numerous chemicals. The load and chronicity of chemical exposure, and the capacity to detoxify the burden, dictate the extent of cell membrane damage, following which there may be breakdown of protective barriers:

- Damage to the skin barrier results in dominant TH2 allergic responses (Callard and Harper 2007).

- The blood brain barrier is a tightly regulated and immune-privileged unit. When its function is disrupted, humoral immunity is altered and autoimmune mechanisms can be induced, causing neurodegenerative disorders (El-Fawal *et al.* 1999). Chemicals can then alter the integrity of nerve cell membranes, affecting neuronal excitability, neurotransmitter systems and synaptic activity in the entire nervous system.

- Intestinal and brain barriers provide us with complex immune protection and communicate between themselves extensively. Thus gut function significantly impacts on neurological function. Enteric glial cells (star-shaped immune system cells) regulate the gut in a functionally similar way to how astroglial cells regulate the blood brain barrier (Savidge, Sofroniew and Neunlist 2007). This extensive network of gut neural cells is constantly interacting with its environment, such as viruses and food molecules, conveying messages back to the autonomic nervous system. This in turn controls all of the body's automatic organ responses, such as gut motility, bladder function, vascular circulation, thermoregulation, cardiac function, emotions and hormonal control. Disruption can occur anywhere along this autonomic pathway, causing symptoms at varying levels of the autonomic system (Monro 2005). It is observed that patients with loss of oral tolerance to foods may present with a wide range of symptoms relating to these organ systems. Therefore toxic overloads and/or compromised detoxification, due both to the direct action of chemicals on the nervous system and their damaging effects on protective barriers, are states which predispose individuals to allergies and autonomic dysfunction. (See Chapter 8 for a further discussion of this topic.)

Induction of immune reactions by hapten-induced adducts

Chemicals can act as a hapten (see Table 3.9). Haptens do not cause antigenic responses on their own, as they are too small to be recognised by antibodies. Only when they are linked to an immunologic carrier, such as a larger protein, by the formation of adducts, will an antibody response occur (Gunther *et al.* 2007). The antibody formed can then attack the body's cell that is presenting the hapten antigen, leading to an altered immune response, known as autoimmunity.

Direct suppression of immune function by chemicals

Solvents and chemicals can directly decrease populations of immune cells. Natural killer cells (NK) and T lymphocytes decrease following toluene exposure (Tanigawa *et al.* 2001). (Toluene is found in many paints and solvents, such as domestic cleaners and nail polish.) Low levels of cytotoxic NK cell activity are associated with increased risk of cancer (Imai *et al.* 2000).

Table 3.10 Examples of haptens

Medication		Environmental chemicals	
Non-steroidal anti-inflammatory drugs	Tricyclic antidepressants	Azo-dyes	Nickel sulphate
Paracetamol	Diazepam	Tartrazine	Mercuric chloride
Beta blockers	Omeprazole	Formaldehyde	Benzenes

14. Conclusion

With the exponentially increasing number of chemicals being released into the environment, healthcare practitioners should consider detoxification pathways, whatever the presenting situation of their client. The functional medicine approach involves reducing toxic exposures through lifestyle modification, using nutrients to allow cellular reparative and homeostatic processes to operate, and applying specific treatments to reduce the total body burden of toxicants.

Compromised detoxification is a major cause of an increased body burden of toxins. The higher the toxic load, the higher the risk of allergic, autoimmune and neurological disorders. The more sensitive a person is to xenobiotics, the higher the priority for detoxification.

Always bear in mind that people have enormous variation in their ability to detoxify. This helps to explain the wide range of clinical responses to treatment, both in terms of the time taken to improve (ranging from days to years) and the variation in side-effects, if any. Caution must be exercised when dealing with a toxic and sensitive client. In such cases, detoxification processes should not be hurried or forced, or undertaken without prior testing of detoxification capacity.

In all cases, nutritional programmes for detoxification should always start with a good diet. The importance of a clean, broad-based whole food diet will, for many, remain life long.

References

Anderson, O. and Aaseth, J. (2002) 'Molecular mechanisms of in vivo metal chelation: Implications for clinical treatment of metal intoxications.' *Environmental Health Perspective 110*, suppl. 5, 887–890.

Angstwurm, M.W., Engelmann, L., Zimmermann, T., Lehmann, C. *et al.* (2007) 'Selenium in intensive care (SIC): Results of a prospective randomized, placebo-controlled, multiple-center study in patients with severe systemic inflammatory response syndrome, sepsis, and septic shock.' *Critical Care Medicine 35*, 1, 118–126.

Auborn, K., Fan, S., Rosen, E., Goodwin, L. *et al.* (2003) 'Indole-3-carbinol is a negative regulator of estrogen.' *Journal of Nutrition 133*, 7 suppl., 2470S–2475S.

Baker, B.P., Benbrook, C.M., Groth, E. IIIrd and Benbrook, K.L. (2002) 'Pesticide residues in conventional, integrated pest management grown and organic foods: Insights from three US data sets.' *Food Additives and Contaminants 19*, 5, 427–446.

Bennet, P. (2006) 'Managing biotransformation: The metabolic, genomic, and detoxification balance points.' *Proceedings from the 13th International Symposium of The Institute for Functional Medicine*. Available at www.alternative-therapies.com/at/web_pdfs/ifm_proceedings_low.pdf.

Biswas, S.K. and Rahman, I. (2009) 'Environmental toxicity, redox signalling and lung inflammation: The role of glutathione.' *Molecular Aspects of Medicine 30*, 1–2, 60–76.

Borghesi, L.A. and Lynes, M.A. (1996) 'Stress proteins as agents of immunological change. Lessons from metallothionein.' *Cell Stress and Chaperones 1*, 2, 99–108.

Bosma, P.J., Chowdhury, J.R., Bakker, C., Gantla, S. *et al.* (1995) 'The genetic basis of the reduced expression of bilirubin UDP-Glucuronosyl transferase 1 in Gilbert's syndrome.' *New England Journal of Medicine 333*, 18, 1171–1175.

Boxshall, G. and Defaye, D. (1994) 'Pathogens of wild and farmed fish: Sea lice.' *Journal of Crustacean Biology 14*, 3, 614–615.

Bralley and Lord (2005) *Laboratory Evaluations in Molecular Medicine – Nutrients, Toxicants and Cell Regulators*. Norcross, GA: Institute for Advances in Molecular Medicine.

Callard, R.E. and Harper, J.I. (2007) 'The skin barrier, atopic dermatitis and allergy: A role for Langerhans cells?' *Trends in Immunology 28*, 289–328.

Cejas, P., Casado, E., Belda-Iniesta, C., De Castro, J. and Espinosa, E. (2004) 'Implications of oxidative stress and cell membrane lipid peroxidation in human cancer.' *Cancer Causes Control 15*, 7, 707–719.

Chow, C.K. (1979) 'Nutritional influence on cellular antioxidant defence systems.' *American Journal of Clinical Nutrition 32*, 5, 1066–1081.

Coughtrie, M.W. (2002) 'Sulphation through the looking glass – recent advances in sulfotransferase research for the curious.' *Pharmacogenomics Journal 2*, 5, 297–308.

Craig, W. (1999) 'Health-promoting properties of common herbs.' *American Journal of Clinical Nutrition 70*, 3 suppl., 491S–499S.

Davison, S. (2002) 'Coeliac disease and liver dysfunction.' *Archives of Disease in Childhood 87*, 293–296.

Devipriya, N., Srinivasan, M., Sudheer, A. and Menon, P. (2007) 'Effect of ellagic acid, a natural polyphenol, on alcohol-induced prooxidant and antioxidant imbalance: A drug dose dependent study.' *Singapore Medicine Journal 48*, 4, 311–318.

Dietrich, C., Geier, A. and Oude Elferink, R. (2003) 'ABC of oral bioavailability: Transporters as gatekeepers in the gut.' *Gut 52*, 12, 1788–1795.

Ditscheid, B., Fünfstück, R., Busch. M., Schubert, R. *et al.* (2005) 'Effect of L-methionine supplementation on plasma homocysteine and other free amino acids: A placebo-controlled double-blind cross-over study.' *European Journal of Clinical Nutrition 5*, 6, 768–775.

Dodd, S., Dean, O., Copolov, D.L., Malhi, G.S. and Berk, M. (2008) 'N-acetylcysteine for antioxidant therapy: Pharmacology and clinical utility.' *Expert Opinion on Biological Therapy 8*, 12, 1955–1962.

Druyan, M.E. (1998) 'Determination of references ranges for elements in human scalp hair.' *Biological Trace Element Research 62*, 3, 183–197.

El-Fawal, H.A.N., Watermann, S.J., De Feo, A. and Shamy, M.Y. (1999) 'Neuroimmunotoxicology: Humoral assessment of neurotoxicity and autoimmune mechanisms.' *Environmental Health Perspective 109*, suppl. 5, 767–775.

Emery, P., Bradley, H., Arthur, V., Tunn, E. and Waring, R. (1992) 'Genetic factors influencing the outcome of early arthritis – the role of sulphoxidation status.' *British Journal of Rheumatology 31*, 7, 449–451.

Exner, R., Wessner, B., Manhart, N. and Roth, E. (2000) 'Therapeutic potential of glutathione.' *Wien Klin Wochenschrift 112*, 14, 610–616.

Fahey, J., Zhang, Y. and Talalay, P. (1997) 'Broccoli sprouts: An exceptionally rich source of inducers of enzymes that protect against chemical carcinogens.' *Proceedings of the National Academy of Science, USA 16*, 94, 19, 10367–10372.

Fetrow, C.W. and Avila, J.R. (2001) 'Efficacy of the dietary supplement S-adenosyl-L-methionine.' *Annals of Pharmacotherapy 35*, 11, 1414–1425.

Fink-Gremmels, J. (2008) 'Mycotoxins in cattle feeds and carry-over to dairy milk: A review.' *Food Additives and Contaminants 25*, 2, 172–180.

Fontana, L. (2009) 'The scientific basis of caloric restriction leading to longer life.' *Current Opinion in Gastroenterology 25*, 2, 144–150.

Food and Agriculture Organisation (2000) 'Food safety and quality as affected by organic farming.' Report of the 22nd regional conference for Europe, Portugal, 24–28 July.

Furst, A. (2002) 'Can nutrition affect chemical toxicity?' *International Journal of Toxicology 21*, 5, 419–424.

Graber, C.D., Goust, J.M., Glassman, A.D., Kendall, R. and Loadholt, C.B. (1981) 'Immunomodulating properties of dimethylglycine in humans.' *Journal of Infectious Disease 143*, 1, 101–105.

Gropper, S., Smith, J. and Groff, J. (2009) *Advanced Nutrition and Human Metabolism.* Belmont, CA: Wadsworth.

Günther, S., Hempel, D., Dunkel, M., Rother, K. and Preissner, R. (2007) 'SuperHapten: A comprehensive database for small immunogenic compounds.' *Nucleic Acids Research 35*, Database issue, D906–D910.

Hayes, W. (2007) 'Chapter 3 Metabolism: A Determinant of Toxicity.' In *Principles and Methods of Toxicology*, 5th edn. Boston: Taylor and Francis.

Hess, E.V. (2002) 'Environmental chemicals and autoimmune disease: Cause and effect.' *Toxicology 27*, 181–182, 65–70.

Hibberd, A.R., Howard, M.A. and Hunnisett, A.G. (1998) 'Mercury from dental amalgam fillings: Studies on oral chelating agents for assessing and reducing mercury burdens in humans.' *Journal of Nutritional and Environmental Medicine 8*, 3, 219–231.

Hites, R.A., Foran, J.A., Carpenter, D.O., Hamilton, M.C. *et al.* (2004) 'Global assessment of organic contaminants in farmed salmon.' *Science 303*, 5655, 226–229.

Hodgson, E. (2004) *A Textbook of Modern Toxicology*, 3rd edn. New York: Wiley and Sons.

Holmes, A.S., Blaxill, M.K. and Haley, B.E. (2003) 'Reduced levels of mercury in first baby haircuts of autistic children.' *International Journal of Toxicology 22*, 277–285.

Hümmerich, J., Zohm, C. and Pfau, W. (2004) 'Modulation of cytochrome P450 1A1 by food–derived heterocyclic aromatic amines.' *Toxicology 199*, 2–3, 231–240.

Ide, T., Horii, M., Kawashima, K. and Yamamoto, T. (1989) 'Bile acid conjugation and hepatic taurine concentration in rats fed on pectin.' *British Journal of Nutrition 62*, 3, 539–550.

Imai, K., Matsuyama, S., Miyake, S., Suga, K. and Nakachi, K. (2000) 'Natural cytotoxic activity of peripheral-blood lymphocytes and cancer incidence: An 11-year follow-up study of a general population.' *Lancet 356*, 1795–1799.

James, L.P., Mayeux, P.R. and Hinson, J.A. (2003) 'Acetaminophen-induced hepatotoxicity.' *Drug Metabolism and Disposition 31*, 12, 1499–1506.

Johns Cupp, M. and Tracy, T.S. (1998) 'Cytochrome P450: New nomenclature and clinical implications.' *American Academy of Family Physicians 57*, 1, 107–111.

Kaminsky, L.S. and Fasco, M.J. (1992) 'Small intestinal Cytochromes P450.' *Critical Reviews in Toxicology 21*, 6, 407–422.

Kather, H., Bieger, W., Michel, G., Aktories, K. and Jakobs, K. (1985) 'Human fat cell lipolysis is primarily regulated by inhibitory modulators acting through distinct mechanisms.' *Journal of Clinical Investigation* *76*, 1559–1565.

Kelly, G. (2009) 'Inulin-type prebiotics: A review (part 2).' *Alternative Medicine Review 14*, 1, 38–55.

Kimura, Y., Nagata, Y. and Buddington, R. (2004) 'Some dietary fibers increase elimination of orally administered polychlorinated biphenyls but not that of retinol in mice.' *Journal of Nutrition 134*, 1, 135–142.

Kiruthiga, P.V., Shafreen, R.B., Pandian, S.K. and Devi, K.P. (2007) 'Silymarin protection against major reactive oxygen species released by environmental toxins: Exogenous H2O2 exposure in erythrocytes.' *Basic and Clinical Pharmacology and Toxicology 100*, 6, 414–419.

Kuchroo, V.K. and Nicholson, L.B. (2003) 'Immunology: Fast and feel good?' *Nature 422*, 27–28.

Lammers, K., Lu, R., Brownley, J., Lu, B. *et al.* (2008) 'Gliadin induces an increase in intestinal permeability and zonulin release by binding to the chemokine receptor CXCR3.' *Gastroenterology 135*, 1, 194–204.

Lampe, J.W. (2007) 'Diet, genetic polymorphisms, detoxification, and health risks.' *Alternative Therapeutics in Health Medicine 13*, 2, S108–111.

Lee, B.K., Schwartz, B.S., Stewart, W. and Ahn, K.D. (1995) 'Provocative chelation with DMSA and EDTA: Evidence for differential access to lead storage sites.' *Occupational and Environmental Medicine 52*, 1, 13–19.

Li, Y., Hou, M., Ma, J., Tang, Z. *et al.* (2005) 'Dietary fatty acids regulate cholesterol induction of liver CYP7alpha1 expression and bile acid production.' *Lipids 40*, 5, 455–462.

Liska, D., Lyon, M. and Jones, D. (2006) 'Detoxification and Biotransformation Imbalances.' In D. Jones and S. Quinn (eds) *The Textbook of Functional Medicine*. Gig Harbour, WA: Institute for Functional Medicine.

Lorscheidf, F., Vimy, M. and Summers, A. (1995) 'Mercury exposure from 'silver' tooth fillings: Emerging evidence questions a traditional dental paradigm.' *Journal of the Federation of American Societies for Experimental Biology 9*, 7, 504–508.

Lourenço, R. and Camilo, M.E. (2002) 'Taurine: a conditionally essential amino acid in humans? An overview in health and disease.' *Nutrición Hospitalaria 17*, 6, 262–270.

Lyon, M., Bland, J. and Jones, D. (2006) 'Clinical Approaches to Detoxification and Biotransformation.' In D. Jones and S. Quinn (eds) *The Textbook of Functional Medicine*. Gig Harbour, WA: Institute for Functional Medicine.

Magkos, F., Arvanti, F. and Zampelas, A. (2006) 'Organic food: buying more safety or just peace of mind? A critical review of the literature.' *Critical Reviews in Food Science and Nutrition 46*, 1, 23–56.

Marlow, M. and Vukelja, S. (1988) 'Correlations of metal–metal interactions as measured in hair on childhood intelligence.' *Journal of Advancement in Medicine 1*, 4, 195–203.

Martí, A., Marcos, A. and Martínez, J. (2001) 'Obesity and immune function relationships.' *Obesity Reviews 2*, 131–140.

McCarty, M., Barroso-Aranda, J. and Contreras, F. (2009) 'The low-methionine content of vegan diets may make methionine restriction feasible as a life extension strategy.' *Medical Hypotheses 72*, 2, 125–128.

McCarver, D. and Hines, R. (2002) 'The ontogeny of human drug metabolizing enzymes: Phase II conjugation enzymes and regulatory mechanisms.' *Journal of Pharmacology and Experimental Therapeutics 300*, 2, 361–366.

McLaren Howard, J. (2002) 'The detection of DNA adducts (risk factors for DNA damage). A method for genomic DNA, the results and some effects of nutritional intervention.' *Journal of Nutritional and Environmental Medicine 12*, 19–31.

Meakins, T., Persaud, C. and Jackson, A. (1998) 'Dietary supplementation with L-Methionine impairs the utilization of urea-nitrogen and increases 5-L-Oxoprolinuria in normal women consuming a low protein diet.' *Journal of Nutrition 128*, 720–727.

Minich, D. and Bland, J. (2007) 'Acid-alkaline balance: Role in chronic disease and detoxification.' *Alternative Therapies in Health and Medicine 13*, 4, 62–65.

Monograph (2003) (no listed authors) 'Methylsulfonylmethane (MSM).' *Alternative Medicine Review 8*, 4, 438–441.

Moore, M.R. (2003) 'A commentary on the impacts of metals and metalloids in the environment upon the metabolism of drugs and chemicals.' *Toxicology Letter 148*, 3, 153–158.

Monro, J. (2005) 'Man's sense of awareness.' Lecture presentation at 23rd American Environmental Health Foundation, Dallas, Texas.

Naurath, H.J., Riezler, R., Pütter, S. and Ubbink, J.B. (2001) 'Does a single vitamin B-supplementation induce functional vitamin B-deficiency?' *Clinical Chemistry and Laboratory Medicine 39*, 8, 768–771.

Olthof, M.R. and Verhoef, P. (2005) 'Effects of betaine intake on plasma homocysteine concentrations and consequences for health.' *Current Drug Metabolism 6*, 1, 15–22.

Omokhodion, F. and Howard, J. (1994) 'Trace elements in the sweat of acclimatized persons.' *Clinica Chimeca Acta 231*, 1, 23–28.

Osawa T. (2007) 'Nephroprotective and hepatoprotective effects of curcuminoids.' Review. *Advances in Experimental Medicine and Biology 595*, 407–423.

Parcell, S. (2002) 'Sulfur in human nutrition and applications in medicine.' *Alternative Medicine Review 7*, 1, 22–44.

Piñeiro-Carrero, V. and Piñeiro, E. (2004) 'Liver.' *Paediatrics 113*, suppl. 4, 1097–1106.

Prasad, A.S., Bao, B., Beck, F.W., Kucuk, O. and Sarkar, F.H. (2004) 'Antioxidant effect of zinc in humans.' *Free Radical Biology and Medicine 37*, 8, 1182–1190.

Reeves, G., Tonelli, L., Anthony, B. and Postolache, T. (2007) 'Precipitants of adolescent suicide: Possible interaction between allergic inflammation and alcohol intake.' Review. *International Journal of Adolescent Medical Health 19*, 1, 37–43.

Roth, E., Zellner, M., Wessner, B., Strasser, E. *et al.* (2003) 'Glycine – an inert amino acid comes alive.' *Nutrition 19*, 9, 817–818.

Ruiz-Gutiérrez, V., Pérez-Espinosa, A., Vázquez, C. and Santa-María, C. (1999) 'Effects of dietary fats (fish, olive and high-oleic-acid sunflower oils) on lipid composition and antioxidant enzymes in rat liver.' *British Journal of Nutrition 2*, 3, 233–241.

Saka, S., Aouacheri, W. and Abdennour, C. (2002) 'The capacity of glutathione reductase in cell protection from the toxic effect of heated oils.' *Biochimie 84*, 7, 661–665.

Savidge, T.C., Sofroniew, M.V. and Neunlist, M. (2007) 'Starring roles for astroglia in barrier pathologies of gut and brain.' *Laboratory Investigation 87*, 731–736.

Scadding, G.K., Ayesh, R., Brostoff, J., Mitchell, S.C., Waring, R.H. and Smith, R.L. (1988) 'Poor sulphoxidation ability in patients with food sensitivity.' *British Medical Journal 297*, 6641, 105–107.

Schnabel, R., Lubos, E., Messow, C.M., Sinning, C.R. *et al.* (2008) 'Selenium supplementation improves antioxidant capacity in vitro and in vivo in patients with coronary artery disease: The selenium therapy in coronary artery disease patients (SETCAP) study.' *American Heart Journal 156*, 6, 1201.e1–1201. e11.

Sher, A, and Rahman, A. (1994) 'Role of diet on the enterohepatic recycling of estrogen in women taking contraceptive pills.' *Journal of Pakistan Medical Association 44*, 9, 213–215.

Siems, W., Brenke, R., Sommerburg, O. and Grune, T. (1999) 'Improved antioxidative protection in winter swimmers.' *Quarterly Journal of Medicine 92*, 193–198

Slavin, J., Martini, M., Jacobs Jr, D. and Marquart, L. (1999) 'Plausible mechanisms for the protectiveness of whole grains.' *American Journal of Clinical Nutrition 70*, suppl., 459S–463S.

Song, C., Killeen, A.A. and Leonard, B.E. (1994) 'Catalase, superoxide dismutase and glutathione peroxidase activity in neutrophils of sham-operated and olfactory-bulbectomised rats following chronic treatment with desipramine and lithium chloride.' *Neuropsychobiology 30*, 1, 24–28.

Song. J-H., Fujimoto, K. and Miyazawa, T. (2000) 'Polyunsaturated (n-3) fatty acids susceptible to peroxidation are increased in plasma and tissue lipids of rats fed docosahexaenoic acid-containing oils.' *Journal of Nutrition 130*, 3028–3033.

Steventon, G., Williams, A.C., Waring, R.H., Pall, H.S. and Adams, D. (1988) 'Xenobiotic metabolism in motor neuron disease.' *Lancet 2*, 8612, 644–647.

Steventon, G.B., Heafield, M.T., Sturman, S., Waring, R.H. and Williams, A.C. (1990) 'Xenobiotic metabolism in Alzheimer's disease.' *Neurology 40*, 7, 1095–1098.

Swagerty Jr, D.L., Walling, A.D. and Klein, R.M. (2002) 'Lactose intolerance.' *American Family Physician 65*, 1845–1850, 1855–1856.

Szczurek, E.I., Bjornsson, C.S., Noto A.D. and Taylor, C.G. (2009) 'Renal metallothionein responds rapidly and site specifically to zinc repletion in growing rats.' *Journal of Trace Elements in Medicine and Biology 23*, 3, 176–182.

Takahashi, M., Tsuboyama-Kasaoka, N., Nakatani, T., Ishii, M. *et al.* (2002) 'Fish oil feeding alters liver gene expressions to defend against PPAR-alpha activation and ROS production.' *American Journal of Gastrointestinal Liver Physiology 282*, G338–348.

Tanigawa, T., Araki, S., Nakata, A., Yokoyama, K. *et al.* (2001) 'Decreases of natural killer cells and T-lymphocyte subpopulations and increases of B lymphocytes following a 5-day occupational exposure to mixed organic solvents.' *Archives of Environmental Health 1*, 443–448.

Trent, R.J. (2005) *Molecular Medicine: An Introductory Text*, 3rd edin. Amsterdam: Elsevier.

Venkatraman, J., Poomchai, A., Satsangi, N. and Fernandes, G. (1998) 'Effects of dietary n-6 and n-3 lipids on antioxidant defense system in livers of exercised rats.' *Journal of the American College of Nutrition 17*, 6, 586–594.

Vognild, E., Elvevoll, E., Brox, J., Olsen, R. *et al.* (1998) 'Effects of dietary marine oils and olive oil on fatty acid composition, platelet membrane fluidity, platelet responses, and serum lipids in healthy humans.' *Lipids 33*, 4, 427–436.

Wahab, P., Peters, W., Roelofs, H. and Jansen, J. (2005) 'Glutathione S-transferases in small intestinal mucosa of patients with coeliac disease.' *Cancer Science 92*, 3, 279–284.

Wander, R., Du, S-H., Ketchem, S. and Rowe, K. (1996) 'Alpha-tocopherol influences in vivo induces of lipid peroxidation in postmenopausal women given fish oil.' *Journal of Nutrition 126*, 643–652.

Waring, R. (2004) *Absorption of Magnesium Sulphate through the Skin* (republished by the Epsom Salt Council).

Williams, E., Leyk, M., Wrighton, S., Davies, P. *et al.* (2004) 'Estrogen regulation of the Cytochrome P450 3A subfamily in humans.' *Journal of Pharmacology and Experimental Therapeutics 311*, 2, 728–735.

Wu, G. (2009) 'Amino acids: Metabolism, functions, and nutrition.' *Amino Acids 37*, 1, 1–17.

Xu, H., Zhou, Y.L., Zhang, J.M., Liu, H., Jing, L. and Li, G.S. (2007) 'Effects of fluoride on the intracellular free Ca2+ and Ca2+-ATPase of kidney.' *Biological Trace Element Research 116*, 3, 279–288.

Yang, C., Brady, J. and Hong, J. (1992) 'Dietary effects on cytochromes P450, xenobiotic metabolism, and toxicity.' *Journal of the Federation of American Societies for Experimental Biology 6*, 2, 737–744.

Yasko, A. (2005) 'Genetic bypass: Using nutrition to bypass genetic mutations.' Payson, AZ: Matrix Development Publishing.

Yehuda, S. and Carrasso, R.L. (1993) 'Modulation of learning pain thresholds and thermoregulation in the rat by preparations of free purified alpha linolenic and linoleic acids: Determination of the optimal w-3-to-w-6 ratio.' *Proceedings of the National Academy of Sciences of the USA 90*, 21, 10345–10349.

Yehuda, S., Rabinovitz, S. and Mostofsky, D.I. (1997) *Handbook of Essential Fatty Acid Biology: Biochemistry, Physiology and Behavioural Neurobiology*, 1st edn. New York: Humana Press.

Yu, M-H. (2005) *Environmental Toxicology: Biological and Health Effects of Pollutants*, 2nd edn, London: CRC Press.

Recommended Further Reading

Bryson, C. (2004) The Fluoride Deception. New York: Seven Stories Press.

Griem, P., Wulferink, M., Sachs, B., González, J.B. and Gleichmann, E. (1998) 'Allergic and autoimmune reactions to xenobiotics: How do they arise?' *Immunology Today 19*, 133–141.

Gorden, B.R. (2003) 'Approaches to testing for food and chemical sensitivities. Review.' *Otolaryngology Clinics of North America 36*, 5, 917–940.

Honor, A., Birtwistle, S., Eaton, K. and Maberly, J. (1997) *Environmental Medicine in Clinical Practice.* Southampton: BSAENM Publications.

MacDonald Baker, S. (1997) *Detoxification and Healing: The Key to Optimal Health.* Connecticut: Keats Publishing.

Pangborn, J.B. (1994) *Mechanisms of Detoxication and Procedures for Detoxification.* DDI-Bionostics Handbook. Chicago: Doctors Data Inc.

Rea, W. (1992–1996) Chemical Sensitivity Volume 1: Chemical Sensitivity, Volume 2: Sources of total body load, Volume 3: Clinical Manifestations of pollutant overload, Volume 4: Tools of diagnosis and methods of treatment. Chelsea, MI: Lewis.

Resources for toxicological data

Agency for Toxic Substances and Disease Registry

www.atsdr.cdc.gov

The National Institute for Occupational Safety and Health

www.cdc.gov/NIOSH

Chapter 4

POLYUNSATURATED FATTY ACID (PUFA) IMBALANCES

Part 1 The health effects of imbalances in PUFA status and metabolism

Lorraine Nicolle and Ada Hallam

1. What are essential fatty acids?

The association between dietary fat and chronic ill health has been studied for many years, especially with regard to the excessive intake of animal and man-made fats and, conversely, deficiencies of the essential fatty acids (EFAs).

Strictly speaking, there are only two true EFAs, namely linoleic acid (LA) and alpha-linolenic acid (ALA). However, because many of their derivatives may become essential under certain conditions (see below), this chapter covers EFAs and their metabolites.

EFAs are polyunsaturated fatty acids (PUFAs). Each PUFA type is named according to the location of the first double bond when counting from the methyl (-CH$_3$) or omega (n) end of the hydrocarbon chain. Omega-3 fatty acids (ALA and its derivatives) and omega-6 fatty acids (LA and its derivatives) have double bonds located in the third and sixth position respectively from the omega (n) end of the molecule.

The clinician should take note that while some *non*-essential fats are used therapeutically (such as certain saturated (SFAs) and monounsaturated fatty acids (MUFAs)), a discussion of these is beyond the scope of this chapter. These fats can be synthesised in the body. For example, SFAs can be made from glucose and can then be desaturated to n-5, n-7 and n-9 MUFAs (Lord and Bralley 2008, p.281).

Aside from being used as energy in beta-oxidation, EFAs and their derivatives are important to human health because:

- they have valuable cell membrane functions

- o structure and fluidity
- o hormone and neurotransmitter receptor function
- o gene expression
- they are precursors to short-lived local hormones called eicosanoids.

Many of these mechanisms will be elaborated upon in the sections below, with an emphasis on eicosanoid modulation in chronic disease.

2. EFA metabolism and eicosanoid synthesis

Figure 4.1 shows the metabolism of the EFAs LA and ALA into their immuno-modulating derivatives (eicosapentaenoic acid (EPA), docosahexaenoic acid (DHA), arachidonic acid (AA), gamma-linolenic acid (GLA) and dihomo-gamma-linolenic acid (DGLA)) via a series of elongation and desaturation reactions. These are then released from cell membranes by the enzymes phospholipase A2 (PLA2) and C (PLC) and metabolised to short-lived signalling molecules known as eicosanoids:

- prostaglandins, thromboxanes and others (via the cyclo-oxygenase (COX) enzyme), and
- leukotrienes and others (via lipooxygenase (LOX)).

(Roynette *et al.* 2004)

Recently, some new eicosanoids have been described, such as:

- the EPA- and DHA-derived resolvins, docosatrienes and neuroprotectins, which dampen inflammation (Calder 2009)
- the endocannabinoids, which interact with regulators of appetite and weight gain.

Eicosanoids balance each other with opposing effects in order to control many physiological processes, such as arterial constriction, platelet aggregation, tumour growth, innate immunity and inflammation (discussed below).

3. Changes in dietary fat intake over time

The advent of agriculture and industrialisation has led to significant changes in our intake of dietary fats over the last 10,000 years and this is thought to have contributed to the rise of chronic ill health (Cordain *et al.* 2005). Compared with pre-agricultural times, today's diet is characterised by:

- high SFAs, as intensively farmed livestock has a higher fat content
- an excessively high ratio of n-6:n-3 PUFAs. This is due to the introduction of vegetable oils, to livestock being fed a grain-based diet and to a sharp reduction in wild meat and fish, which contain some n-3 FAs

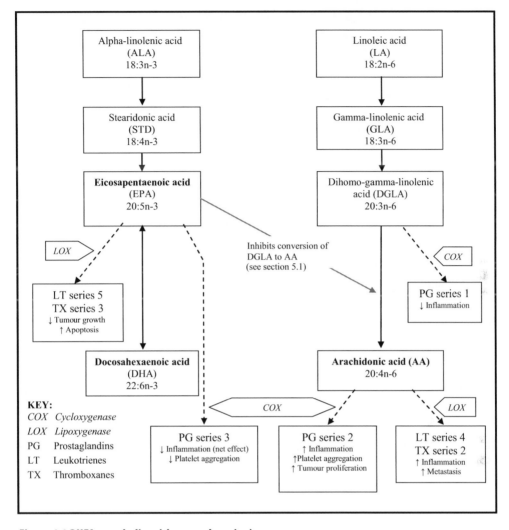

Figure 4.1 PUFA metabolism (shortened version)

- the introduction of artificial *trans* fats, due to the industrial hydrogenation of vegetable oils in processed foods, margarines and reduced fat spreads (Cordain *et al.* 2005).

3.1 The n-6:n-3 FA ratio

The current ratio of n-6: n-3 is estimated to range from 10:1 to 18:1, versus the estimated ratio in hunter-gatherer diets of 1:1 to 3:1 (Cordain *et al.* 2005; Simopoulos 2008). The UK government recommends a n-6:n-3 ratio of 5:1 (Committee on the Medical

Aspects of Food Policy 1991). A ratio more in line with that of the hunter-gatherer diets does indeed seem warranted, given its effect in studies on many chronic diseases (see section 6 below), although the precise optimal ratio is likely to vary, according to the following:

- *the geno- and phenotype of the individual patient*: For example, Simopoulos (2008) describes how individuals with genetic variants at 5-lipoxygenase (5-LOX) may benefit, more than those without the allele, from a higher intake of EPA and DHA.

- *the disease being treated*: For example, the proliferation of rectal cells in patients with colorectal cancer was found to respond to a 2.5:1 ratio, but not to a 4:1 ratio; in rheumatoid arthritis (RA) a ratio of 2–3:1 reduced inflammation; while in asthma a ratio of 5:1 was beneficial (Simopoulos 2008) (some of these variations could be due to inter-study design differences).

- *the existing levels and weightings of EFAs and metabolites in the individual's cell membranes*: Assumptions can be made from dietary (and supplemental) history but a blood test may be more accurate (see below).

Such a range of clinical considerations exemplifies the multifactorial aetiology of chronic disease and the bio-individual nature of therapeutic ratios of n-6:n-3.

3.2 Trans *fats*

Trans fatty acids (TFAs) are unsaturated fatty acids that have been altered so that at least one double bond is in the *trans* configuration. A hydrogen atom moves from the same side to the opposite side of the molecule, thus straightening the molecule and making it rigid (see Figure 4.2).

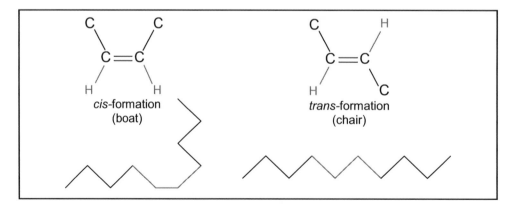

Figure 4.2 The effect of changing from cis *to* trans *on the shape of a PUFA*

TFAs are less prone to oxidation than their original PUFAs but epidemiological data links their consumption with conditions such as cardiovascular disease (CVD) and cancer (Chajes *et al.* 2008; Ros and Mataix 2006) (see the sections on these conditions in section 6 below). It is suggested that TFAs alter cell membrane structure and cellular signalling, and induce pro-inflammatory responses and endothelial cell dysfunction (Harvey *et al.* 2008). However, data is often limited and conflicting, due to inconsistencies regarding the TFA content of certain foods and variability within similar food products (Chajes *et al.* 2008).

While TFAs occur naturally in some meat and dairy products, due to biohydrogenation by bacteria in the first stomach of ruminants, the primary dietary source is via the industrial production of partially hydrogenated vegetable oils in products like margarines, reduced-fat spreads, cakes, sweets, biscuits, chocolate, crisps, baked goods and fast foods (Chajes *et al.* 2008).

The clinician should also note that, in addition to the industrial production of TFAs, PUFAs can be detrimentally altered in other ways. As PUFAs' double bonds are vulnerable to oxidation, these fats can easily be damaged by excessive light or heat, as occurs in frying, grilling, baking at high temperatures or being left in the sun.

3.2.1 CONJUGATED LINOLEIC ACID

Conjugated linoleic acid (CLA) is a TFA that may have some health benefits. CLA refers to a mixture of LA isomers containing conjugated double bonds (that is, the single and double bonds alternate in the molecule), found mainly in the meat and dairy products from cows and sheep. The two main isomers are *cis*-9, *trans*-11, providing more than 80 per cent of dietary CLA, and *trans*-10, *cis*-12.

Animal studies indicate that these two isomers have different effects on health. While the *cis*-9, *trans*-11 isomer appears to have an anti-carcinogenic effect, beneficial effects on body fat and blood lipids are attributed to the *trans*-10, *cis*-12 isomer (Churruca, Fernandez-Quintela and Portillo 2009). However, results are inconsistent when the two isomers are supplemented together and there have been some reports of the two-isomer CLA being deleterious, by increasing inflammation, lipid peroxidation and insulin resistance (Gaullier *et al.* 2007; Poirier *et al.* 2006; Salas-Salvadó, Márquez-Sandoval and Bulló 2006).

Researchers have called for long-term human trials (mice display greater sensitivity) into the mechanisms of CLA and for formulations containing single isomers to be thoroughly assessed *in vivo* for safety and efficacy before recommendations can be made (Gaullier *et al.* 2007; Poirier *et al.* 2006; Salas-Salvadó *et al.* 2006).

4. Signs and symptoms of PUFA deficiency

Table 4.1 lists some common signs and symptoms associated with PUFA deficiency.

Table 4.1 Some signs, symptoms and conditions commonly associated with PUFA deficiency

Possible n-3 deficiency	General PUFA deficiency	Possible n-6 deficiency
• Behavioural issues[1]: aggression, violence, anxiety • Fatigue[3] • Depression[3] • Schizophrenia[3] • Allergies[2] • Immune dysregulation[3] • Rheumatoid arthritis[3] • Inflammatory conditions • Cardiovascular complications[3]: heart and circulatory problems	• Dermatological problems[3]: itchy, dry, flaky skin and hair • Brittle nails[2] • Eczema[2] • Follicular keratosis[2] • Excessive thirst and urination[2] • ADHD[1,3] (trials show most significant results using a mix of EFAs high in EPA and DHA) • Exacerbation of certain cancers[3]: breast, prostate. Other studies link this to EPA/DHA deficiency – see 6.3 below • Mild to moderate asthma[3]	• Growth retardation[3] • Pre-eclampsia[3] • Impaired wound healing • Hair loss

1. Hallahan and Garland 2004; 2. Sinn 2007; 3. Yehuda, Rabinovitz and Mostofsky 2005

Although deficiency signs related to specific PUFAs have been suggested for some conditions, due to inconsistencies in EFA trial designs it is sometimes difficult to establish whether a specific PUFA deficiency correlates with a particular sign or symptom or whether there is an increased need for PUFAs in general. When considering any treatment protocol the clinician should be mindful of the patient's *individual* need, based on the issues discussed below.

5. A closer look at some of PUFAs' mechanisms

5.1 The role of eicosanoids

Eicosanoid synthesis constitutes one of the PUFAs' most profound effects on human health. One of the eicosanoids' most well-researched roles is that of their control of local inflammation. In general, the AA-derived eicosanoids mediate local inflammation and the n-3 derivatives counter this effect (see Figure 4.1).

The FA content of immune cells of people consuming a typical Western diet is approximately 20% AA, 2.5% DHA and 1% EPA. As a result, inflammatory eicosanoids, such as prostaglandin E2 (PGE2), tend to dominate (Calder 2007).

Although inflammation is a vital physiological function, the intensity and duration of such a response often becomes pathophysiological. Indeed, inflammation is now recognised as an important component of many of today's chronic diseases. Conditions like multiple sclerosis (MS), rheumatoid arthritis (RA), osteoarthritis (OA), neurological disorders, depression, inflammatory bowel disease (IBD), cancer and cardiovascular disease (CVD) involve AA-derived PGE2 and leukotriene B4 (LTB4), as well as various combinations of inflammatory cytokines (like tumour necrosis factor-α (TNF-α) and interferon-γ (IFN-γ)), interleukins (IL), transcription factors, (such as nuclear factor kappa B (NF-κB)) and the plasma protein C-reactive protein (CRP).

Due to competition for enzymes at every step of the n-3/n-6 cascade (see Figures 4.1 and 4.2), eicosanoid production can be modified by changing the balance of their precursors (AA, DGLA and EPA) in the cell membrane phospholipids. This is influenced by dietary and supplemental intake (see Figure 4.3). The delta-6-desaturase (d6D) enzyme (see Figure 4.3) has a greater affinity for n-3 than n-6 PUFAs. Hence a greater intake of ALA competitively inhibits LA's metabolism and may thus help to moderate inflammation (Lord and Bralley 2008, p.281).

Studies show that excessive AA can exacerbate the sorts of disorders mentioned above (Calder 2006), while EPA/DHA supplementation tends to show an inverse relationship between clinical benefit and the ratio of AA:EPA (see section 6 below).

5.1.1 ANTI-INFLAMMATORY MECHANISMS OF N-3 PUFAS

N-3 PUFAs are anti-inflammatory not only, as mentioned above, via their competitive inhibition of the n-6 pathway at d6D, but also through:

- EPA and DHA partially replacing AA in the cell membrane

- EPA inhibiting conversion of DGLA to AA

- n-3 FAs having a greater affinity for COX and LOX than n-6 FAs

- EPA influencing cytokine production through direct effects on transcription factors (see 5.2 below).

Note that it cannot be assumed that such attributes of EPA and DHA necessarily apply to ALA (Anderson and Ma 2009) (see 7.2.3 below).

5.1.2 THE IMPORTANCE OF N-6 PUFAS

The clinician should keep in mind that, although AA is generally inflammatory, this is not necessarily always the case for other n-6 PUFAs.

For example, although GLA is a precursor for inflammatory AA, its elongation to dihomo-γ-linolenic acid (DGLA) occurs more rapidly than does DGLA's subsequent desaturation to AA (see Figure 4.2) (Johnson *et al.* 1997). DGLA-derived PGE1 is potently anti-inflammatory and is thus another pathway that the body can use to moderate the effects of the AA cascade. The importance of maintaining the ability to produce adequate series 1 eicosanoids can also be seen from some of their other vital roles, such as:

- maintaining the integrity of the gastric mucosa (as witnessed by the increased risk of gastric ulceration with the regular use of non-steroidal anti-inflammatory drugs (NSAIDs), most of which are non-selective COX inhibitors)

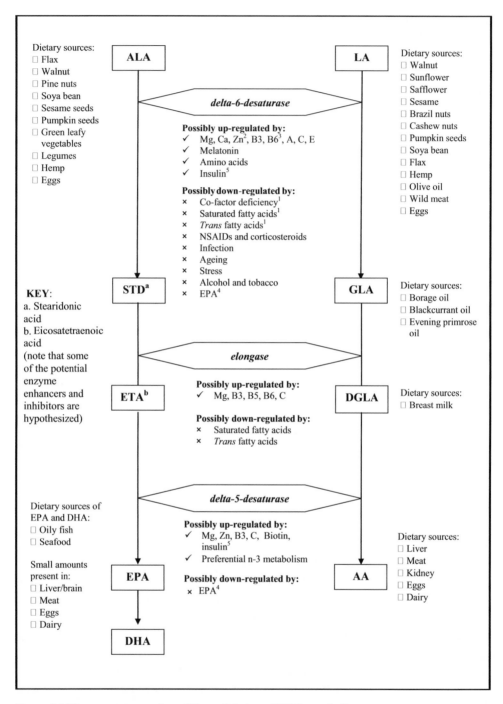

Figure 4.3 Dietary sources and possible modulators of PUFA metabolism

1. Lord and Bralley 2008; 2. Huang et al. 1982; 3. Tsuge, Hotta and Hayakawa 2000; 4. Parsons 1995; 5. see the discussion in 5.1.2 below and in Chapter 5, section 5.3.5.

- maintaining healthy renal function

- guarding against excessive bleeding or haemorrhage.

GLA may also increase transforming growth factor-β (TGF-β □)-mediated responses (Harbige *et al.* 2000). TGF-β □ down-regulates pro-inflammatory TH1 responses and is vital in maintaining optimal gut function (Biassi, Mascia and Poli 2007), itself a key factor in maintaining immune and inflammatory balance in the body. See Chapter 8 for a discussion on gut-immune system links.

In general, it is worth keeping in mind that the extent to which n-6 PUFAs are converted to the inflammatory AA-derived eicosanoids depends on the relative activity of the conversion enzymes. Some experts believe that d5D may generally be of low activity and that most AA may therefore come from dietary sources like meat and dairy (Lerman in Jones 2005, p.419). Even if this is the case, d5D (and d6D) can be up-regulated in certain situations, such as excessive insulin in insulin-sensitive individuals (see Chapter 5, section 5.3.5). There is also some evidence for a possible up-regulation of d5D in type 2 diabetes patients with poor metabolic control (Sartore *et al.* 2008). Hence a diet high in sugars and/or refined carbohydrates may have an inflammatory effect in many individuals. (Figure 4.3 summarises key factors that may modulate PUFA metabolism by affecting the conversion enzymes.)

Other data, however, indicates that unlike GLA (as described above), LA is normally rapidly converted to AA (see Chapter 5's discussion of Horrobin *et al.* 1991). It would therefore be wise for practitioners to be on the look-out for evidence of excessive LA intake in patients' diets. LA has also been shown to induce inflammatory genes in human endothelial cells (Toborek *et al.* 2002), to increase the oxidation of low density lipoprotein cholesterol (LDL-C) and to inhibit the incorporation of EPA (from fish oil supplements) into the cell membrane (Simopoulos 2008).

However, in a recently described 'new twist to an old tale', Calder (2009) proposes that some actions of PGE2 may actually be *anti*-inflammatory. The proposed mechanism is the inhibition of some inflammatory cytokines and leukotrienes and the inducement of the inflammation-resolving eicosanoid lipoxin A(4). Thus it now seems that the general premise of AA being an inflammatory FA may not hold true in all cases.

5.2 Cellular signalling and transcription

Another area of current research is that of the PUFAs' ability to regulate gene expression. For example, by altering certain signalling pathways, AA can up-regulate the inflammatory transcription factor NF-κB, while EPA has an opposing effect (Wahle, Rotondo and Heys 2003). (EPA's mechanism here is via down-regulated phosphorylation of NF-κB's inhibitory subunit IκB.) NF-κB regulates inflammatory gene expression (Calder 2009) by inducing various inflammatory cytokines and the COX and LOX enzymes, all of which are associated with disease progression (Wahle *et al.* 2003).

Similarly, PUFAs and their eicosanoids can interact with nuclear receptors known as peroxisome proliferator-activated receptors (PPARs), in order to turn off and on certain genes that govern lipid metabolism. Activation of specific PPARs leads to increases in FA and glucose metabolism, increased insulin sensitivity (Duan, Usher and Mortensen 2008), reduced inflammatory responses, reduced rates of FA and cholesterol synthesis (Konig *et al.* 2007) and modifications in cell growth and differentiation (Hamakawa *et al.* 2008). Thus regulation of PPAR activation is relevant to diseases like CVD, diabetes and cancer.

Conversely, failure of such PPAR activation can lead to high blood triglycerides and cholesterol. FA:PPAR interaction is now hypothesised to be one of the main mechanisms by which the traditional mediterranean diet reduces the risk of many chronic diseases (Clarke *et al.* 2002). PPAR ligand drugs have now been developed, such as the new class of insulin-sensitisers, the thiazolidinediones (also known as glitazones).

5.3 Membrane structure and organisation

Although the scope of this chapter does not allow for a comprehensive discussion of membrane structure and function, the clinician should never underestimate the importance of optimum membrane fluidity in the regulation of information that is received by the membrane-resident receptors, such as hormone and neurotransmitter receptors. Membrane fluidity thus has a significant effect on the cell's function. Fluidity increases with n-3 FAs and decreases with n-6 FAs, SFAs and *trans* fats (Lord and Bralley 2008, p.274).

An emerging area of research is that of the PUFAs' ability to modify a type of membrane microdomain known as a lipid raft. Such research is still clarifying the size, structure and function of lipid rafts but recent findings indicate that they may play important roles in the development of cancer, insulin resistance and other degenerative diseases (Yaqoob 2009).

6. PUFA modulation of some specific disease processes

The plethora of research studies on PUFAs in specific disease states means that a chapter of this length cannot provide a truly comprehensive discussion. As EPA and DHA seem to have been the most studied PUFAs, this text focuses primarily on their role in some of the most common chronic diseases. (The importance of PUFAs in brain and behavioural conditions is discussed in Part 2, section 9 of this chapter.)

6.1 Cardiovascular disease (CVD)

There are strong associations between dietary fats and CVD. For example, fish consumption is correlated with reduced CVD risk (Tziomalos, Athyros and Mikhailidis 2007), whereas the incidence of CVD seems to rise with higher TFA intake. Indeed,

TFAs may be more of a problem than SFAs (Stender and Dyerberg 2004). Long-held beliefs that CVD is caused primarily by the consumption of animal fat are now being challenged (Ottoboni and Ottoboni 2004). Among the TFAs' detrimental effects is their propensity to increase arterial inflammation (Lopez-Garcia et al. 2005). Denmark experienced a greater than 50 per cent reduction in deaths from ischaemic heart disease in the 20-year period between 1976 and 1996, in which the average TFA intake was reduced from 6g/day to 1g (Stender and Dyerberg 2004).

When it comes to intervention studies, there is good evidence that n-3 FAs are effective in the secondary prevention of heart attack. Most of the current available evidence is for EPA and DHA. For example, Lee et al. (2008) reviewed three randomised controlled trials (RCTs), comprising a total of 32,000 participants, and found that EPA and DHA supplementation led to a significant reduction in CV events. But there is also some indication that ALA may have an effect. Singh, Dubnov and Niaz (2002), for example, found that patients on a high ALA diet had significantly fewer cardiac events and deaths than controls.

Not all the data is positive and a 2004 Cochrane meta-analysis failed to establish evidence for the use of n-3 PUFAs in either cardiac health or cancer in the general population, or in those with CVD (Hooper et al. 2004). However, this null conclusion has since been refuted by scientific societies and most reputable cardiac agencies continue to advocate oily fish as helpful in reducing the risk of CVD.

There is also accumulating evidence for fish oil's efficacy as an additive treatment, for example as an adjunct to statins, in primary and secondary CVD (Tziomalos et al. 2007).

6.1.1 LIKELY MECHANISMS

The possible mechanisms for n-3 PUFAs' effects on CVD may involve the modulation of:

- plasma lipids
- thrombosis
- LDL oxidation
- vasodilation
- platelet aggregation
- plaque stabilisation
- arrhythmias
- inflammation.

Some of these are discussed here.

Perhaps surprisingly, in trials that find CVD benefits, fish oil (FO) does not necessarily lower LDL-C but there is evidence that it lowers triglycerides (Lee et al. 2008; Tziomalos et al. 2007). At higher doses (3–4g) EPA/DHA is effective as both a monotherapy and an additive treatment in hypertriglyceridaemia, despite LDL levels remaining the same, or even rising (Balk *et al.* 2006; Milte *et al.* 2008).

Other studies have found that, although FO may not lower the overall level of LDL, it may still have a beneficial effect on cholesterol, by changing the concentrations of the lipoprotein subclasses (such as very low density lipoprotein (VLDL) and small LDL) (Mostad *et al.* 2008), such that the overall LDL composition is less atherogenic.

PUFAs also appear to influence the process of LDL oxidation. Oxidated LDL-C is thought to have a significant atherogenic impact (Ishigaki *et al.* 2008). High LA intake increases the LA content of LDL and its susceptibility to oxidation (Simopoulos 2006). However, n-3 PUFAs may prevent excessive LA accumulation in cells. Moreover, Lee and Wander (2005) propose that the oxidised lipid metabolites from n-3-rich LDL are less reactive (and thus less disease-promoting) than the metabolites formed from the oxidation of n-6-rich LDL. Note that oleic acid (found in olive oil) appears to be the principal lipid that increases LDL's resistance to oxidation (Parthasarathy *et al.* 1990).

High LA intakes can also lower levels of protective apolipoprotein A-1 and result in reduced high density lipoprotein (HDL) (Cunnane *et al.* 2004).

One of EPA/DHA's most important mechanisms in CVD may be the synthesis of anti-inflammatory eicosanoids (see above). Studies have shown that inflammation in CVD is reduced with increased fish consumption (Zampelas *et al.* 2005), an increased EPA:AA ratio (Wada *et al.* 2008), consumption of FO (Cleland *et al.* 2006) and supplementation of DHA (Kelley *et al.* 2009).

An anti-inflammatory effect may also be seen in n-3 FAs' effect on gene expression. An example is that of a variation in the 5-LOX genotype associated with increased CVD risk. 5-LOX is responsible for the regulation of inflammatory leukotrienes derived from AA. Dwyer *et al.* (2004) identified two variant alleles displaying a two-fold increase in plasma levels of CRP and separately associated with an increased risk of atherosclerosis and diabetes. Dietary AA and LA promoted the atherogenic effect in this subpopulation, whereas n-3 PUFAs reduced the effect.

6.1.2 CLINICAL CONSIDERATIONS

Studies support the use of 0.5–1.8g/day mixed EPA/DHA in CVD (Kris-Etherton, Harris and Appel 2002; Lee *et al.* 2008; von Shacky and Harris 2007), although occasionally higher doses have been used with good results (von Shacky *et al.* 1999) and doses of 3–4g have been most successful in treating hypertriglyceridaemia (Lee *et al.* 2008). Moreover, evidence points to doses of at least 2.7g being required for anti-inflammatory effects (Cleland, James and Proudman 2006). There is far less evidence for the use of ALA but 1.5–3g/day has been suggested (Kris-Etherton *et al.* 2002).

Cardiac societies generally recommend between 500 and 1000mg/day. Mild gastro-intestinal symptoms have been reported at doses greater than 3g/day (Wang *et al.* 2006).

Based on the wealth of scientific evidence, von Schacky and Harris (2007) propose that, rather than generalised recommendations for a standard minimum intake, a better population goal would be to aim for a specific 'omega-3 FA index', that is, red blood cell membrane percentage of EPA and DHA. They propose that an n-3 FA index of more than 8 per cent is associated with a 90 per cent less risk of sudden cardiac death, compared with an n-3 FA index of less than 4 per cent (Europe's current average index being 3.3%). Such an individualised treatment goal could allow for genetic variations.

6.2 Insulin resistance, obesity and metabolic syndrome

In direct opposition to SFAs, n-3 PUFAs improve insulin sensitivity by up-regulating insulin receptors and their binding affinity (Das 2003), and by activating adipocyte glucose transporter 4 (GLUT4) (Simopoulos 2006).

A 2007 review found that a combination of EPA and DHA reduces the risk of metabolic syndrome progressing to type 2 diabetes and reduces death rates from both conditions, primarily due to these PUFAs' reduction of two of the CVD risk factors that are elevated in metabolic syndrome, namely high triglycerides and platelet aggregation (Barre 2007). The same review concluded that the impact of EPA and DHA on the other biochemical imbalances in metabolic syndrome are less well established. It also found that the only published evidence for ALA in type 2 diabetes is for the reduction of platelet aggregation.

In contrast, TFAs have been found to reduce insulin sensitivity in animal studies (Ibrahim, Natrajan and Ghafoorunissa 2005). See Chapter 5 for a discussion of insulin resistance and metabolic syndrome.

As mentioned above, new eicosanoids have been described, such as the endocannabinoids, which interact with regulators of appetite and weight gain. From a clinical perspective, it appears that certain AA-containing molecules (such as 2-arachidonoylglycerol) bind to the CB1 cannabinoid receptor, where they act as agonists (Sugiura 2009) to increase appetite. This is useful knowledge for the nutrition practitioner, given that CB1 receptor *antagonist* drugs are being developed for obesity (Lord and Bralley 2008, p.288). Natural AA antagonists, in the form of EPA and DHA, already exist. Anecdotally, these PUFAs may have a useful role in weight loss programmes.

6.3 Cancer

Much of the observational data shows a negative correlation between n-3 FA intake and cancer incidence and a positive correlation with n-6 FAs, SFAs and TFAs. For example, colorectal cancer (CC) is positively associated with red and processed meat intake and negatively associated with fish intake (World Cancer Research Fund 2007). Chajes *et al.* (2008) report a two-fold increase in the risk of developing invasive breast cancer (BC) in women with higher serum levels of TFAs. Having said this, however, it appears that some human studies of prostate cancer (based on dietary questionnaires) show correlations between tumour growth and higher ALA intake (Anderson and Ma 2009).

When it comes to intervention studies, several *in vitro* and animal studies indicate that n-3 PUFAs may offer some protection against certain types of cancer, especially colon and breast cancer. However, human clinical trials have had mixed results (Chajes *et al.* 2008), possibly due to the presence of so many confounding factors. For example, Poole *et al.* (2007) suggest that the beneficial effects of n-3 PUFA intake may occur only in subjects with a particular genetic polymorphism in eicosanoid synthesis, the COX-1 P17L polymorphism. Thus, there is a need for RCTs to be undertaken that overcome such confounding factors. A 2008 review of n-3 PUFAs and cancer (Berquin, Edwards and Chen 2008) lists 22 trials underway or recently completed that had not been published at the time of writing. In the meantime, this same review concludes that, according to the human trials already published:

- at high doses, n-3 FAs may reduce cachexia for patients with advanced malignancies

- n-3 FAs may improve the effects of surgery and chemotherapy

- increasing the n-3:n-6 FA ratio may reduce rectal cell proliferation and PGE2 release (inflammation) in people at risk of colon cancer

- there are promising results in prostate cancer (but see the concern with ALA above).

Study results for n-6 FAs in cancer also remain inconsistent. For example, despite the significant correlations between intake and disease that have been found in observational studies, Chavarro *et al.* 2007 found inverse correlations between LA and breast and prostate cancer incidence. With regard to GLA and DGLA, Shannon *et al.* 2007 found these PUFAs to be directly associated with cancer risk, while Kenny *et al.* 2000 found in a small pilot study that the addition of GLA led to a faster clinical response in elderly breast cancer patients taking tamoxifen.

6.3.1 POSSIBLE MECHANISMS

Despite the inconsistency of human clinical trials, *in vitro* and animal studies have described a number of possible mechanisms by which n-3 PUFAs may be beneficial in cancer, such as via:

- reduced inflammation through resolvins and competitive inhibition of PGE2 (Maclean *et al.* 2005)

- an anti-angiogenic role via a decrease in the number of tumour microvessels and reduced synthesis of nitric oxide (Calviello *et al.* 2004; Roynette *et al.* 2004)

- a decrease in vascular endothelial growth factor (VEGF) (Calviello *et al.* 2004); VEGF is associated with malignant and pre-malignant colorectal tumours

- a down-regulation of the cell proliferation mediator protein kinase C (PKC), which is implicated in colon and breast cancer (Roynette *et al.* 2004)

- an increase in cancer cell apoptosis via intracellular n-3 lipid peroxidation and the inducement of specific PPARs (Berquin *et al.* 2008). In addition, fascinating studies have been carried out by Kang (2003) showing human breast cancer cells in culture committing apoptosis, after converting n-6 PUFAs to n-3 PUFAs. In order to make this conversion possible, the cells were given a gene that encodes for the enzyme omega-3 fatty acid desaturase. The enzyme converted the PUFAs until the n-6:n-3 FA ratio was little more than 1:1, leading to apoptosis

- encouraging a preferential uptake of cytotoxic chemotherapy drugs into malignant versus normal cells (Pardini 2006).

Conversely, from observational, *in vitro* and animal studies, n-6 PUFAs are proposed to enhance tumour growth, by way of such mechanisms as:

- their up-regulation of NF-κB, regarded as anti-apoptotic (Wahle *et al.* 2003)

- increased PGE2 and lipid peroxidases

- the inhibition of cellular gap junctions, leading to altered signalling and cell proliferation (Saadatian-Elahi *et al.* 2004).

6.3.2 CLINICAL CONSIDERATIONS

Studies have used dosages ranging from 2.5 to 7.7g mixed EPA/DHA per day with varying inter-individual responses; highlighting the need for further research (Bourre 2007; Roynette *et al.* 2004) but also implying that a therapeutic dose is likely to be quite high. Given the possible detrimental effects of excessive n-6 PUFAs in cancer, the clinician should take steps to address any imbalance. It would not be wise to supplement n-6 PUFAs without first checking the individual's membrane EFA status (see section 7.1 below).

6.4 Multiple sclerosis (MS)

As is generally the case with chronic diseases, the development of MS is multi-factorial. However, there seems to be an element of fatty acid imbalance, given that the condition is positively associated with high SFA intake and PUFA deficiency. Whether diet is a trigger or a risk factor, is an important consideration but the potential of PUFAs to modulate the disease's progression appears well founded (Harbige and Sharief 2007; Weinstock-Guttman *et al.* 2005).

It has been postulated that MS patients have an inborn mishandling of EFAs. For example, Harbige and Sharief (2007) found disturbed bioconversion of LA to both DGLA and AA. They suggest this could in part be due to genetic polymorphisms in the COX or LOX families of enzymes. Their double-blind RCT using a very high dose (14g/day) of GLA-rich borage oil over 18 months showed a reduction in relapses and disease progression and attenuation of:

- the rise of inflammatory cytokines TNF-α and IL-1β

- the decline of anti-inflammatory TGF-β (such a decline is associated with MS relapses)

- the reduction of LA and AA levels, both of which are important for the healthy composition of white brain matter.

Other studies have found that newly diagnosed MS patients display a lower ratio of n-3:n-6 FAs when compared to healthy controls. Nordvik *et al.* (2000) found that neurological symptoms improved with fish oil (and vitamin) supplementation, which increased the plasma phospholipid n-3:n-6 FA ratio. Studies trialling EPA/DHA interventions have also reported:

- significant reductions in MS-associated cytokines (IL-1, IL-2, TNF-α, IFN-γ, PGE2 and LTB4), relapse rate, and disease progression (Gallai *et al.* 1995; Nordvik *et al.* 2000)

- an improvement in physical and emotional well-being with the concomitant use of a low fat diet, EPA/DHA supplementation and current drug therapies (Weinstock-Guttman *et al.* 2005).

However, an earlier two-year double-blind RCT, using 1.71g EPA and 1.14g DHA, showed increased PUFA serum and tissue levels, but no significant beneficial trend in overall disability and relapse rates (Bates *et al.* 1989). (Note that interpretation of these results may have been compromised by the control group being advised to reduce SFA and increase LA intake.)

MS is a notoriously difficult disease to study, due to its long and unpredictable nature. Early research focused mainly on n-6 PUFAs, while more recent trials (although Harbige and Sharief 2007 is an exception) have looked at n-3 PUFAs. Some of the findings appear contradictory.

Thus the clinician needs to be aware of the need for individual assessment, encompassing both dietary and lifestyle considerations and, where possible, FA testing, with the ultimate aim of achieving adequate PUFA levels and an n-6:n-3 FA ratio closer to that of the Paleolithic diet. Yehuda (2003) found that a 4:1 ratio optimised PUFA uptake into the brain.

6.5 Other chronic inflammatory disorders

There is a wealth of evidence surrounding the benefits of the longer chain PUFAs in auto-immune inflammatory diseases, such as rheumatoid arthritis and other chronic conditions like osteoporosis.

6.5.1 RHEUMATOID ARTHRITIS (RA)

Many people with RA report marked improvement in symptoms with EPA supplementation (Calder 2008; Stamp, James and Cleland 2005). GLA has also been effective in controlled trials (Belch and Hill 2000; Zurier *et al.* 1996). However, as Lerman (in Jones 2005, p.422) points out, most studies have used rather high doses, such as 2.6–7.1g/day fish oil; or 2.8g/day GLA. See Chapter 11 for a case discussion of RA.

6.5.2 OSTEOPOROSIS

There is some evidence that EPA/DHA may help to reduce bone loss in low oestrogen conditions (Sun *et al.* 2003; Terano 2001). EPA/DHA combined with GLA has also been found to be effective, although there are far fewer studies that include the n-6 PUFAs (Schlemmer *et al.* 1999). However, not all studies have been positive (Bassey *et al.* 1999) and it would also appear that excessive EPA dosing (1g/kg body weight) could be detrimental to bone loss (Poulsen and Kruger 2006).

Moreover, direct evidence of the beneficial effects of n-3 FAs on human osteoporosis is still scarce. Most of the research thus far has been *in vitro* or on animals and the time periods are usually too short to be able to give an idea of the likely long-term effects of treatment, despite the fact that osteoporosis is a slow-progressing, long-term condition. Nevertheless, such research does indicate that, as Salari *et al.* say in their 2008 systematic review, the role of n-3 PUFAs warrants further investigation in human trials. Many possible mechanisms have been postulated, including the anti-inflammatory effects of EPA/DHA and GLA, especially in the light of the more recent understanding of post-menopausal osteoporosis being associated with high levels of inflammatory cytokines (Roggia *et al.* 2004).

6.5.3 BRAIN AND BEHAVIOURAL CONDITIONS

Please see section 9 in Part 2 of this chapter for a discussion of PUFAs in the brain.

7. General recommendations and therapeutic considerations

7.1 Patient testing

An individual's sensitivity to the biological effects of altering PUFA intake will depend on a number of factors, such as:

- dietary and lifestyle patterns
- stress levels
- existing PUFA levels and ratios in membrane phospholipids
- his/her genetic profile.

Thus the optimum PUFA intake, both in terms of overall levels and the n-6:n-3 FA ratio, should be assessed on an individual basis. This will involve taking a detailed case history, including dietary and lifestyle information, and in most cases undertaking laboratory tests.

The most commonly used functional test measures levels of individual FAs in the cell membranes of packed erythrocytes. More than 30 analytes of PUFAs, MUFAs, SFAs and TFAs are indexed. However, the real value of the test is derived from assessing patterns of abnormalities within FA families, especially regarding FA ratios, rather than looking separately at the level of each individual FA. Lord and Bralley (2008) put forward various patterns of abnormality to look for, such as:

- *general FA (including EFA) deficiency*: Endogenous FA synthesis may be stepped up to help compensate but EFAs will be lacking and the patient's ability to produce eicosanoids will suffer.

- *n-3 FA deficiencies*: This is the most common area of clinical concern, as seen from the studies above. One can also see imbalances within the n-3 family (such as adequate ALA but low EPA/DHA), which can indicate suboptimal function of the desaturase and/or elongase enzymes, possibly due to insufficient co-factors (see Figure 4.3 above), or to genetic polymorphisms.

- *ALA or EPA excess*: A possibility with long-term supplementation of flax or fish oil (see Box 4.1).

- *n-6 FA deficiencies*: This may be relatively uncommon, due to the popular Western diet (see above) but see Box 4.1. Such deficiencies manifest as skin conditions, as n-6 FAs are the most abundant and necessary EFA class in skin cells. Impairment of d6D (see Figure 4.3) can be considered if there is an excessively high LA:DGLA ratio.

- *n-6 FA excess*: This is a relatively common finding and is implicated in many diseases (see above), primarily due to AA's conversion to series 2 eicosanoids.

- *TFA toxicity*: Implicated in chronic disease, as discussed above.

7.2 General dietary recommendations

General UK and international guidelines recommend that total FA intake should range from 15 to 35 per cent of daily energy intake (DEI) – in other words, calories. SFAs should account for no more than 10 per cent DEI; total PUFAs should equal 6–10 per cent DEI (n-6 FAs 5–8%: n-3 FAs 1–2% DEI) and TFAs should constitute a maximum of 1–2 per cent DEI, with the remainder consisting of oleic acid (n-9) (Graham *et al.* 2007; Wahlqvist 2005; Williams *et al.* 2007). However, it has also been suggested that desirable LA levels may be overestimated and that 2 per cent DEI is adequate (Cunnane *et al.* 2004).

7.2.1 N-3 PUFAS

The daily UK recommended intake for n-3 PUFAs is 450–500mg; with a minimum of 500mg in the presence of CVD (Cunnane *et al.* 2004; Jackson *et al.* 2004). As DHA is vital for foetal visual and cognitive development, pregnant and lactating women should ensure a daily intake of at least 200mg DHA/day (Koletzko, Cetin and Brenna 2007).

RCTs involving pregnant women have used doses of up to 1g DHA and 2.7g n-3 PUFA without significant adverse effects (Koletzko *et al.* 2007).

7.2.2 FISH INTAKE

To achieve n-3 FA guidelines, 2–4 portions of oily fish (depending on the type of fish) should be consumed per week. Table 4.2 lists some types of oily fish and their PUFA content. One can see that eating two 100g salmon or mackerel fillets, three 100g cans of sardines or three 100g tuna fillets a week would more than cover these requirements (Table 4.2).

Table 4.2 Oily fish and their n-3 PUFA content

Type of fish	EPA (g/100g)	DHA (g/100g)	Total n-3 FA (g/100g)
Fresh salmon	0.50–1.2	0.40–1.3	2.7
Fresh mackerel	0.71	0.12–1.10	1.93
Canned sardines	0.55–0.89	0.10–0.86	1.57
Canned and smoked salmon	0.55	0.85	1.54
Fresh tuna	0.3	1.1	1.5
Herring	0.51	0.11–0.69	1.31
Fresh trout	0.23	0.09–0.83	1.15

Source: *Adapted from Jackson et al. 2004 and Massaro et al. 2008*

The fat content of the same type of fish varies, depending on the time of year it is harvested, whether it is farmed or wild and, if farmed, the type of feed used.

Due to concern about the possible contamination of oily fish with methylmercury (MeHg$^+$), dioxins and polychlorinated biphenyls (PCBs), all of which have been associated with CVD, cancer and changes in foetal development (Jackson *et al.* 2004), the UK's Scientific Advisory Committee on Nutrition (SACN) recommends that women who are pregnant or trying to conceive should have a maximum of 1–2 oily fish portions per week.

In line with these recommendations, the UK Committee on Toxicology (COT) (Jackson *et al.* 2004) states that no more than 1.6μg MeHg$^+$/kg bodyweight per week should be consumed by women who are lactating, pregnant or planning pregnancy. Thus shark, swordfish, and marlin should be avoided. Fresh tuna steaks are permitted twice per week and medium-sized tinned tuna four times per week (Jackson *et al.* 2004). For non-reproductive and breastfeeding adults the ceiling is raised to 3.3μg/kg bodyweight per week. Table 4.3 lists the estimated MeHg$^+$ content of certain fish.

Table 4.3 Estimated methylmercury intake from fish

140g portion of fish	Shark (flake)	Swordfish	Marlin	Fresh tuna	Tinned tuna
MeHg[+*]	3.04	2.68	2.20	0.80	0.38

Source: Adapted from Jackson et al. 2004
* amount equates to µg/kg by weight (bw)/week for a 70kg adult (not including estimate from total diet – approximately 0.28µg/kg bw/week)

7.2.3 VEGETARIAN AND VEGAN SOURCES

As would be expected, vegetarians have lower EPA and DHA levels than omnivores (and vegans have lower levels still), with higher plasma LA (Rosell *et al.* 2005).

Due to ALA's poor conversion rate to EPA and DHA (which may be as low as 0.2% and 0.05% respectively), the practitioner should not assume that the health benefits of EPA and DHA extend to their parent PUFAs. It has been found that increasing ALA consumption does not necessarily lead to increased DHA levels in plasma or cell membranes (Berquin *et al.* 2008). Furthermore, a 2009 review of 300 references concluded that, despite the well-studied benefits of EPA and DHA, the relationship between ALA and chronic disease is unclear (Anderson and Ma 2009). Thus, in certain circumstances, it may become essential for a vegan or vegetarian patient to consume EPA and DHA. In recent years, vegan EPA and DHA supplements have become available.

Table 4.4 lists the different FA content of certain nuts and seeds.

7.2.4 SUMMARY OF DIETARY RECOMMENDATIONS

Taking account of the above guidelines, in general terms it would be wise to:

- keep fat intake to a maximum of 35 per cent of caloric intake
- limit intake of saturated fat by using more monounsaturated fats, such as olive oil, nuts and avocados. These can be used in higher quantities than PUFA oils because they are less vulnerable to oxidation
- eat oily fish two to four times a week for EPA and DHA
- eat a handful of mixed seeds a day, or approximately one tablespoon of cold pressed, unadulterated mixed seed oil (including linseed) for ALA and LA
- avoid *trans* and hydrogenated fats
- eat a nutrient-dense, low glycaemic load diet to minimise d5D up-regulation, and to obtain co-factors for d6D and elongase.

Table 4.4 Average fat content of nuts and seeds

Nuts and seeds	LA (g/100g)	ALA (g/100g)	SFA (g/100g)
Almonds	12.2	0.00	3.9
Brazil nuts	20.5	0.05	15.1
Cashews	7.7	0.15	9.2
Hazelnuts	7.8	0.09	4.5
Macadamia nuts	1.3	0.21	12.1
Peanuts	15.6	0.00	6.8
Pecans	20.6	1.00	6.2
Pine nuts	33.2	0.16	4.9
Pistachios	13.2	0.25	5.4
Walnuts	38.1	9.08	6.1
Flaxseed (linseed)	4.32	18.12	3.20
Pumpkin seeds	20.70	0.18	8.67
Sesame seeds (hulled)	23.58	0.42	7.67
Sunflower seeds	32.78	0.07	5.22

Source: *Adapted from* Murray, Pizzorno and Pizzorno 2005, p.802; Ros and Mataix 2006, p.32
(Note that most nuts are also rich in MUFAs.)

7.3 Supplementation

In certain cases, such as pregnant/lactating women, or individuals with particular disease states or at high risk of developing such diseases, supplementation may be considered necessary in order to ensure a therapeutic dose, particularly of EPA, DHA and GLA, due to the poor conversion rates mentioned above. (Note that symptomatic benefits may not be evident for 2–3 months.)

However, the practitioner faces a dilemma, since supplementing single PUFAs at the high doses that have been used in the studies (see above) may, over the long term, lead to an undesirable FA balance in membrane phospholipids (see Box 4.1).

Therefore the best practice would be to undertake a laboratory test (see above) every few months in order to monitor membrane FA ratios. The practitioner must also take into account the full case history, including dietary and lifestyle history, family history, possible drug-nutrient interactions (such as anti-platelet/anticoagulant and antihypertensive agents) and other contraindications, medical conditions and other symptoms.

The clinician should also work on the basis that prescribing high doses of EPA and GLA to reduce inflammation should only be thought of as an interim measure (albeit well warranted if it enables the patient to reduce or avoid NSAIDs or prescription medication), while conducting investigations to put together a comprehensive picture of the antecedents, triggers and mediators of the patient's condition.

The evidence so far indicates that fish oil supplements are safe for general consumption in doses up to 3g EPA/DHA per day. If they are bought from a reputable supplier in the UK they are likely to contain very little methylmercury (Cleland, James and Proudman 2006; Jellin *et al.* 2008). GLA is considered safe at doses up to 2.8g/day for up to one year (Jellin *et al.* 2008).

Box 4.1 Can fish oil supplementation go too far?

The well-publicised message that lowering the n-6:n-3 FA ratio can reduce inflammatory responses that contribute to chronic disease has led to an explosion in the market for flax- and fish oil dietary supplements. While such supplementation may indeed be warranted in many cases, the clinician should take into account that most of the studies on EPA/DHA supplementation have been undertaken over relatively short periods of time. Many do not assess what may happen in long-term supplementation, where not only could the n-3:n-6 FA cell membrane ratio become abnormally high, but n-3 derivatives may also be at excessive levels.

In fact, it has been suggested that excessive fish oil supplementation over the long term could impair innate immunity (Harbige 1998). Later critiques of studies in this area have concluded that while *significant* impairment is unlikely, such unintended consequences need to be considered as possible (Stephensen and Kelley 2006). In a 2007 study significantly higher incidences of flu symptoms, infection and rashes were reported after a relatively short-term (eight-week) dosing of 4g n-3 FA/day compared with those taking a corn oil placebo (Davidson *et al.* 2007).

Thus the clinician needs to evaluate his/her EPA/DHA supplementation strategies for the potential risks, as well as the benefits. Where necessary, the practitioner should consider balancing FO supplementation with a concurrent supplement of GLA, which can be converted to the series 1 eicosanoids.

Gender and hormone treatment also need to be taken into account when prescribing, as women tend to synthesise more DHA from ALA than do men, especially those on oestrogen therapy, while DHA is reconverted to EPA more efficiently in men (Crowe *et al.* 2008).

8. Conclusion

Science has yet to discover more about the mechanisms of PUFAs and, as has been seen in section 6 above, there is still a need for more controlled clinical trials to be undertaken. But PUFAs are vital to health and the evidence to date provides a strong indication that intervening effectively to optimise a patient's intake may make a significant difference to his/her ability to manage his/her chronic disease and/or reduce the risk factors for developing such diseases.

References

Anderson, B.M. and Ma, D.W. (2009) 'Are all n-3 polyunsaturated fatty acids created equal?' *Lipids in Health and Disease 8*, 33 [epub ahead of print].

Balk, E.M., Lichentstein, A.H., Chung, M., Kupelnick, B. *et al.* (2006) 'Effects of omega-3 fatty acids on serum markers of CVD risk: A systematic review.' *Atherosclerosis 189*, 1, 19–30.

Barre, D.E. (2007) 'The role of consumption of alpha-linolenic, EPA and DHA in human metabolic syndrome and type 2 diabetes – a mini-review.' *Journal of Oleo Science 56*, 7, 319–325.

Bassey, J.E., Littlewood, J.J., Rothwell, C.M. and Pye, D.W. (1999) 'Lack of effect of supplementation with essential fatty acids on bone mineral density in healthy pre- and postmenopausal women: Two randomised controlled trials of Efacal v calcium alone.' *British Journal of Nutrition 83*, 629–635.

Bates, D., Cartlidge, N.E.F., French, J.M., Jackson, M.J. *et al.* (1989) 'A double-blind trial of long-chain n-3 polyunsaturated fatty acids in the treatment of multiple sclerosis.' *Journal of Neurology, Neurosurgery, and Psychiatry 52*, 1, 18–22.

Belch, J.J. and Hill, A. (2000) 'EPO and borage oil in rheumatologic conditions.' *American Journal of Clinical Nutrition 71*, 1 suppl., 352S–356S.

Berquin, I.M., Edwards, I.J. and Chen, Y.Q. (2008) 'Multi-targeted therapy of cancer by omega-3 fatty acids.' *Cancer Letters 269*, 2, 363–377.

Biassi, F., Mascia, C. and Poli, G. (2007) 'TGF-b1 expression in colonic mucosa: Modulation by dietary lipids.' *Genes and Nutrition 2*, 2, 233–243.

Bourre, J.M. (2007) 'Dietary omega-3 fatty acids for women.' *Biomedicine and Pharmacotherapy 61*, 2–3, 105–112.

Calder, P.C. (2006) 'n-3 Polyunsaturated fatty acids, inflammation, and inflammatory diseases.' *American Journal of Clinical Nutrition 83*, 6 suppl., 1505S–1519S.

Calder, P.C. (2007) 'Immunomodulation by omega-3 fatty acids.' *Prostaglandins, Leukotrienes and Essential Fatty Acids 77*, 5–6, 327–335.

Calder, P.C. (2008) 'Session 3: Joint Nutrition Society and Irish Nutrition and Dietetic Institute Symposium on nutrition and autoimmune disease PFA, inflammatory processes and RA.' *Proceedings of the Nutrition Society 67*, 4, 409–418.

Calder, P.C. (2009) 'PUFAs and inflammatory processes: New twists in an old tale.' *Biochimie 91*, 6, 791–795.

Calviello, G., Di Nicuolo, F., Gragnoli, S., Piccioni, E. *et al.* (2004) 'n-3 PUFAs reduce VEGF expression in human colon cancer cells modulating the COX-2/PGE2 induced ERK-1 and -2 and HIF-1a induction pathway.' *Carcinogenesis 25*, 12, 2303–2310.

Chajes, V., Thiebaut, A.C.M., Rovital, M., Gauthier, E. *et al.* (2008) 'Association between serum trans-monounsaturated fatty acids and breast cancer risk in the E3N-EPIC study.' *American Journal of Epidemiology 167*, 11, 1312–1320.

Chavarro, J.E., Stampfer, M.J., Li, H. and Campos, H. (2007) 'A prospective study of polyunsaturated fatty acid levels in blood and prostate cancer risk.' *Cancer Epidemiology Biomarkers and Prevention 16*, 7, 1364–1370.

Churruca, I., Fernandez-Quintela, A., Portillo, M.P. (2009) 'Conjugated linleic acid isomers: Differences in metabolism and biological effects.' *Biofactors 35*, 1, 105–111.

Clarke, S.D., Gsperikova, D., Nelson, C., Lapillonne, A. and Heird, W.C. (2002) 'Fatty acid regulation of gene expression.' *Annals of the New York Academy of Sciences 967*, 283–298.

Cleland, L.G., Caughey, G.E., James, M.J. and Proudman, S.M. (2006) 'Reduction of CV risk factors with longterm fish oil treatment in early RA.' *Journal of Rheumatology 33*, 10, 1973–1979.

Cleland, L.G., James, M.J. and Proudman S.M. (2006) 'Fish oil: What the prescriber needs to know.' *Arthritis Research and Therapy 8*, 1.

Committee on the Medical Aspects of Food Policy (1991) *Dietary Reference Values for Food Energy and Nutrients for the UK. Report of the Panel on DRVs of the COMA.* London: Department of Health.

Cordain, L., Boyd Eaton, S., Sebastian, A., Mann, N. *et al.* (2005) 'Origins and evolution of the Western diet: Health implications for the 21st century.' *American Journal of Clinical Nutrition 81*, 2, 341–354.

Crowe, F.L., Skeaff, C.M., Green, T.J. and Gray, A.R. (2008) 'Serum n-3 long-chain PUFA differ by sex and age in a population-based survey of New Zealand adolescents and adults.' *British Journal of Nutrition 99*, 1, 168–174.

Cunnane, S., Drevon, C., Harris, W., Sinclair, A. and Spector, A. (2004) *Recommendations for Dietary Intake of Polyunsaturated Fatty Acids in Healthy Adults.* International Society for the Study of Fatty Acids and Lipids. Available at www.issfal.org.uk/images/stories/pdfs/PUFAIntakeReccomdFinalReport.pdf, accessed on 2 November 2009.

Das, U.N. (2003) 'Is there a role for saturated and long-chain fatty acids in multiple sclerosis?' *Nutrition 19*, 2, 163–168.

Davidson, M.H., Stein, E.A., Bays, H.E., Maki, K.C. *et al.* (2007) 'Efficacy and tolerability of adding prescription omega-3 fatty acids 4g/d to simvastatin 40mg/d in hypertriglyceridemic patients: An 8-week, randomised, double-blind, placebo-controlled study.' *Clinical Therapeutics 29*, 7, 1354–1367.

Duan, S.Z., Usher, M.G. and Mortensen, R.M. (2008) 'Peroxisome proliferator-activated receptor-gamma-mediated effects in the vasculature.' *Circulation Research 102*, 3, 283–294.

Dwyer, J.H., Allayee, H., Dwyer, K.M. and Fan, J. (2004) 'Arachidonate 5-lipoxygenase promoter genotype, dietary arachidonic acid, and atherosclerosis.' *New England Journal of Medicine 350*, 1, 29–37.

Felton, C.V., Crook, D., Davies, M.J. and Oliver, M.F. (1997) 'Relation of plaque lipid composition and morphology to the stability of human aortic plaques.' *Arteriosclerosis, Thrombosis, and Vascular Biology 17*, 7, 1337–1345.

Gallai, V., Sarchielli, P., Trequattrini, A., Franceschini, M. *et al.* (1995) 'Cytokine secretion and eicosanoid production in the peripheral blood mononuclear cells of MS patients undergoing dietary supplementation with n-3 polyunsaturated fatty acids.' *Journal of Neuroimmunology 56*, 2, 143–153.

Gaullier, J-M., Halse, J., Høivik, H.O., Høye, K. *et al.* (2007) 'Six months supplementation with conjugated linoleic acid induces regional-specific fat mass decreases in overweight and obese.' *British Journal of Nutrition 97*, 3, 550–560.

Graham, I., Atar, D., Borch-Johnsen, K., Boysen, G. *et al.* (2007) 'European guidelines on cardiovascular disease prevention in clinical practice: Executive summary.' *Atherosclerosis 194*, 1, 1–45.

Hallahan, B. and Garland, M.R. (2004) 'Essential fatty acids and their role in the treatment of impulsivity disorders.' *Prostaglandins, Leukotrienes and Essential Fatty Acids 71*, 4, 211–216.

Hamakawa, H., Nakashiro, K., Sumida, T., Shintani, S., Myers, J.N., Takes, R.P. *et al.* (2008) 'Basic evidence of molecular targeted therapy for oral cancer and salivary gland cancer.' *Head and Neck 30*, 6, 800–809.

Harbige, L. (1998) 'Dietary n-6 and n-3 fatty acids in immunity and autoimmune disease.' *Proceedings of the Nutrition Society 57*, 4, 555–562.

Harbige, L.S., Layward, L., Morris-Downes, M.M., Dumonde, D.C. and Amor, S. (2000) 'The protective effects of omega-6 fatty acids in experimental autoimmune encephalomyelitis (EAE) in relation to transforming growth factor-beta 1 (TGF-ß1) up-regulation and increased prostaglandin E2 (PGE2) production.' *Clinical and Experimental Immunology 122*, 3, 445–452.

Harbige, L. and Sharief, M. (2007) 'Polyunsaturated fatty acids in the pathogenesis and treatment of multiple sclerosis.' *British Journal of Nutrition 98*, 1, S46–S53.

Harvey, K.A., Arnold, T., Rasool, T., Antalis, C., Miller, S. and Siddiqui, R.A. (2008) 'Trans-fatty acids induce pro-inflammatory responses and endothelial cell dysfunction.' *British Journal of Nutrition 99*, 4, 723–731.

Hooper, L., Thompson, R.L., Harrison, R.A. and Summerbell, C.D. (2004) 'Omega 3 fatty acids for prevention and treatment of cardiovascular disease.' *Cochrane Database of Systematic Reviews 4*:CD003177.

Horrobin, D.F., Ells, K.M., Morese-Risher, N. and Manku, M.S. (1991) 'The effects of evening primrose oil, safflower oil and paraffin oil on plasma fatty acid levels in humans: Choice of an appropriate placebo for clinical studies on evening primrose oil.' *Prostaglandins, Leukotrienes and Essential Fatty Acids 42*, 4, 245–249.

Huang, Y.S., Cunnane, S.C., Horrobin, D.F. *et al.* (1982) 'Most biological effects of zinc deficiency corrected by GLA but not by LA.' *Atherosclerosis 41*, 2–3, 193–207.

Ibrahim, A., Natrajan, S. and Ghafoorunissa, R. (2005) 'Dietary trans-fatty acids alter adipocyte plasm membrane fatty acid composition and insulin sensitivity in rats.' *Metabolism 54*, 2, 240–246.

Ishigaki, H., Katagiri, H., Gao, J., Yamada, T. *et al.* (2008) 'Impact of plasma oxidised LDL removal on atherosclerosis.' *Circulation 118*, 1, 75–83.

Jackson, A., Key, T., Williams, C., Hughes, I. *et al.* (2004) *Scientific Advisory Committee on Nutrition. Advice on Fish Consumption: Benefits and Risks*. Committee on Toxicity. London: Stationery Office.

Jellin, J.M., Gregory, P.J., Batz, F., Hitchens, K. *et al.* (eds) (2008) *Pharmacist's Letter/ Prescriber's Letter Natural Medicines Comprehensive Database*. Stockton, CA: Therapeutic Research Faculty. Available at www.naturaldatabase.com/(S(jqgcwz45jccaru45i0q1laa3))/home.aspx?cs=&s=ND, accessed on 2 November 2009.

Johnson, M.M., Swan, D.D., Surette, M.E., Stegner, J. *et al.* (1997) 'Dietary supplementation with α-linoleic acid alters fatty acid content and eicosanoid production in healthy humans.' *Journal of Nutrition 127*, 8, 1435–1444.

Kang, J.X. (2003) 'The importance of omega-6/omega 3 fatty acid ratio in cell function. The gene transfer of omega-3 fatty acid desaturase.' *World Review of Nutrition and Dietetics 92*, 23–36.

Kelley, D., Siegal, D., Fedor, D., Adkins, Y. and Mackey, B.E. (2009) 'DAH supplementation decreases serum C-reactive protein and other markers of inflammation in hypertriglyceridemic men.' *Journal of Nutrition 139*, 3, 495–501.

Kenny, F.S., Pinder, S.E., Ellis, I.O., Gee, J.M.W. *et al.* (2000) 'Gamma linolenic acid with tamoxifen as primary therapy in breast cancer.' *International Journal of Cancer 85*, 5, 643–648.

Koletzko, B., Cetin, I. and Brenna, T. (2007) 'Dietary fat intakes for pregnant and lactating women.' *British Journal of Nutrition 98*, 5, 873–877.

Konig, B., Koch, A., Spielmann, J., Hilgenfeld, C., Stangl, G.I. and Eder, K. (2007) 'Activation of PPARalpha lowers synthesis and concentration of cholesterol by reduction of nuclear SREBP-2.' *Biochemical Pharmacology 73*, 4, 573–585.

Kris-Etherton, P.M., Harris, W.S. and Appel, L.J. (2002) 'Fish consumption, fish oil, omega-3 fatty acids, and cardiovascular disease.' *Circulation 106*, 21, 2747–2757.

Lee, J.H., O'Keefe, J.H., Lavie, C.J., Marchioli, R. and Harris, W.S. (2008) 'Omega-3 fatty acids for cardioprotection.' *Mayo Clinical Proceedings 83*, 3, 324–332.

Lee, Y.S. and Wander, R.C. (2005) 'Reduced effect on apoptosis of 4-hydroxyhexenal and oxidised LDL enriched with n-3 fatty acids from postmenopausal women.' *Journal of Nutritional Biochemistry 16*, 4, 213–221.

Lerman, R.H. (2005) 'Essential Fatty Acids.' In D. Jones (2005) *The Textbook of Functional Medicine*. Gig Harbour, USA: IFM.

Lopez-Garcia, E., Schulze, M., Meigs, J.B., Manson, J. *et al.* (2005) 'Consumption of transfatty acids is related to plasma biomarkers of inflammation and endothelial dysfunction.' *Journal of Nutrition 135*, 3, 562–566.

Lord, R. and Bralley, J. (2008) 'Fatty Acids.' In R. Lord and J. Bralley (2008) *Laboratory Evaluations for Integrative and Functional Medicine.* 2nd edn. Georgia: Metametrix Institute.

Maclean, C., Newberry, S., Mojica, W., Issa, A. *et al.* (2005) 'Effects of omega-3 fatty acids on cancer.' *Evidence/Report Technology Assessment 113*, 1–4.

Massaro, M., Scoditti, E., Carluccio, M.A., Montinari, M.R. and De Caterina, R. (2008) 'Omega-3 fatty acids, inflammation and angiogenesis: Nutrigenomic effects as an explanation for anti-atherogenic and anti-inflammatory effects of fish and fish oils.' *Journal of Nutrigenetics and Nutrigenomics 1*, 4–23.

Milte, C., Coates, A., Buckley, J.D, Hill, A.M. *et al.* (2008) 'Dose-dependent effects of DHA-rich fish oil on erythrocyte DHA and blood lipid levels.' *British Journal of Nutrition 99*, 5, 1083–1088.

Mostad, I.L., Bjerve, K.S., Lyderson, S., Grill, V. *et al.* (2008) 'Effects of marine n-3 FA supplementation on lipoprotein subclasses measured by nuclear magnetic resonance in subjects with type II diabetes.' *European Journal of Clinical Nutrition 62*, 3, 419–429.

Murray, M., Pizzorno, J. and Pizzorno, L. (2005) *The Encyclopedia of Healing Foods.* New York: Atria Books.

Nordvik, I., Myhr, K.M., Nyland, H. and Bjerve, K.S. (2000) 'Effect of dietary advice and n-3 supplementation in newly diagnosed MS patients.' *Acta Neurologica Scandinavica 102*, 3, 143–149.

Ottoboni, A. and Ottoboni, F. (2004) 'The Food Guide Pyramid: Will the defects be corrected?' *Journal of American Physicians and Surgeons 9*, 4, 109–113.

Pardini, R.S. (2006) 'Nutritional intervention with omega-3 fatty acids enhances tumor response to anti-neoplastic agents.' *Chemico-Biological Interactions 162*, 2, 89–105.

Parsons, H.G. (1995) 'Modulation in delta 9, delta 6 and delta 5 fatty acid desaturase activity in the human intestingal CaCo-2 cell line.' *Journal of Lipid Research 36*, 3, 552–563.

Parthasarathy, S., Khoo, J.C., Miller, E., Barnett, J. *et al.* (1990) 'Low density lipoprotein rich in oleic acid is protected against oxidative modification: Implications for dietary prevention of atherscloerosis.' *Proceedings of the National Academy of Sciences USA 87*, 10, 3894–3898.

Poirier, H., Shapiro, J.S., Kim, R.J. and Lazar, M.A. (2006) 'Nutritional supplementation with trans-10, cis-12–conjugated linoleic acid induces inflammation of white adipose tissue.' *Diabetes 55*, 6, 1634–1641.

Poole, E.M., Bigler, J., Whitton, J. and Sibert, J.G. (2007) 'Genetic variability in prostaglandin synthesis, fish intake and risk of colorectal polyps.' *Carcinogenesis 28*, 6, 1259–1263.

Poulsen, R.C. and Kruger, M.C. (2006) 'Detrimental effect of EPA supplementation on bone following ovariectomey in rats.' *Prostaglandins, Leukotreines and Essential Fatty Acids 75*, 6, 419–427.

Roggia, C., Tamone, C., Cenci, S., Pacifici, R. and Isaia, G.C. (2004) 'Role of TNF-alpha producing T-cells in bone loss induced by oestrogen deficiency.' *Minerva Medicine 95*, 2, 125–132.

Ros, E. and Mataix, J. (2006) 'Fatty acids composition of nuts – implications for cardiovascular health.' *British Journal of Nutrition 96*, 2, S29–S35.

Rosell, M.S., Lloyd-Wright, Z., Appleby, P.N., Sanders, T.A.B., Allen, N.E. and Key, T.J. (2005) 'Long-chain n–3 polyunsaturated fatty acids in plasma in British meat-eating, vegetarian, and vegan men.' *American Journal of Clinical Nutrition 82*, 2, 327–334.

Roynette, C.E., Calder, P.C., Dupertuis, Y.M. and Pichard, C. (2004) 'n-3 Polyunsaturated fatty acids and colon cancer prevention.' *Clinical Nutrition 23*, 2, 139–151.

Saadatian-Elahi, M., Norat, T., Goudable, J. and Riboli, E. (2004) 'Biomarkers of dietary fatty acid intake and the risk of breast cancer: A meta-analysis.' *International Journal of Cancer 111*, 4, 584–591.

Salari, P., Rezaie, A., Larijani, B. and Abdollahi, M. (2008) 'A systematic review of the impact of n-3 fatty acids in bone health and osteoporosis.' *Medical Science Monitor 14*, 3, RA37–44.

Salas-Salvadó, J., Márquez-Sandoval, F. and Bulló, M. (2006) 'Conjugated linoleic acid intake in humans: A systematic review focusing on its effect on body composition, glucose, and lipid metabolism.' *Critical Reviews in Food Science and Nutrition 46*, 6, 479–488.

Sartore, G., Lapolla, A., Reitano, R., Zambon, S. *et al.* (2008) 'Desaturase activities and metabolic control in type 2 diabetes.' *Prostaglandins, Leukotreines and Essential Fatty Acids 79*, 1–2, 55–58.

Schlemmer, C.K., Coetzer, H., Claassen, N. and Druger, M.C. (1999) 'Oestrogen and essential fatty acid supplementation corrects bone loss due to ovariectomy in the female Sprague Dawley rat.' *Prostaglandins, Leukotrienes and Essential Fatty Acids 61*, 6, 381–390.

Shannon, J., King, I.B., Moshofsky, R., Lampe, J.W. *et al.* (2007) 'Erythrocyte fatty acids and breast cancer risk: A case-control study in Shanghai, China.' *American Journal of Clinical Nutrition 85*, 4, 1090–1097.

Simopoulos, A.P. (2006) 'Evolutionary aspects of diet, the omega 6/omega 3 ratio and genetic variation: Nutritional implications for chronic disease.' *Biomedicine and Pharmacotherapy 60*, 9, 502–507.

Simopoulos, A.P. (2008) 'The importance of the omega-6/omega-3 fatty acid ratio in cardiovascular disease and other chronic diseases.' *Experimental Biology and Medicine 233*, 6, 674–688.

Singh, R.B., Dubnov, G. and Niaz, M.A. (2002) 'Effect of an Indo-Mediterranean diet on progression of CAD in high-risk patients (Indo-Mediterranean Diet Heart Study): A randomised, single-blind trial.' *Lancet 360*, 9344, 1455–1461.

Sinn, N. (2007) 'Physical fatty acid deficiency signs in children with ADHD symptoms.' *Prostaglandins, Leukotrienes and Essential Fatty Acids 77*, 2, 109–115.

Stamp, L.K., James, M.J. and Cleland, L.G. (2005) 'Diet and RA: A review of the literature.' *Seminars in Arthritis and Rheumatism 35*, 2, 77–94.

Stephensen, C.B. and Kelley, D.S. (2006) 'The innate immune system: Friend and foe.' *American Journal of Clinical Nutrition 83*, 2, 331–342.

Stender, S. and Dyerberg, J. (2004) 'Influence of trans fatty acids on health.' *Annals of Nutrition and Metabolism 48*, 2, 61–66.

Sugiura, T. (2009) 'Physiological roles of 2-arachidonoylglycerol, an endogenous cannabinoid receptor ligand.' *Biofactors 25*, 1, 88–97.

Sun, D.X., Krishnan, A., Zama, K., Lawrence, R., Bhattacharya, A. and Fernandes, G. (2003) 'Dietary n-3 FAs decrease osteoclastogenesis and loss bone mass in ovariectomized rats.' *Journal of Bone and Mineral Research 18*, 7, 1206–1216.

Terano, T. (2001) 'Effect of omega-3 polyunsaturated fatty acid ingestion on bone metabolism and osteoporosis.' In *Fatty Acids and Lipids: New Findings. 4th Congress of the International Society for the Study of Fatty Acids and Lipids 88*, 141–147.

Toborek, M., Lee, Y.W., Garrido, R., Kaiser, S. and Hennig, B. (2002) 'Unsaturated fatty acids selectively induce an inflammatory environment in human endothelial cells.' *American Journal of Clinical Nutrition 75*, 1, 119–125.

Tsuge, H., Hotta, N. and Hayakawa, T. (2000) 'Effects of vitamin B6 on (n-3) PUFA metabolism.' *Journal of Nutrition 130*, 2S suppl., 333S–334S.

Tziomalos, K., Athyros, V.G. and Mikhailidis, D.P. (2007) 'Fish oils and vascular disease prevention: An update.' *Current Medicinal Chemistry 14*, 24, 2622–2628.

von Schacky, C. and Harris, W.S. (2007) 'Cardiovascular benefits of omega-3 fatty acids.' *Cardiovascular Research 73*, 2, 310–315.

von Schacky, C., Angerer, P., Kothny, W., Theisen, K. and Mudra, H. (1999) 'The effect of dietary v-3 fatty acids on coronary atherosclerosis. A randomized, double-blind, placebo-controlled trial. '*Annals of Internal Medicine 130*, 7, 554–562.

Wada, M., DeLong, C., Hong, Y., Rieke, C.J. *et al.* (2007) 'Enzymes and receptors of prostaglandin pathways with arachidonic acid-derived vs EPA-derived substrates and products.' *Journal of Biological Chemistry 282*, 31, 22254–22266.

Wahle, K.W.J., Rotondo, D. and Heys, S.D. (2003) 'Polyunsaturated fatty acids and gene expression in mammalian systems.' *Proceedings of the Nutrition Society 62*, 2, 349–360.

Wahlqvist, M.L. (2005) 'Dietary fat and the prevention of chronic disease.' *Asia Pacific Journal of Clinical Nutrition 14*, 4, 313–318.

Wang, C., Harris, W.S., Chung, M., Lichtenstein, A.H. *et al.* (2006) 'n-3 fatty acids from fish or fish-oil supplements, but not α-linolenic acid, benefit cardiovascular disease outcomes in primary- and secondary-prevention studies: A systematic review.' *American Journal of Clinical Nutrition 84*, 1, 5–17.

Weinstock-Guttman, B., Baier, M., Park, Y., Feichter, J. *et al.* (2005) 'Low fat intervention with n-3 fatty acid supplementation in multiple sclerosis patients.' *Prostaglandins, Leukotrienes and Essential Fatty Acids 73*, 5, 397–404.

Williams, C., Thompson, A.K., Shaw, D.I., Minihane, A.M. *et al.* (2007) *Update on Trans Fatty Acids and Health. Position Statement by the Scientific Advisory Committee on Nutrition.* London: Stationery Office.

World Cancer Research Fund (2007) *Food, Nutrition, Physical Activity and the Prevention of Cancer: A Global Perspective.* Available at www.dietandcancerreport.org, accessed on 2 November 2009.

Yaqoob, P. (2009) 'The nutritional significance of lipid rafts.' *Annual Review of Nutrition 29*, 257–282.

Yehuda, S. (2003) 'Omega-6/omega-3 ratio and brain-related functions.' *World Review of Nutrition and Dietetics 92*, 37–56.

Yehuda, S., Rabinovitz, S. and Mostofsky, D.I. (2005) 'Essential fatty acids and the brain: From infancy to aging.' *Neurobiology of Aging 26*, 1 suppl., S98–S102.

Zampelas, A., Panagiotakos, D.B., Pitsavos, C., Das, U.N. *et al.* (2005) 'Fish consumption among healthy adults is associated with decreased levels of inflammatory markers related to cardiovascular disease: The ATTICA study.' *Journal of the American College of Cardiology 46*, 1, 120–124.

Zurier, R.B., Rossetti, R.G., Jacobson, E.W., De Marco, D.M. *et al.* (1996) 'GLA treatment of RA. A randomized, placebo-controlled trial.' *Arthritis Rheum. 39*, 11, 1808–1817.

Part 2 PUFAs in the brain

Smita Hanciles and Zeller Pimlott

9. PUFAs in the brain

9.1 The role of fatty acids in brain development and function

PUFAs comprise about 60 per cent of the brain, affecting its growth and connectivity, and are essential for the maintenance of optimal brain function throughout life. Adequate supplies of highly unsaturated fatty acids (HUFAs) are crucial for increasing the fluidity of neuronal membranes (which is reduced by saturated fats and cholesterol). The optimal functioning of neurotransmitter receptors and ion channels, as well as other membrane-associated proteins, is dependent on this fluidity.

Four PUFAs are particularly important for brain development and function: DGLA and AA from the omega-6 series, and EPA and DHA from the omega-3 series. AA and DHA are major structural components of neuronal membranes and make up 20 per cent of the dry mass of the brain. These PUFAs are so essential during prenatal development that the placenta acts to double the levels circulating in maternal plasma. The transfer of DHA from the mother to the foetus is greatest during the third trimester, when the foetus's brain is growing rapidly. The brain continues to experience rapid growth until two years of age and studies have suggested that higher DHA levels in the mother during pregnancy and lactation affords behavioural benefits for the child and accounts for the enhanced brain functioning and cognitive advantage observed in breastfed infants (Helland *et al.* 2008; Hibbeln *et al.* 2007).

Whereas AA and DHA play a structural role, EPA and DGLA are important for brain function and cell signalling. EPA and DGLA are also converted into anti-inflammatory eicosanoids, which promote an increase in neural connectivity. The inflammation, narrowed blood vessels and reduced blood coagulation time that occur where there is an excess of AA relative to EPA and DGLA also have potential effects on mental health and performance (Richardson 2006). In addition, the AA-derived endocannabinoids act at specific receptors on the blood vessel wall to produce vasodilation, thus influencing many aspects of mood, cognition and behaviour. They therefore have significance for psychiatric disorders (Bradshaw and Walker 2005).

Brain magnocellular neurones provide rapid signalling and fast conduction, important for rapid responses and tracking changes in light, sound and position. These are found throughout the brain and require high membrane flexibility, which is provided by a local environment of EFAs, particularly omega-3 fatty acids (FAs). Thus they are particularly vulnerable to omega-3 FA deficiency. DHA speeds up neuronal responses by increasing membrane flexibility and thus improving magnocellular neuronal timing functions. Impaired development of magnocellular neurones is found in many neuro-developmental disorders, such as developmental dyslexia, dyspraxia, attention deficit hyperactivity disorder (ADHD) and autistic spectrum disorders (ASD) and has also been found in schizophrenia, depression and antisocial behaviour. In all these conditions the ability to focus attention precisely is reduced (Taylor and Richardson 2000).

There is constant replacing and recycling of PUFAs during the normal turnover of membrane phospholipids, as well as in the cell signalling cascades. Phospholipase A2 (PLA2) enzymes remove PUFAs from membrane phospholipids, creating potentially damaging interim products, including free fatty acids (FFAs), which are susceptible to oxidation. Over-activity of PLA2 enzymes has been implicated in schizophrenia (Richardson and Ross 2000); and elevated PLA2 levels, potentially causing FA deficiency, have been reported in dyslexia (MacDonell *et al.* 2000).

Membrane FA composition is also affected by the altering of gene expression via PPARs (see section 5.2 above). Accumulating evidence suggests that PPAR agonists may have therapeutic potential in brain disorders by controlling neuroinflammation and neurodegeneration. Several unsaturated FAs bind to PPAR isoforms, whereas SFAs are generally poor PPAR ligands. However, experimental studies require high concentrations of lipids to activate PPARs and their role *in vivo* as PPAR ligands remains controversial (Bernardo and Minghetti 2008).

9.2 PUFAs in ADHD, dyslexia and dyspraxia

Evidence suggests that PUFAs may play a role in three common developmental disorders of learning and behaviour – dyslexia, dyspraxia and ADHD. ADHD is characterised by overactivity, impulsiveness and inattentiveness. There is considerable overlap between these three disorders, as well as with ASDs, and each can occur with differing degrees of severity. Impaired magnocellular function in these children may make them vulnerable to omega-3 FA deficiency and trials have been conducted to test supplementation with EPA, DHA, GLA (as evening primrose oil) and vitamin E.

In children diagnosed with dyslexia who displayed symptoms of ADHD, trials have shown an improvement of ADHD behaviours when supplemented with both omega-3 and omega-6 FAs and this correlated with measurements of red blood cell fatty acid concentrations (Richardson 2004; Stevens *et al.* 2003). The largest trial (though still small) was the Oxford-Durham trial including 117 underachieving children, aged 5–12, with developmental coordination disorder. Significant improvements for those taking the supplements were seen for learning, behaviour and working memory. Reading improved at three times the normal rate and spelling improved at twice the normal rate. Similarly significant reductions in ADHD-type symptoms were observed. The trial used a combination of high-EPA fish oil and evening primrose oil, providing 558mg EPA, 174mg DHA and 60mg GLA daily (Richardson and Montgomery 2005).

Trials such as these have led to much public interest in the idea that parents can improve their child's IQ and performance at school by giving them a daily fish oil supplement. A large number of products targeted at this market can be found on supermarket shelves, with names strongly suggestive of such a role. However, there have been few adequately controlled trials on healthy children without neurodevelopmental conditions. Thus the existing trial results cannot necessarily be extended to the general population.

Evidence suggests that EPA may be more important than DHA for reducing the problems with attention, perception and memory associated with ADHD, dyslexia and dyspraxia; and this is supported by other findings. Voight *et al.* (2001) concluded that a four-month period of DHA supplementation (345mg/day) did not decrease symptoms of ADHD and results from a recent study showed no benefit from DHA on the cognitive performance of healthy school children (Kennedy *et al.* 2009). Supplements with a high ratio of EPA to DHA are therefore required for effectiveness but there is a need for larger scale studies to determine optimal treatment formulations and doses.

Observations within studies show that it is often a subgroup that shows an improvement with FA supplementation and therefore individuality needs to be taken into account. A trial with 75 children and adolescents (8–18 years) found that only 26 per cent responded with more than 25 per cent reduction of ADHD symptoms after three months' supplementation with omega-3 and 6 FAs (Johnson *et al.* 2009). There is a need to develop methods of identifying individuals most likely to benefit from FA supplementation, as the causes of behavioural disorders are so varied.

Richardson (2002) proposes that an initial dosage of fish oil supplying around 500mg daily of EPA is probably most appropriate for dyslexia and related conditions, along with 50mg per day of GLA (if included). Inclusion of vitamin E with PUFA supplements is advised as an antioxidant to protect these FAs from oxidation. See section 7.2 in Part 1 of this chapter for general and governmental guidelines on PUFA intake. Unlike medication, FAs do not work rapidly to alter mental function and it can take up to three months for the maximum benefits from supplementation to be achieved, as there is slow turnover of these FAs in the brain.

9.3 The role of PUFAs in depression

The idea that omega-3 FAs could play a role in the treatment of depression is suggested by tissue composition evidence and also by epidemiological evidence that higher fish consumption is associated with a lower prevalence of depression (Freeman *et al.* 2006). In a review of trials up to March 2007, Ross, Seguin and Sieswerda (2007) identified nine placebo-controlled trials of omega-3 FA supplementation in major depressive and bipolar disorders. The trials were small in general, with five trials including less than 50 subjects, and of short duration, from 4 to 18 weeks, and in most cases the subjects were also on conventional antidepressant medication during the trial. An antidepressant effect was observed in six of the nine trials and meta-analysis indicates that omega-3 FA supplementation was significantly more effective than placebo. The evidence from the small number of trials on bipolar disorder suggests a beneficial effect of omega-3 FAs on depressive, but not manic, symptoms.

Similar results were obtained for depression and bipolar disorder in a meta-analysis carried out by Freeman *et al.* (2006). Larger and longer trials are needed before definite conclusions can be reached but the available evidence indicates that omega-3 FAs could be an effective adjunctive treatment for patients with treatment-resistant depression. Several mechanisms have been proposed to explain how omega-3 FAs could modulate depression, including their effects on membrane fluidity, levels of pro-inflammatory cytokines, levels of neurotrophins (such as brain-derived neurotrophic factor) and gene expression (Owen, Rees and Parker 2008).

9.3.1 WHAT DOES THE RESEARCH TELL US ABOUT THE DAILY INTAKE OF OMEGA-3 FAS THAT IS LIKELY TO BE MOST EFFECTIVE?

Based upon evidence from trials, and the fact that no serious side-effects were observed, a nutrition practitioner may decide to advise clients with depression to increase their omega-3 FA intake, either through diet or by supplementation. Ross, Seguin and

Sieswerda (2007) concluded that a combined intake of EPA and DHA of approximately 1–2g per day is effective and that higher doses were actually less effective in most cases. After reviewing the evidence base the American Psychiatric Association (APA) concluded that patients with depression should consume 1g/day of EPA and DHA combined, as an adjunct to conventional antidepressant treatment (Freeman *et al.* 2006). There is no equivalent recommendation in the UK.

9.3.2 WHAT DOES THE RESEARCH TELL US ABOUT THE RATIO OF EPA TO DHA THAT IS MOST LIKELY TO BE EFFECTIVE?

Ross *et al.* (2007) found that EPA is likely to play more of a role in the antidepressant effect than DHA. However, some evidence suggests that a mixture of EPA and DHA is more effective than EPA alone (Keck *et al.* 2006). An interesting study also suggests that krill oil, which contains more EPA per gram than fish oil (240mg/g versus 180mg/g) as well as naturally occurring phospholipids, significantly improved depressive symptoms of pre-menstrual syndrome (PMS) when compared to fish oil (Logan 2004). Bringing together the available evidence, including the APA recommendation (Freeman *et al.* 2006) and the slightly higher dosage suggested in the review by Ross *et al.* (2007), a suitable starting point for treatment would be a daily dosage of approximately 1g EPA and 0.2g DHA.

9.3.3 IS THERE A ROLE FOR OMEGA-6 FAS?

Although there seems to be a relative lack of research on omega-6 FAs in depression, Peet and Horrobin (2002) have interpreted the results of their study on EPA as showing a possible role for AA. They found that 1g/day EPA had a mood elevating effect in patients with depression whereas 4g/day EPA did not. As their earlier work had shown that supplementation of 4g/day EPA decreases AA levels in erythrocyte membranes, they suggested that the balance between omega-3 and omega-6 FAs is important. Further research using mixtures of different omega-3 and omega-6 FAs is warranted.

9.4 PUFAs and schizophrenia

Ross *et al.* (2007) also reviewed trials of omega-3 FA supplementation in schizophrenia. Five trials, mostly of high quality, were reviewed. Any beneficial effects observed were small and the interpretation of results was complicated by different concurrent treatments, so that the authors conclude that the available data does not support a role for omega-3 FAs in the treatment of schizophrenia. Peet (2008) suggests that single nutrient studies may be unsuccessful because patients tend to have multiple deficiencies, due to very poor diets. On the basis of both preliminary findings from trials looking at combinations of nutrients, and several studies showing that homocysteine-lowering and antioxidant vitamins are important for omega-3 FA metabolism, Peet (2008) suggests that combinations of these vitamins with omega-3 FAs may be required to alleviate symptoms.

9.5 Cognition, behaviour and mood in the general population

9.5.1 COGNITION

A much debated possible use for omega-3 FAs is in the slowing down of cognitive decline in the elderly and the prevention of dementia, including Alzheimer's disease. The evidence is contradictory. On reviewing the results of three prospective cohort studies, Issa *et al.* (2006) found an association between total dietary omega-3 FA consumption and a reduced risk of dementia. A trial on 174 patients with mild to moderate Alzheimer's disease has reported that supplementation of 1.7g DHA and 0.6g EPA daily for six months did not delay the rate of cognitive decline. However, the results suggest that supplementation may be more effective in prevention than in treatment, since a beneficial effect was observed in the subgroup of patients with the mildest disease (Freund-Levi *et al.* 2006). A recent trial found that supplementation of 1.8g of combined EPA and DHA had no overall effect on cognitive performance (Van de Rest *et al.* 2008).

For the practitioner, this raises the question of whether, while conclusive trial data is unavailable, routine supplementation of omega-3 FAs for adult clients is justified on the basis that it may prevent cognitive decline and dementia in later life. One consideration would be the age at which supplementation would have to start to be effective, since Richards *et al.* (2004) suggest that cognitive decline may start earlier in mid-life than is commonly assumed. Another consideration is dosage; the Freund-Levi *et al.* (2006) trial used a combined DHA and EPA dosage that is roughly five times higher than general population recommendations and a preventative dose would have to be taken over a long time period, raising concerns over safety. Further insight may be gained with the results of a large ongoing trial of cognitively normal 70–79-year-old adults to investigate the effect of supplementation with 0.5g DHA and 0.2g EPA daily on mental decline over a two-year period (Dangour *et al.* 2006). The dosage used in this study is not significantly different from general population recommendations. Thus positive results would suggest that the practitioner need only recommend moderate consumption of oily fish, of between two and four portions per week, to maintain cognitive function (Dangour *et al.* 2006).

9.5.2 BEHAVIOUR

Epidemiological and clinical studies have suggested an association between low levels of omega-3 FAs and behavioural problems, including aggression, hostility and antisocial and criminal behaviour. A well-designed large double-blind placebo-controlled trial on 231 young adult prison inmates found that supplementation with a mixture of FAs, including EPA and DHA, in addition to a range of vitamins and minerals, reduced incidents involving antisocial behaviour or violence by 35.1 per cent (Gesch *et al.* 2002). For those behaviours associated with a lack of impulse control, the most well-researched mechanism by which EFAs are believed to exert an effect is by altering the fluidity of the synaptic membrane in monoamine neurotransmitter systems, particularly the serotonergic system (Garland and Hallahan 2006). After reviewing the evidence base, the APA has recommended that patients with impulse-control disorders should consume 1g/day of EPA and DHA combined (Freeman *et al.* 2006).

Is there any evidence that FA supplementation could help with everyday behavioural problems in the general population, for example with aggressive behaviour at work or at home, or disruptive behaviour in the classroom?

Hamazaki *et al.* (1996) found that daily supplementation of 1.5–1.8g DHA, along with small amounts of a range of other FAs, produced a significant prevention of the increase in aggression against others during the period before examinations. The same group has also studied aggression in schoolchildren in a large controlled intervention study of 166 9–12-year-old subjects, using fish oil-fortified foods to deliver an average of 514mg DHA and 120mg of EPA per day (Itomura *et al.* 2005). The results were mixed, although a significant decrease in physical aggression and impulsivity in girls was observed.

Can the practitioner use omega-3 FAs in a treatment plan to help a client with no diagnosed behavioural disorder but suffering from feelings of aggression or hostility in everyday life?

The reduction in antisocial behaviour observed in the prison study conducted by Gesch *et al.* (2002) was impressive. However, how far these results can be applied to the general population is debatable; although the inmates were not selected on the basis of any diagnosed condition, it is perhaps unlikely that their behaviour reflects that of the general population, and the authors comment that behaviour in institutions is atypical (Gesch *et al.* 2002). The current evidence base on the use of omega-3 FAs, mainly DHA, for those in the general population, as described above, is not sufficient to warrant a specific recommendation for supplementation; however, the intake recommended by the APA for those with diagnosed impulse-control disorders (1g/day EPA and DHA combined) is well within safety limits and could be beneficial in some cases.

9.5.3 MOOD

There is a growing body of evidence that omega-3 FAs, in particular EPA and DHA, can help as an adjunctive treatment in patients with diagnosed mood disorders, as described in the section on depression, above.

What is the evidence that it could be a useful treatment for sub-clinical depressive symptoms in the general population?

Some positive results have been obtained. For example, in a small study, Fontani *et al.* (2005) found an increase in vigour and general wellbeing in subjects after five weeks of supplementation with 2.8g omega-3 FAs including 1.6g EPA and 0.8g DHA. On the other hand, Rogers *et al.* (2008) found no beneficial effect from supplementation of 850mg DHA and 630mg EPA per day on depressed mood, among 190 subjects with mild to moderate depression, although the amount of EPA used was less than that in the positive trials. Furthermore, associations have not been found between plasma concentrations of omega-3 FAs and depressed mood in a non-clinical population (Appleton *et al.* 2008). The currently proposed mechanisms by which omega-3 FAs could alleviate depression cannot explain why sub-clinical depression would not be similarly helped, unless different aetiologies are involved (Appleton *et al.* 2008).

Overall, the evidence for the use of omega-3 FAs in the treatment of mild depressive symptoms is less convincing than that for their use in the treatment of diagnosed depression; further research is needed in this area. Meanwhile, the intake recommended by the APA for those with diagnosed depression (1g/day EPA and DHA combined) is well within safety limits and could be beneficial for some people with mood disorders in the general population.

9.6 Conclusion

Adequate supplies of PUFAs play a key role in brain structure and function and cell signalling. Evidence suggests that PUFAs may also play a role in developmental disorders of learning and behaviour, as well as in some psychiatric conditions, such as depression. Small supplementation trials show the effectiveness of some PUFAs in reducing the symptoms of some of these conditions, but larger scale studies are required to determine optimal doses and ratios for treatment. As the causes of the disorders discussed above can be varied, and often only a subgroup of the study population will show improvement, methods of identifying individuals most likely to benefit from supplementation also need to be developed.

References

Appleton, K.M., Gunnell, D., Peters, T.J., Ness, A.R., Kessler, D. and Rogers, P.J. (2008) 'No clear evidence of an association between plasma concentrations of n-3 long-chain polyunsaturated fatty acids and depressed mood in a non-clinical population.' *Prostaglandins, Leukotrienes and Essential Fatty Acids 78,* 6, 337–342.

Bernardo, A. and Minghetti, L. (2008) 'Regulation of glial cell functions by PPAR natural and synthetic agonists.' *PPAR Research Volume* 2008 ID 864140.

Bradshaw, H.B. and Walker, J.M. (2005) 'The expanding field of cannabimimetic and related lipid mediators.' *British Journal of Pharmacology 144,* 4, 459–465.

Dangour, A.D., Clemens, F., Elbourne, D., Fasey, N. *et al.* (2006) 'A randomised controlled trial investigating the effect of n-3 long-chain polyunsaturated fatty acid supplementation on cognitive and retinal function in cognitively healthy older people: The older people and n-3 long-chain polyunsaturated fatty acids (OPAL) study protocol [ISRCTN72331636].' *Nutrition Journal 5,* 20.

Fontani, G., Corradeschi, F., Felici, A., Alfatti, F., Migliorini, S. and Lodi, L. (2005) 'Cognitive and physiological effects of omega-3 polyunsaturated fatty acid supplementation in healthy subjects.' *European Journal of Clinical Investigation 35,* 11, 691–699.

Freeman, M.P., Hibbeln, J.R., Wisner, K.L., Davis, J.M. *et al.* (2006) 'Omega-3 fatty acids: Evidence basis for treatment and future research in psychiatry.' *Journal of Clinical Psychiatry 67*, 12, 1954–1967.

Freund-Levi, Y., Eriksdotter-Jönhagen, M., Cederholm, T., Basun, H. *et al.* (2006) 'Ω-3 fatty acid treatment in 174 patients with mild to moderate Alzheimer disease: OmegAD study.' *Archives of Neurology 63*, 10,1402–1408.

Garland, M.R. and Hallahan, B. (2006) 'Essential fatty acids and their role in conditions characterised by impulsivity.' *International Review of Psychiatry 18*, 2, 99–105.

Gesch, C.B., Hammond, S.M., Hampson, S.E., Eves, A. and Crowder, M.J. (2002) 'Influence of supplementary vitamins, minerals and essential fatty acids on the antisocial behaviour of young adult prisoners: Randomised, placebo-controlled trial.' *British Journal of Psychiatry 181*, 1, 22–28.

Hamazaki, T., Sawazaki, S., Itomura, M., Asaoka, E. *et al.* (1996) 'The effect of docosahexaenoic acid on aggression in young adults. A placebo-controlled double-blind study.' *Journal of Clinical Investigation 97*, 4, 1129–1133.

Helland, I.B., Smith, L., Blomén, B., Saarem, K., Saugstad, O.D. and Drevon, C.A. (2008) 'Effect of supplementing pregnant and lactating mothers with n-3 very-long-chain fatty acids on children's IQ and body mass index at 7 years of age.' *Pediatrics 122*, 2, 472–479.

Hibbeln, J.R., Davis, J.M., Steer, C., Emmett, P. *et al.* (2007) 'Maternal seafood consumption in pregnancy and neurodevelopmental outcomes in childhood (ALSPAC study): An observational cohort study.' *Lancet 369*, 9561, 578–585.

Issa, A.M., Mojica, W.A., Morton, S.C., Traina, S. *et al.* (2006) 'The efficacy of omega-3 fatty acids on cognitive function in aging and dementia: A systematic review.' *Dementia and Geriatric Cognitive Disorders 21*, 2, 88–96.

Itomura, M., Hamazaki, K., Sawazaki, S., Kobayashi, M. *et al.* (2005) 'The effect of fish oil on physical aggression in schoolchildren – a randomized, double-blind, placebo-controlled trial.' *Journal of Nutritional Biochemistry 16, 3*, 163–171.

Johnson, M., Ostlund, S., Kadesjo, B. and Gillberg, C. (2009) 'Omega-3/omega-6 fatty acids for attention deficit hyperactivity disorder: A randomised placebo controlled trial in children and adolescents.' *Journal of Attention Disorders 12*, 5, 394–401.

Keck, P.E., Mintz, J., McElroy, S.L., Freeman, M.P. *et al.* (2006) 'Double-blind, randomized, placebo-controlled trials of ethyl-eicosapentanoate in the treatment of bipolar depression and rapid cycling bipolar disorder.' *Biological Psychiatry 60*, 9, 1020–1022.

Kennedy, D.O., Jackson, P.A., Elliott, J.M., Scholey, A.B. et al. (2009) 'Cognitive and mood effects of 8 weeks' supplementation with 400 mg or 1000 mg of the omega-3 essential fatty acid docosahexaenoic acid (DHA) in healthy children aged 10–12 years.' *Nutritional Neuroscience 12*, 2, 48–56.

Logan, A.C. (2004) 'Omega-3 fatty acids and major depression: A primer for the mental health professional.' *Lipids in Health and Disease 3*, 25.

MacDonell, L.E.F., Skinner, F.K., Ward, P.E., Glen, A.I.M. *et al.* (2000) 'Increased levels of cytosolic phospholipase A2 in dyslexics.' *Prostaglandins, Leukotrienes and Essential Fatty Acids 63*, 1–2, 37–39.

Owen, C., Rees, A. and Parker, G. (2008) 'The role of fatty acids in the development and treatment of mood disorders.' *Current Opinion in Psychiatry 21*, 1, 19–24.

Peet, M. (2008) 'Omega-3 polyunsaturated fatty acids in the treatment of schizophrenia.' *Israel Journal of Psychiatry and Related Sciences 45*, 1, 19–25.

Peet, M. and Horrobin, D.F. (2002) 'A dose-ranging study of the effects of ethyl-eicosapentaenoate in patients with persistent schizophrenic symptoms.' *Journal of Psychiatric Research 36*, 1, 7–18.

Richards, M., Shipley, B., Fuhrer, R. and Wadsworth, M.E.J. (2004) 'Cognitive ability in childhood and cognitive decline in mid-life: Longitudinal birth cohort study.' *British Medical Journal 328*, 552–554.

Richardson, A.J. (2002) 'Fatty acids in dyslexia, dyspraxia and ADHD. Can nutrition help.' *Dyspraxia Foundation Professional Journal.* Available at Food and Behaviour Research, www.fabresearch.org, accessed on 2 November 2009.

Richardson, A.J. (2004) 'Long-chain polyunsaturated fatty acids in childhood developmental and psychiatric disorders.' *Lipids 39,* 12, 1215–1222.

Richardson, A.J. (2006) 'Omega-3 fatty acids in ADHD and related neurodevelopmental disorders.' *International Review of Psychiatry 18,* 2, 155–172.

Richardson, A.J. and Montgomery, P. (2005) 'The Oxford-Durham study: A randomized controlled trial of dietary co-ordination disorder supplementation with fatty acids in children with developmental co-ordination disorder.' *Pediatrics 115,* 5, 1360–1366.

Richardson, A.J. and Ross, M.A. (2000) 'Fatty acid metabolism in neurodevelopmental disorder: A new perspective on associations between attention-deficit /hyperactivity disorder, dyslexia, dyspraxia and the autistic spectrum.' *Prostaglandins, Leukotrienes and Essential Fatty Acids 63,* 1/2, 1–9.

Rogers, P.J., Appleton, K.M., Kessler, D., Peters, T.J. *et al.* (2008) 'No effect of n-3 long-chain polyunsaturated fatty acid (EPA and DHA) supplementation on depressed mood and cognitive function: A randomised controlled trial.' *British Journal of Nutrition 99,* 2, 421–431.

Ross, B.M., Seguin, J. and Sieswerda, L.E. (2007) 'Omega-3 fatty acids as treatments for mental illness: Which disorder and which fatty acid?' *Lipids in Health and Disease 6,* 21.

Stevens, L., Zhang, W., Kuczek, T., Grevstad, N. *et al.* (2003) 'EFA supplementation in children with inattention, hyperactivity, and other disruptive behaviours.' *Lipids 38,* 10, 1007–1021.

Taylor, K.E. and Richardson, A.J. (2000) 'Visual function, fatty acids and dyslexia.' *Prostaglandins, Leukotrienes and Essential Fatty Acids 63,* 1–2, 89–93.

Van de Rest, O., Geleijnse, J.M., Kok, F.J., van Staveren, W.A. *et al.* (2008) 'Effect of fish oil on cognitive performance in older subjects.' *Neurology 71,* 6, 430–438.

Voight, R.G., Llorente, A.M., Jensen, C.L., Kennard Fraley, J., Berretta, M.C. and Heird, W.C. (2001) A randomised, double-blind, placebo-controlled trial of docosahexaenoic acid supplementation in children with attention-deficit/hyperactivity.' *Journal of Paediatrics 139,* 2, 189–196.

Chapter 5

THE METABOLIC SYNDROME: INSULIN RESISTANCE, DYSGLYCAEMIA AND DYSLIPIDAEMIA

T. Michael Culp

1. Imbalances of affluence

Metabolic syndrome refers to a cluster of specific conditions and diseases, previously thought to be unconnected, that share a causal aetiology in the dysregulation of insulin and glucose metabolism. This fundamental functional imbalance leads to subsequent metabolic changes that result in putatively non-pathological changes (like increased stature, central obesity and male pattern baldness) but can also lead to increasingly problematic pathological changes like hyperkeratosis skin conditions, acne vulgaris, myopia (short-sightedness), high blood pressure, atherosclerosis, coronary artery disease (CAD), type 2 diabetes (NIDDM), and possibly breast, colon and prostate cancer.

The underlying fundamental causes of these various diseases lie in dietary, lifestyle and behavioural changes characteristic of civilisation and especially of modern, industrialised society, specifically eating too much, eating too many refined carbohydrates and moving too little. Metabolic syndrome is fundamentally a condition of impaired energy throughput – too much supply and too little demand. To call it 'affluence syndrome' is perfectly apt.

Our ancestors regularly engaged in hard labour trying to eke out of their environment enough food to enable them to survive. In the space of a few generations, we have managed to turn this situation on its head. In an age of abundance, we eat all that we like and much more than we need. An increasingly mechanised society has reduced the need for manual labour to such an extent that we had to invent 'exercise' to try and counterbalance our institutionalised indolence. The greatest threat to our ancestors was starvation; ours is death from gluttony.

Undeniably, modern life has increased lifespan and created an easier life, but the survival mechanisms that evolved over countless millennia of famine and hardship are still operating today. Metabolic syndrome and the diseases that come in its wake are a direct outgrowth of our evolutionary success. Evolution has given us the desire to eat more and do less, while modernity has given us more to eat and less to do. The combination is nothing short of deadly. Most of the classic 'diseases of civilisation', like heart disease, type 2 diabetes, obesity and hypertension are direct outgrowths of our own survival 'success'.

1.1 Feast or famine

Survival of any organism or species depends on its ability to adapt to a changing environment. One of the most frequently changing variables in nature is the availability or lack of food – the proverbial 'feast or famine' cycle. The best time for growth and reproduction is when there is a sustained availability of food. By contrast, when food becomes scarce, it is essential to reduce energy expenditures in order to increase the likelihood of surviving until such time as food becomes available once more.

The coordination of our physiology is mediated by hormones, and the secretion of many hormones in the body is linked to the bioavailability of food. Increased food intake in modern times has caused significant and persistent changes in hormone patterns of individuals. These altered hormone patterns account for alterations in our metabolism (hence the term 'metabolic syndrome') that lead invariably to the development of the 'diseases of civilisation'.

1.2 Xenohormesis

In 2006 Yun, Lee and Doux proposed that signals from the exterior world, including food, toxins, temperature and stress, for example, turn on and turn off specific metabolic processes. They claim that environmental stress, especially the coming of autumn, stimulates plants to convert complex starches to simple sugars and stimulates animals to increase the proportion of higher-energy saturated storage fats and to reduce the production of more metabolically active polyunsaturated fats. The increase of simple sugars, saturated fats, salt and complex polyphenols within an organism reflects its stress experience in responding to factors like winter, drought, pestilence or infection.

Xenohormesis is the idea that we can read, interpret and borrow the stress response of the plants and animals that we eat. We respond to the stress-induced alterations in the nutritional composition of the foods we eat by altering our own physiology, hoarding calories in order to contend better with the ecological challenges we are about to face.

Yun and Doux (2007) carried this idea further to propose that taste preferences themselves evolved as a means of improving stress adaptation and not, as has been commonly assumed, to ensure adequate intake of essential nutrients. We have no particular taste preference for any of the specific vitamins, minerals, amino acids or fats that are essential for health, but we do have them for sugar, fat and salt.

Xenohormesis is a two-edged sword. If the total amount of food consumed is low (as in a traditional winter experience) these embedded stress signals would be advantageous to survival, since they would encourage hoarding of energy reserves better enabling us to survive. However, the regular excess consumption of sugar, fat and salt, characteristic of contemporary dietary habits would convey embedded stress signals in an illegitimate way. Our genetically driven response to these types of food is to hoard calories in preparation for winter but, in our case, the winter of deprivation never comes, and the stage is set for the development of metabolic syndrome.

2. Physiological responses to food intake

Increased intake of carbohydrates (and to a lesser extent of protein) results in increased blood sugar levels and a responsive, proportional increase in insulin secretion. Increases in blood sugar levels are dependent on the total number of calories ingested and the *glycaemic load* (GL) (see below) of the carbohydrate consumed (Ludwig 2002). The higher the GL of a particular food, the more rapid the rise in blood glucose and the greater the release of insulin. In healthy individuals this promotes more rapid uptake of glucose in peripheral tissues.

Adding protein and/or fat to a meal reduces total glycaemic and insulinaemic response (Wolever and Jenkins 1986), but 24-hour blood glucose and insulin levels remain significantly less in isocaloric mixed meals that include lower-GL carbohydrates (Miller 1994). Habitual consumption of higher GL carbohydrates, especially in a high-calorie diet, causes greater insulin secretion over time, and this chronic acute hyperinsulinaemia leads to a reduction in the sensitivity of insulin receptors, resulting in cellular insulin resistance.

2.1 Glycaemic index and glycaemic load

The glycaemic index (GI) is measure of the rise in blood sugar after eating a specific type of food. In creating the GI, scientists hoped to verify the theory that higher fibre content of foods would reduce the rate of rise in blood sugar. Accordingly, the GI is a relative scale comparing the rise in blood glucose from 50g of carbohydrate in a test food versus 50g of carbohydrate from either glucose or white bread. The rise in blood glucose from glucose or white bread is set at 100 and test foods are compared as a percentage of that rise.

Unfortunately, GI does not tell you how much carbohydrate is in a typical serving of the test food, and this leads to some unrealistic GI values. For example, carrots have a GI of 72, implying that carrots produce 72 per cent of the response as pure glucose. What is not revealed is that one would have to consume 700g of carrot to get a 50g dose of carbohydrate.

To overcome these limitations, the 'GL' was created. GL is defined as the GI of any particular food multiplied by the carbohydrate content per serving. For example, carrots have a GL of 5, reflecting the reality that eating a serving of carrots would only produce a minimal rise in blood glucose. For many vegetables and for nearly all fruits, the GL better reflects the known epidemiological benefits of their regular consumption.

2.2 Insulin resistance and blood sugar control

Insulin resistance refers to a decrease in the sensitivity of body tissues to the metabolic action of insulin. Insulin resistance is associated with at least four biochemical changes, including chronic elevations of blood glucose (McClain 2002), insulin (Del Prato *et al.* 1994), very low density lipoproteins (VLDL) (Zammit *et al.* 2001) and free fatty acids (Boden and Shulman 2002). Excessive caloric intake and consumption of high GL carbohydrates promote all four proximal changes associated with insulin resistance.

Important tissues that typically become resistant include:

- adipose tissue
- liver – the impaired sensitivity to insulin results in an increase in hepatic glucose production
- skeletal muscle – insulin resistance leads to a decrease in glucose uptake.

This combination contributes to a net rise in blood glucose. In response, the pancreatic beta-cells secrete more insulin, which, by the law of mass action, is able to overcome the cellular receptors' resistance, and glucose can enter the cells and normal physiology is restored, at least temporarily.

In skeletal muscle cells decreased uptake of glucose creates a local energy crisis once the intracellular reserves of glucose have been exhausted. In response, muscle cells increase the conversion of amino acids into organic acids and subsequently into glucose (local gluconeogenesis). However, this process creates an intracellular nitrogen excess that is controlled by the cellular excretion of the amino acid alanine. Pancreatic alpha-cells are exquisitely sensitive to circulating alanine levels and as they rise, the alpha cells secrete the hormone glucagon. Glucagon exerts its main action on liver cells, stimulating glycogenolysis and gluconeogenesis, both of which serve to increase blood sugar levels, which, in turn, leads to further increased insulin secretion.

This cycle of compensatory hyperglycaemia and hyperinsulinaemia can continue to control blood sugar and energy metabolism reasonably effectively for many years. However, given enough time and an excessive burden on the beta cells to produce ever-increasing quantities of insulin, the beta cells will begin to fail and become unable to produce sufficient insulin to stabilise the high blood glucose levels. When this happens, it results in a sudden and dramatic rise in blood glucose levels and to the development of overt type 2 diabetes.

3. Consequences of dysglycaemia

3.1 Diabetes and more

Diabetes is the most direct linear pathology that arises from metabolic syndrome. Indeed, as far back as 1936, H.P. Himsworth postulated that the central problem with type 2 diabetes was insulin receptor resistance rather than insulin deficiency, as was clearly the case in type 1 diabetes. Yet it was not until 1988 that Gerald Reaven proposed a unified theory of peripheral cellular insulin receptor resistance, which results not only in type 2 diabetes, but also contributes to a wide array of seemingly disparate disease processes, including dyslipidaemia, coronary artery disease (CAD), hypertension and central obesity.

3.2 Dyslipidaemia

In addition to its effects on blood glucose levels, glucagon activates hormone-sensitive lipase and stimulates the release of free fatty acids (FFAs) from peripheral adipose tissue into the bloodstream (Ludwig 2002). This is part of the body's attempt to deliver energy in any form possible to putatively starving cells due to their insulin receptor resistance. In the liver, glucagon stimulates triglyceride synthesis and also shifts the balance of cholesterol carrier molecules towards more VLDL and LDL cholesterol synthesis and less high density lipoprotein (HDL) cholesterol synthesis, and toward smaller and denser fragments of each cholesterol type. This is associated with significantly increased risk of cardiovascular disease.

While this physiologic response would increase one's chances for survival in an environment in which food is scarce, it becomes pathological when stimulated by excess and high-GL food. Indeed, high-GL meals are known to cause increased hepatic secretion of VLDL particles during both fasting and post-absorptive states (Mittendorfer and Sidossis 2001). Not, surprisingly, Lakka *et al.* (2002) found that middle-aged men with metabolic syndrome were more than three times as likely to die of coronary artery or heart disease, even after adjusting for all other known risk factors.

3.3 Hyperinsulinaemia and heart disease/CAD

Consistently, hyperinsulinaemia itself has been shown to be a risk factor for ischaemic heart disease (Despres *et al.* 1996). For each standard deviation increase in fasting insulin levels, the risk of heart disease increases by 170 per cent. Experimental evidence demonstrates that insulin stimulates proliferation of smooth muscle cells and augments lipid synthesis in vascular smooth muscle cells (Stout 1990). Thus, insulin appears to contribute directly to imbalances in blood lipids and to the formation of fibrolipid plaques and atherosclerosis, both essential components of the pathogenesis of CAD.

Fat cells in the abdomen and omentum do not express hormone-sensitive lipase but do remain sensitive to the action of increased levels of insulin, which causes them to take up and store more FFAs and triglycerides. This phenomenon has the evolutionary advantage of preserving abdominal and omental fat, which structurally anchor and protect the vital abdominal organs in times of starvation. In metabolic syndrome, however, the net result over time is a translocation of fat from the extremities to the abdomen, resulting in ever-increasing central obesity.

Indeed, the waist-to-hip ratio (WHR) is the best anthropometric measure of insulin resistance. The WHR is a much better measure of risk for heart attack than body mass index (BMI) or waist circumference alone (Yusuf *et al.* 2005). In a meta-analysis of risk for CAD, de Koning *et al.* (2007) found that for every 1cm increase in waist circumference, the relative risk of a cardiovascular event increased by 2 per cent, yet for a 0.01 unit increase in WHR, the relative risk increased by 5 per cent. Likewise, the WHR is also the best anthropometric predictor of stroke and transient ischaemic attack (Winter *et al.* 2008) and of death from all causes (Pischon *et al.* 2008).

Despite the epidemiological evidence that WHR is significantly superior to waist circumference alone in predicting risk, the National Cholesterol Education Project Adult Treatment Panel III (NCEP ATPIII) and the International Diabetes Federation recommend using only waist circumference in screening for disease risk, for the ostensible reason that its reproducibility is better.

3.4 Insulin's effects on IGF-1 and other hormones

Of course insulin does not act alone in the body but synergistically with many hormones, including growth hormone (GH), insulin-like growth factor-1 (IGF-1), testosterone, oestrogen and other androgens, all geared towards coordinating growth and reproduction with the bioavailability of food. Alterations in insulin secretion affect other hormone secretion patterns and the combination can lead to a variety of health problems.

3.4.1 CANCER RISK

Compensatory hyperinsulinaemia has been shown to decrease hepatic synthesis of IGF binding protein-1 (IGFBP-1). This increases the circulating levels of free IGF-1, the biologically active fraction that acts to increase cellular protein synthesis and promote cellular hypertrophy and cell proliferation, and thus leads to an increased risk of cancer. High free IGF-1 levels also suppress GH secretion via a negative feedback loop. Lower GH secretion results in decreased hepatic production of IGFBP-3 (and also, ironically, of total IGF-1) (Attia *et al.* 1998). Normally, IGFBP-3 prevents IGF-1 binding to its receptor and thereby inhibits cellular proliferation. Low IGFBP-3 levels also cause epithelial cells to be less sensitive to retinoic acid, a major inhibitor of cellular proliferation. Moreover, retinoic acid plays a key role in the regulation of apoptosis, or programmed cell death, in which cells commit suicide rather than become cancerous. Thus hyperinsulinaemia contributes to cellular proliferation and increased cancer risk via a number of pathways.

Box 5.1 Summary of hyperinsulinaemia's effects on cell proliferation

- Hyperinsulinaemia → decreased liver production of IGFBP-1
- IGFBP-1 binds IGF-1 and prevents its action
- IGF-1 promotes growth, hypertrophy and hyperplasia
- High IGF-1 → lower GH → decreased liver production of IGFBP-3 and IGF-1
- IGFBP-3 prevents IGF-1 binding to receptor, inhibiting action of IGF-1
- Low IGFBP-3 → decreased sensitivity to retinoic acid in epithelial cells
- Retinoic acid inhibits cell proliferation and helps regulate apoptosis

---

3.4.2 SKIN TAGS AND ACNE VULGARIS

Both insulin and free IGF-1 stimulate the synthesis of androgens in the ovaries (Cara 1994) and testes (Bebakar *et al.* 1990), and both inhibit hepatic synthesis of sex hormone binding globulin (SHBG), allowing for higher levels of free, biologically active androgens, which directly contribute to the pathophysiology of acne vulgaris, male pattern vertex balding, cutaneous papillomas (skin tags), acanthosis nigricans, polycystic ovary syndrome (PCOS) and certain epithelial cell carcinomas, specifically, colon, breast and prostate cancer (Cordain, Eades and Eades 2003).

Cutaneous papillomas (skin tags) are pigmented, hyperproliferative lesions on the skin that tend to appear on the neck, under the axilla and in the groin area. They are frequently observed in obese individuals and are a known marker for type 2 diabetes. Out of 200 outpatients with skin tags, Kahana *et al.* (1987) found that 26 per cent had overt type 2 diabetes (8% were unaware of this) while another 8 per cent had significantly impaired glucose tolerance tests. The association between skin tags and diabetes is so strong (over 62% in Thappa 1995) that the presence of skin tags in any patient should initiate testing to rule out type 2 diabetes.

Acne vulgaris is caused by the interaction of three causal factors: follicular hyperkeratinisation contributes to blocked sebum glands, increased androgen increased sebum production, and an overgrowth of the bacteria *Propionibacterium acnes* on the skin causes local inflammation (Thiboutot 1996). The first two of these causal factors are exacerbated by hyperinsulinaemia. Most acne vulgaris occurs at puberty when androgen levels increase dramatically, increasing sebum production. However, minimising hyperinsulinaemia through dietary and lifestyle changes (see below) provides a theoretical approach to effective treatment.

Both skin tags and acne vulgaris are characterised by hyperkeratinisation. Chronic hyperinsulinaemia leads to chronic elevation of non-esterified FFAs, which causes increased production of epidermal growth factor, and a decreased production of IGFBP-3 locally, allowing an increase in free IGF-1 that promotes the proliferation of keratinocytes. Furthermore, decreased IGFBP-3 reduces the binding affinity of retinoic acid for its receptors, thus reducing the normal inhibition of cellular proliferation.

In summary, a high-calorie, high-GL diet generates a consistent metabolic cascade: hyperinsulinaemia → insulin resistance → decreased IGFBP-1 production → increased circulating free IGF-1 → cellular hypertrophy and cell proliferation.

Indeed, this diet-driven hormone cascade helps to explain the steady trend in the last 200 years in industrialised countries towards increased stature (Malina 1990) and earlier age of menarche (Tanner 1973). Zeigler (1967) demonstrated that the increase in stature correlates highly with the increase in sucrose consumption in Denmark, England, Japan, the Netherlands, New Zealand, Norway and Sweden. Consistent with this observation, Koo *et al.* (2002) demonstrated in a prospective cohort that high fibre consumption (lower GL) correlates with later age of menarche. Increased stature has long been recognised as an independent risk factor for many cancers (Albanes *et al.* 1988), but this association is likely due to hyperinsulinaemia rather than to stature *per se*.

4. Metabolic syndrome – contributory factors to consider

4.1 The 'chicken and egg' conundrum

While it has been generally thought that insulin receptor resistance represents the primary disturbance in metabolic syndrome and that hyperinsulinaemia is a compensatory response, Del Prato *et al.* (1994) demonstrated the reverse. They demonstrated that hyperinsulinaemia caused significant drops in glucose disposal in healthy young adults. Indeed chronic high insulin levels decreased cellular glucose utilisation by 18 per cent after 48 hours and by a further 28 per cent after the next 24 hours. These results suggest that insulin resistance increases progressively and is a result of chronic hyperinsulinaemia, rather than just a cause of it. Also, although basal glucose oxidation remained elevated after 72 hours, glycogen synthesis was reduced by 66 per cent. Not only is insulin resistance associated with impaired glycogen synthesis, but it appears to be a consequence of hyperinsulinaemia, rather than of hyperglycaemia.

The central message here is that insulin resistance causes compensatory hyperinsulinaemia *and* chronic hyperinsulinaemia contributes directly to peripheral insulin resistance.

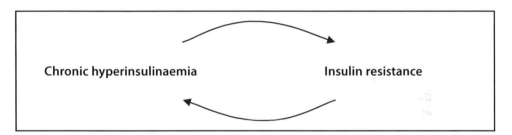

Chronic hyperinsulinaemia   **Insulin resistance**

Figure 5.1 Chronic hyperinsulinaemia and insulin resistance

Further, hyperglycaemia and hyperinsulinaemia separately and jointly contribute not only to central obesity (as described in 3.2 above) but also to general obesity. In Del Prato's study, both chronic insulin infusion and chronic glucose infusion led to suppression of basal lipid oxidation, with the combination of hyperglycaemia and hyperinsulinaemia causing the most profound suppression. Ironically, lipid oxidation is increased, not decreased, in full-blown diabetes (NIDDM), but this represents a more profound state of cellular starvation, and lipid oxidation changes vary depending on the degree of dysfunction and pathology.

In animal models every time a cell is exposed to insulin the production of the insulin-regulated glucose receptor on the cell's membrane, GLUT4, is decreased (Flores-Riveros *et al.* 1993). Exposure to even physiological levels of insulin lowers GLUT4 mRNA production by 70–80 per cent within ten hours. A 90 per cent suppression of

GLUT4 was also found with exposure to physiological levels of arachidonic acid (AA) (Tebbey *et al.* 1994). By contrast, exercise increased GLUT4 transcription (MacLean *et al.* 2002).

Thus a diet rich in high glycaemic load carbohydrates and in animal fat and omega-6 vegetable oil, combined with a sedentary lifestyle, would theoretically be an ideal recipe for promoting insulin resistance.

4.2 Insulin and oxidative stress

Lipid accumulation in skeletal muscle is also associated with the development of insulin resistance. Anderson *et al.* (2009) have observed that the intracellular redox environment, reflected by the reduced-to-oxidised glutathione ratio, is sensitive to nutritional intake, shifting to a more oxidised state acutely with increased ingestion of carbohydrates and chronically with increased ingestion of fats. Increased consumption of carbohydrates and fats contributes to intracellular oxidative stress and reduces cellular capacity to neutralise reactive oxygen species (ROS) and other free radicals. Increased levels of ROS have been shown to play a significant role in both tumour necrosis factor-α (TNF-α) and glucocorticoid-induced insulin resistance (Houstis *et al.* 2006). The rate at which hydrogen peroxide (H_2O_2) is emitted from mitochondria is considered an important barometer of mitochondrial function and of the overall cellular redox environment (Schafer and Buettner 2001). The rate of mitochondrial H_2O_2 emission is significantly greater on a high fat diet (Anderson, Yamazaki and Neufer 2007). Increased mitochondrial H_2O_2 emission may be another primary factor in the aetiology of insulin resistance.

The glucose-driven increase in free radical production may also contribute to vascular endothelium dysfunction and hypertension by causing disturbances in nitric oxide (NO) pathway regulation. Insulin is known to stimulate production of nitric oxide in the endothelium (endothelial NO synthase, or eNOS) leading to peripheral vasodilation, increased blood flow, and cellular insulin-mediated glucose uptake (Assumpcao *et al.* 2008). Insulin resistance thus leads to reduced NO-mediated vasodilation. This is associated with excessive superoxide and peroxynitrite production, which in turn activates inducible NO synthase (iNOS) and stimulates the release of pro-inflammatory mediators (Wellen and Hotamisligil 2005). Furthermore, visceral adipose tissue produces and secretes a number of pro-inflammatory adipocytokines, such as TNF-α, interleukin-6 (IL-6), non-esterified fatty acids, angiotensin II and leptin, all of which induce insulin resistance, oxidative stress and contribute to hypertension (Katagiri, Yamada and Oka 2007).

4.3 High risk carbohydrates

4.3.1 PROCESSED FLOUR AND SUGARS

White table sugar – sucrose – is a disaccharide containing one molecule each of glucose and fructose. Consumption in the UK remained at less than 10kg per person per year until 1860. Thereafter, sugar consumption rose more or less steadily to over 50kg per year in 1970 (Cleave 1974), then accelerated even more rapidly. According to the United States Department of Agriculture (USDA) (2002), Americans consumed an annual average of 55.5kg sugar per person in 1970, rising to 69.1kg per year by 2000, thanks in part to the introduction of high-fructose corn syrup (HFCS) as a new and cheaper form of sugar.

However, increased GL is not just due to increased consumption of refined sugar. The introduction of steel roller mills in the 1880s allowed for the mass production of fibre-depleted wheat flour (Cleave 1974), ground into such uniformly small particles that there is no significant difference in glycaemic response between wholegrain or refined flour.

According to the USDA report in 1997 the typical American diet consisted of approximately 16 per cent sugars and 20 per cent high-GL refined cereal grains, suggesting that at least 36 per cent of total energy in the US diet directly promotes reactive hyperinsulinaemia and compensatory insulin resistance. The data is even worse in the UK, since, based on data from *The Dietary and Nutrition Survey of British Adults* from 1986–7, the average British adult consumed approximately 20 per cent of calories from sugars and a further 30 per cent of calories from starches (Pryer *et al.* 2001).

4.3.2 FRUCTOSE: FRIEND OR FOE?

Unlike glucose, pure fructose exhibits a very low GI (19) and GL (2) (Foster-Powell, Holt and Brand-Miller 2002). Despite this, fructose is used experimentally to induce insulin resistance in rats when fed at 35–65 per cent of energy intake levels (Zavaroni *et al.* 1980). High fructose feeding in healthy humans (normal diet + 1000kcal fructose) also causes impaired insulin sensitivity (Beck-Nielsen, Pedersen and Lindskov 1980). Even 20 per cent of calories from fructose worsened insulin sensitivity in hyperinsulinaemic men (Reiser *et al.* 1989).

Fructose exhibits a strong insulinogenic effect when blood glucose levels are even modestly elevated, as would occur in a typical postprandial state (Reiser *et al.* 1987). Animal studies suggest that fructose is the primary nutrient mediator of sucrose-induced insulin resistance and glucose intolerance. Rats fed a high-starch diet (68% of calories) were switched to either an isocaloric sucrose (glucose/fructose) diet or a starch/fructose diet. In both groups glucose and insulin areas under the curves increased by 61 and 29 per cent respectively, suggesting that fructose is a primary element responsible for the development of insulin resistance (Thresher *et al.* 2000).

Fructose consumption causes elevations in serum levels of triglycerides and VLDL cholesterol (Hallfrisch, Reiser and Prather 1983). Seventeen per cent of energy from fructose, typical for the modern Western diet, has been shown to elevate serum triglyceride concentrations in healthy individuals (Bantle *et al.* 2000). Fructose consumption has also been shown to increase non-esterified serum FFAs, which in itself may further contribute to hepatic and peripheral insulin resistance (Mayes 1993).

Sucrose remains the most common sweetener used in the Western diet but HFCS is not far behind. HFCS is now the least expensive form of sweetener added to processed foods and, not surprisingly, HFCS is now the major source of fructose in the US diet, far exceeding the amounts from honey or fruits (Park and Yetley 1993).

Honey, the major source of sweetener before 1800, is often suggested as a healthy alternative to sugar for diabetics, but there is little clinical evidence to support this view. Since honey contains approximately 52 per cent fructose and 34 per cent glucose, it could potentially cause similar problems in regard to promoting insulin resistance. However, consumption of honey has always been limited and remains so today, largely because it is significantly more expensive to produce than sucrose or HFCS (Foster-Powell and Miller 1995).

Most fruits typically contain 50–70 per cent fructose as a combination of free fructose and sucrose (USDA Food Composition 2009), and could theoretically pose significant risk, especially if consumed in the concentrated form of fruit juice. However, a typical serving of whole fruit (80g) contains less than 10g of total carbohydrate and accordingly only 5–7g of fructose. In addition, whole fruits frequently contain soluble fibre that slows sugar absorption. Whole fruit consumption should be encouraged as part of a healthy diet, whereas excessive fruit juice, sugar, HFCS and honey consumption should be avoided.

5. Preventing and reversing insulin resistance and metabolic syndrome

There is a tendency in allopathic medicine toward a reductionist bias, tacitly assuming that each disease will have only a single cause and that there will likely be only one treatment to best eradicate the disease. In fact there are myriad diseases whose aetiologies lie in complex networks of genetic susceptibility, environmental influences and dietary and lifestyle choices that combine to create physiological and biochemical imbalances. Such imbalances can persist for many years without degenerating into a well-classified disease process. Metabolic syndrome is a case in point. Functional disturbances can exist for decades before the onset of overt type 2 diabetes, CAD or hypertension. Since the aetiology is multi-factorial, so too will be the most successful treatment regimen.

A more holistic approach to nutritional therapy sees specific 'nutrients' as only part of a complex information system that constitutes any living organism. Inherent in any food is an information code that we 'read' and 'interpret' by eating, digesting and assimilating that food. Although that information includes specific 'active nutrients', the efficacy of a good diet cannot be limited to any such specific nutrients. It is essential to bear in mind that all macro- and micro-nutrients will be more effective in the framework of an overall healthier diet and lifestyle.

The primary stimulus for dysregulation of the insulin axis in metabolic syndrome is a diet too high in total calories and high GL carbohydrates, and a lifestyle that is too sedentary. While specific substances may be found to ameliorate the multiple physiological dysfunctions, the core of any effective treatment must lie with fundamental changes to diet and lifestyle.

5.1 The role of physical activity

When the problem is energy throughput, a comprehensive treatment regimen must address not only what is going into the system but what is being expended. A recent Cochrane Review of diet and exercise intervention trials (Orozco *et al.* 2008) demonstrated a 37 per cent reduction in the risk of developing diabetes in susceptible individuals when modest increases in physical activity, such as walking 20 minutes a day, were added to standard recommendations of reduced caloric intake. The meta-analysis also demonstrated additional benefits in terms of body weight, waist circumference and blood pressure, all key components of metabolic syndrome. These trials support the central importance of increasing energy throughput in order to reverse metabolic syndrome. Reducing caloric intake alone is just not enough.

The importance of physical activity may be illustrated by the Amish communities in the United States. Old Order Amish have eschewed many of the conveniences of modern life, including electricity, automated farm machinery and automobiles. They consume roughly the same diet as other white Americans, have similar body composition, and even the same incidence of impaired glucose tolerance, but they have a 50 per cent lower incidence of diabetes (Hsueh *et al.* 2000).

In a review of the efficacy of physical exercise on preventing and treating individuals with diabetes, Clark (1997) showed evidence that regular, moderate-intensity physical activity is associated with a 33–67 per cent lower incidence of type 2 diabetes over a 4–14 year period and a 15–20 per cent lower glycosylated haemoglobin (HbA1c), a marker of long-term blood glucose levels, in people with type 2 diabetes. As a therapeutic option, regular moderate exercise remains a critically important clinical intervention since, as Clark observed, 60–70 per cent of the general population is physically inactive.

Increasing obesity is associated with increasing risk of fatigue, back pain, need for cholecystectomy, need for hysterectomy, hypertension, heart disease, diabetes and death (Folsom *et al.* 2000). However, losing weight, rather than improving health, may significantly increase one's risk of death (Gaesser 1999). Comparing overweight individuals who lost more than 15 per cent of their body weight with those who lost less than 5 per cent, the former had twice the risk of death (Pamuk *et al.* 1992). The simplest explanation of this phenomenon may be that most weight loss is typically accomplished by reducing caloric intake *without* increasing protein consumption and exercise. Dieting alone results in an increased loss of lean muscle mass instead of fat mass, whereas isocaloric diets that increase protein and decrease sugar consumption appear to preserve muscle mass, encourage more fat loss, and maintain basal metabolic rate (BMR) (Allison *et al.* 2003). Loss of lean muscle mass during periods of dieting serves to reduce the BMR and make the individual's metabolism less efficient. Resumption of old eating habits or a 'normal' diet would promote weight gain, since the BMR has been reduced as a result of the lean muscle loss. This process explains the weight cycling commonly observed among dieters. With each period of calorie restriction, the dieter becomes less healthy.

By contrast, exercise training has been shown to preserve lean muscle mass in individuals during diet-induced weight loss (Ballor and Poehlman 1994). Individuals who exercise during reduced-calorie diets also maintain their weight loss longer than those who diet alone (Johannsen, Redman and Ravussin 2007).

Insulin sensitivity correlates to the degree of unsaturation of fatty acids in cell membrane phospholipids. Andersson *et al.* (1998) found that placing middle-aged men on a moderate exercise programme without any change in diet decreased the levels of saturated fat (palmitic acid), linoleic and arachidonic acids, and increased the level of monounsaturated oleic acid. Overall, exercise alone increased the degree of unsaturation and improved insulin sensitivity.

5.2 The roles of calorie restriction and sirtuins

5.2.1 CALORIE RESTRICTION

While *periodic* calorie restriction lowers metabolic efficiency and increases the risk of death, *consistently* reducing caloric intake by at least 25 per cent has been shown to greatly extend healthy lifespan. In the 1930s Clive McCay found that restricting caloric intake in rats could substantially increase both their average and extreme life expectancy. Calorie restriction also delays senile infertility and tumour formation and preserves the capacity for efficient stress adaptation and homeostasis.

The metabolic benefits accrued by calorie restriction appear to be due in part to lowering insulin levels. Lower cellular insulin exposure in turn lowers overall growth factor exposure, improves age-related decline of mitochondrial function, and helps to maintain a longer-term favourable balance of the insulin-to-growth hormone antagonism (Parr 1997).

The role of growth hormone changes, depending on calorie intake:

- in a calorie-replete individual, growth hormone stimulates the production and release of IGF-1, stimulating cell mitosis and growth

- in a calorie-restricted individual, growth hormone secretion increases but IGF-1 levels decline. In this case, growth hormone might be better called 'repair hormone' since it stimulates increased synthesis of proteins that repair cellular DNA.

Thus calorie repletion alone alters the metabolic effects of growth hormone.

5.2.2 RESVERATROL AND SIRT-1

Recent discoveries have demonstrated that some stress response molecules found in plants may override normal environmental signalling in mammals and may provide a novel therapeutic approach for correcting metabolic syndrome, even in the presence of a diet high in carbohydrates and fat.

Resveratrol is a polyphenol produced by grapes in response to the stress of fungal infections common in autumn. Baur and colleagues (2006) found that giving resveratrol to mice could reverse nearly all of the detrimental metabolic effects of a high-GL diet and sedentary lifestyle, apart from obesity, which did not change. Administering oral resveratrol led to increased insulin sensitivity, reduced IGF-1 and increased peroxisome proliferator-activated receptor-1 (PPAR-1) activity. (See Chapter 4 for more on PPARs.) These signalling changes stimulated the growth of significant quantities of new mitochondria and improved motor function. Resveratrol was found to oppose the effects of the high-calorie diet in 144 out of 153 biochemical pathways known to be adversely affected by a high-calorie diet.

Box 5.2 SIRTs

SIRT-1 is a sirtuin gene, of which there are now known to be at least seven in mammals, all of which may be involved in different aspects of adapting our physiology to food availability and other environmental stressors.

All SIRTs appear to be activated by calorie restriction but resveratrol appears to focus on activating SIRT-1 (whose role is described within the text).

SIRT-3 regulates mitochondrial function and thermogenesis in brown fat. Its discovery may change our understanding of certain types of obesity (Shi *et al.* 2005).

SIRT-4 appears to modulate insulin secretion (Argmann and Auwerx 2006).

Su and Hung (2006) found that diabetic rats treated with resveratrol had a 25 per cent drop in plasma glucose concentration by day 14, and the triglyceride concentration was reduced by 50 per cent. The blood sugar-lowering effect of resveratrol appears to be independent of insulin, and up-regulates transcription of the gene SIRT-1 (silent information regulator transcript), which in turn alters the production of several other transcription factors (Elliott and Jirousek 2008).

These include:

- increased PPAR-γ-coactivator 1-α (PGC-1α) (induces mitochondrial biogenesis and increases fatty acid oxidation; controls gluconeogenesis and glycogenolysis)

- increased FoxO (increases catalase activity and reduces the concentration of ROS); reduces the inflammatory response to FFAs by down-regulating inflammatory mediators (IL-6, C-reactive protein (CRP) and monocyte chemotactic protein (MCP-1))

- decreased NF-$\kappa\beta$ (lowers chronic inflammatory responses).

Even though resveratrol is a naturally occurring signalling molecule, it is unlikely that such effects as were seen in the mice in Baur *et al.*'s study could be achieved in humans through food alone. Those mice were fed 24mg/kg of resveratrol daily. For a 70kg person, this would equal ~1700mg of resveratrol/day. As the best red wine contains approximately 10mg/L resveratrol, one would need to consume about 250 standard bottles of red wine a day to have a therapeutic effect. Resveratrol and its mimetics are a promising area of research but clinically effective supplements or drugs that activate SIRT-1 are years or decades away.

For humans, eating less, or combining eating less with exercising more, would appear to still be the best way to activate SIRT-1 genes. A 25 per cent calorie restriction or a 12.5 per cent calorie restriction combined with a 12.5 per cent increased energy expenditure via exercise have both been shown to increase mitochondria numbers in skeletal muscle while decreasing whole body oxygen consumption and DNA damage, thereby demonstrating improved mitochondrial function (Civitarese *et al.* 2007).

5.3 The role of diet and nutrients

5.3.1 THE MEDITERRANEAN DIET

Box 5.3 The Mediterranean diet

- Abundant plant foods, including fruits, vegetables, potatoes, pulses, nuts, seeds and minimally refined whole grains

- Dessert: fruit, often accompanied with small amounts of cheese

- Main fat source: olive oil

- Main animal protein source: fish; poultry, eggs, lamb and goat consumed in moderate amounts

- Beef and pork: consumed sparingly

- Wine: consumed with most meals in low to moderate amounts

The 'Mediterranean diet' is characterised by food patterns typical of Crete, Greece and southern Italy catalogued in the early 1960s, where adult life expectancy was among the highest in the world and where rates of coronary heart disease, hypertension, obesity and certain cancers were among the lowest. The Mediterranean diet first studied also included significant physical work in the field or kitchen on a daily basis, thereby increasing energy throughput (Willett *et al.* 1995).

The vast majority of data from large epidemiological studies supports the notion that the Mediterranean diet is useful in preventing and treating the central diseases associated with metabolic syndrome. Serra-Majem *et al.* (2006) review a growing number of clinical intervention trials that are beginning to elucidate the mechanisms by which this simple dietary approach is effective. They conclude that the Mediterranean diet showed favourable effects on lipoprotein levels, endothelium vasodilation, insulin resistance and antioxidant capacity, resulting in reduced CAD mortality and reduced cancer incidence in healthy and obese individuals, and was cardioprotective in patients with documented CAD.

Recently, Fung *et al.* (2009) reported on the Nurses' Health Study, a 20-year follow-up on 85,000 women, showing that those on the Mediterranean diet had reductions of 29 per cent in CAD, 19 per cent in stroke and 39 per cent in death from CAD or stroke. Esposito *et al.* (2004) demonstrated that in individuals with documented metabolic syndrome, after two years following a Mediterranean diet, only 44 per cent of participants still met metabolic syndrome criteria, compared to 87 per cent who followed the American Heart Association recommended diet (high carbohydrate, low fat, low cholesterol). Appel *et al.* (1997) demonstrated that the Mediterranean diet lowered blood pressure in people with or without high blood pressure.

The moderate-fat Mediterranean diet also appears to be superior to low-fat diets in losing weight and keeping weight off. McManus, Antinoro and Sacks (2001) showed that, over 18 months, the Mediterranean diet group lost an average of 4.1kg and had a reduction of waist circumference (a marker of insulin resistance) of 6.9cm, while the low-fat diet group *gained* 2.9kg in body weight and their waist circumference *increased* by 2.6cm.

5.3.2 RED WINE REVISITED

Red wine is an essential component of the typical Mediterranean diet and it may benefit individuals via a number of mechanisms, including antioxidant status, blood viscosity and endothelial relaxation, quite apart from its potential role is SIRT-1 activation (see above) (Liu *et al.* 2008). In a three-month randomised trial with 21 healthy men, half stayed on a standard Western diet while the other half were placed on a Mediterranean diet. The Western diet group had lower vitamin C levels and increased levels of damaged DNA. The Mediterranean group had 28 per cent increased total antioxidant capacity. In the second month red wine was added to both groups. In both groups vitamin C levels and total antioxidant reactivity increased, while vitamin E levels and DNA damage decreased. The addition of wine also was able to restore normal endothelial reactivity in the Western diet group (Leighton *et al.* 1999)

5.3.3 OLIVE OIL

Sarkkinen *et al.* (1996) compared the effectiveness of a high-monounsaturated fat (MUFA) diet (olive oil) to a high-polyunsaturated fat (PUFA) diet (mostly linoleic acid) in individuals with documented insulin resistance who previously ate a high saturated fat (SFA) diet. While the high PUFA diet decreased total cholesterol, the high MUFA diet reduced total cholesterol, LDL cholesterol, apolipoprotein B and fasting glucose, suggesting that factors other than membrane fluidity alone may be playing a role in metabolic syndrome.

Madigan *et al.* (2000) compared the addition of 30ml per day of olive oil to 30ml of sunflower oil (a high omega-6 PUFA) over two weeks in diabetics. On the sunflower arm of the trial, fasting glucose, insulin, total and LDL cholesterol, fasting and postprandial chylomicron components (apoB48 and abpB100) and VLDL phospholipids were all higher than on the olive oil arm, suggesting that sunflower oil may contribute to cardiovascular disease. In addition, olive oil has been shown to make LDL cholesterol more resistant to oxidation than a high PUFA diet (Baroni *et al.* 1999), probably due to less unsaturation and the presence of potent antioxidant phenolic compounds in olive oil, shown to reduce markers for increased thrombotic risk (Ruano *et al.* 2007).

A longer, two-month, randomised trial showed that an olive oil-rich Mediterranean diet reduced fasting insulin levels and the fasting insulin/glucose ratio, with improved insulin-mediated glucose transport, while a high-vegetable oil diet did not (Ryan *et al.* 2000). Salas-Salvadó *et al.* (2008) found that adherence to an *ad libitum* Mediterranean diet in insulin resistant individuals could reduce the prevalence of metabolic syndrome by 6.7 per cent. Incredibly, adding one whole litre of extra virgin olive oil per week in addition to the Mediterranean diet reduced the prevalence by 13.7 per cent.

Olive oil consumption has long been associated with decreased cardiovascular disease risk (Lairon 2007). One recent case-matched control study concluded that after adjusting for all other known risk factors, use of olive oil as the main dietary fat was associated with a 47 per cent lower risk of having an acute myocardial event.

5.3.4 WALNUTS

The health benefits of olive oil may be improved by the addition of walnuts. Walnuts are known to be high in omega-3 alpha-linolenic acid (ALA). Zambon *et al.* (2000) found that replacing 35 per cent of MUFA calories with walnuts improved lipid parameters in hypercholesterolaemic subjects on a Mediterranean diet. Total cholesterol, LDL cholesterol and lipoprotein (a) were reduced additionally by 9.0 per cent, 11.2 per cent and 9.2 per cent. There was no effect on HDL, VLDL, triglycerides or susceptibility to oxidation.

The putative mechanism is increased efficiency in the hepatic uptake and clearance of LDL cholesterol. This increased activity correlated linearly with the increased ALA content of plasma triglycerides in the walnut phase of the trial. Vasodilation and hypertension also improved on replacing 32 per cent of energy intake from MUFA with walnuts (Ros *et al.* 2004). Interestingly, mixed nuts produced no additional benefits over an olive oil-rich diet (Salas-Salvadó *et al.* 2008), probably because most nuts are rich in omega-6 linoleic acid, whereas walnuts also contain omega-3 ALA.

5.3.5 OTHER DIETARY FATS

Dietary fats play a complex role in glucose metabolism and consequently in the pathophysiology of metabolic syndrome. During the twentieth century, total per capita energy consumption in the United States increased by 9 per cent, sugar by 64 per cent and fat by 32 per cent. Much of the increased fat consumption has come from increased vegetable oil (omega-6). Given that the consumption of fat and sugar increased in the same time period, it is difficult to separate their metabolic effects.

The balance of fatty acids (FAs) in the diet is important in part because it affects the balance of FAs in cell membranes. It appears that, in general, the more unsaturated FAs in any membrane, the more flexible and fluid that membrane is, and the more responsive insulin receptors are to insulin signalling (Borkman *et al.* 1993). Docosahexaenoic acid (DHA) is the longest and most unsaturated FA found in human membranes and therefore contributes more than any other single fat to membrane fluidity and function but it is the balance of all membrane fats that is most important.

In terms of dietary fat consumption, fish, shellfish and wild game contain a greater percentage of 'structural' fat and less 'storage' fat. By contrast, domesticated livestock contains more storage fat per unit weight. Structural fat tends to be significantly more unsaturated than storage fat, which may help explain why the consumption of fish and game appears to be protective against metabolic syndrome, while excess consumption of domesticated meat increases risk (Crawford *et al.* 1970).

Most data suggests that short-term isocaloric substitution of dietary fat for dietary carbohydrate does not cause insulin resistance (Swinburn 1993), but a chronically high-fat diet is known to increase triglyceride accumulation in skeletal muscle, which, in turn, directly contributes to insulin resistance in those muscles (Pan *et al.* 1995). Triglyceride accumulation in the skeletal muscle correlates inversely with insulin sensitivity, as does a high ratio of omega-6 to omega-3 fats, while the percentage of long-chain omega-3 FAs, EPA and DHA, in membrane phospholipids correlates extremely highly with insulin sensitivity (Storlien *et al.* 1996). The cell membranes of diabetics contain much higher relative levels of SFAs and MUFAs and much lower levels of both omega-3 and omega-6 PUFAs compared to non-diabetics. The percentage of linoleic acid (LA) compared with longer chain PUFAs was also higher in diabetics (Horrobin 1988).

This imbalance may be due in part to a disruption in the metabolic efficiency of the delta-6 desaturase (d6D) and delta-5-desaturase (d5D), enzymes that are responsible for the conversion of the shorter omega-6 LA and omega-3 ALA into their more unsaturated and metabolically active long-chain PUFAs (see Figure 4.1 in Chapter 4). These enzymes are stimulated by insulin (and d5D is inhibited by glucagon) but only if insulin binds efficiently to its cellular receptors. In a healthy individual, insulin increases d6D and d5D activity but, as insulin resistance develops, the insulin is less effective in binding to its cellular receptors and therefore less effective in increasing d6D and d5D activity. Gradually, the relative percentage of long-chain PUFAs declines in cell membranes and the resulting decrease in membrane fluidity further contributes to insulin resistance (Anderson 1995). Consistent with these findings, Horrobin (1997) found that he could improve neuropathy in diabetics by supplementing evening primrose oil (EPO) containing gamma-linolenic acid (GLA) (a metabolic product of d6D activity on LA) thus bypassing this metabolic block.

David Horrobin and his colleagues (1991) had previously found that even in healthy individuals EPO and safflower oil had significantly different effects on plasma fatty acid concentrations. Evening primrose oil raised the level of dihomo-gamma-linolenic acid (DGLA) but had no significant effect on arachidonic acid (AA) levels, whereas safflower oil (high in LA) raised the levels of LA and AA, without raising DGLA. This suggests that LA may be rapidly converted to AA by a tightly linked enzyme sequence in healthy humans and that GLA, found in EPO, may be rapidly converted to DGLA but then only slowly on to AA. If true, this would have significant implications for management of neuropathy and other pro-inflammatory complications of diabetes, especially since 85 per cent of our current dietary PUFA intake is estimated to be from linoleic acid (Mann *et al.* 1995).

Storlien *et al.* (1991) found that diets high in saturated, monounsaturated (omega-9), or polyunsaturated (omega-6) FAs led to severe insulin resistance in rats. Substituting 11 per cent of FAs in the high omega-6 fat diet with long-chain omega-3 FAs from fish oils normalised insulin action, but short-chain omega-3 FAs (ALA from flax oil) had no effect. However, the flax oil substitution was effective in preventing the insulin resistance induced by the high-saturated fat diet. The implication here is that increasing dietary long-chain omega-3 fats is universally beneficial in improving insulin sensitivity, but short-chain omega-3 fats are beneficial only when replacing saturated fats in the diet. Even olive oil, which has been shown to be so protective against metabolic syndrome in the overall context of a healthy Mediterranean diet, can induce insulin resistance if long-chain omega-3 fats are excluded from the diet.

South Asians living in the United Kingdom have a far higher incidence of diabetes than native European Caucasians (19% versus 4%). They also exhibit higher blood pressure, higher insulin levels, higher plasma triglycerides, lower HDL cholesterol concentrations and significantly higher death rates from CAD. While there is no significant difference in obesity rates between the two groups, South Asians have a much higher WHR (McKeigue *et al.* 1991). Interestingly, South Asians have much less saturated fat in their diets but more PUFA in the form of omega-6 vegetable oils and consequently, a far higher omega 6:3 ratio. Das (1995) demonstrated that South Asians with diabetes have significantly lower plasma phospholipid levels of GLA, DGLA, AA, EPA and DHA than non-diabetic controls, consistent with findings in diabetic whites.

While reducing dietary fat consumption has been shown to promote weight loss, it has also been shown that individuals on a low-calorie, low-fat diet typically gain weight and waist circumference, whereas those placed on a low-calorie, moderate-fat diet reduce their weight and waist circumference (McManus *et al.* 2001). Moreover, Walker *et al.* (1996) found that a high-olive oil diet is more beneficial than a high-fibre, high-carbohydrate, low-fat diet. Both groups lost similar amounts of fat, but the high-olive oil diet promoted fat loss from the abdomen, whereas the low-fat diet resulted in a disproportionate loss of lower body fat, worsening the WHR and worsening insulin resistance.

The clinical inference from research on the effects of dietary fat on metabolic syndrome suggests a potential hierarchy of benefits for individuals:

- Fish oils appear universally beneficial for metabolic syndrome when replacing any other type of dietary fat. Both EPA and DHA directly and profoundly increase membrane fluidity and receptor sensitivity, and EPA contributes to an increase in anti-inflammatory eicosanoid production, as does DGLA from GLA-containing oils.

- Reducing saturated and *trans* fats is prudent for all individuals.

- Olive oil appears more beneficial than high-LA vegetable oils, but the inclusion of moderate vegetable sources of ALA in walnuts provides additional benefits.

Altered eicosanoid production may also help explain why olive oil is better than vegetable oil as an intervention for metabolic syndrome prevention and treatment. As an omega-9 fat, olive oil cannot easily be made into any eicosanoid and therefore remains neutral in terms of inflammation. According to Horrobin's (1991) research, outlined above, in healthy individuals, omega-6 vegetable oil rapidly converts to AA, the metabolic precursor for pro-inflammatory cytokines. It is logical to infer that this conversion would proceed even more rapidly with a high GL diet since this would initiate increased insulin release which in turn would up-regulate delta-5-desaturase activity in insulin-sensitive individuals.

See Chapter 4 for a general discussion of the role of PUFAs in human health.

5.3.6 PROTEIN

Increased lean protein consumption has been shown to increase diet-induced thermogenesis (DIT), the number of calories used to digest and metabolise macronutrients. Dauncey and Bingham (1983) found that a high-protein, low-carbohydrate diet increased total energy expenditure by 12 per cent compared to the same individuals when they consumed a high-carbohydrate, low-protein diet. Crovetti *et al.* (1998) found that the DIT associated with a high-protein meal (69% of calories from protein) is about 275 per cent greater than the DIT of a high-fat or high-carbohydrate meal. The DIT of a high protein meal correlates highly with meal satiety, and individuals eating more protein are likely therefore to consume fewer calories and to burn a higher percentage of those calories in the process of digestion.

Low-calorie diets that maintain a higher percentage of protein (45%) have been shown to improve insulin sensitivity when compared to an isocaloric high-carbohydrate diet (60%). Glucose disposal and oxidation increased with the higher protein diet and decreased with the higher carbohydrate diet. However, opposite results were found with lipid oxidation (Piatti *et al.* 1994). Despite this, increasing lean protein consumption while keeping calorie intake constant appears to be one effective recommendation for improving metabolic syndrome risk and treatment.

5.3.7 RATE OF GLUCOSE ABSORPTION, LOW GI/GL DIETS

An experiment done by Jenkins *et al.* (1990) on the rate of absorption of glucose showed that sipping a fixed amount of a glucose solution over four hours was markedly less stressful on the body than drinking the same amount in ten minutes. Insulin secretion was 54 per cent lower in the sipping group, C-peptide was 47 per cent lower, and cortisol, glucagon and growth hormone levels were all reduced. This suggests that slow absorption of glucose, by reducing the impact on insulin production, reduces the risk of hyperinsulinaemia and therefore of insulin resistance.

Frost *et al.* (1998) found that women placed on a low versus a high GI diet for three weeks had improved *in vivo* insulin sensitivity and improved *in vitro* adipocyte insulin sensitivity, and that these effects were greater in women who had a family history of CAD or higher baseline insulin levels. Similar results were found by Peirera *et al.* (2002) who placed overweight hyperinsulinaemic non-diabetic adults on either a whole- or refined-grain isocaloric diets for six weeks. The wholegrain diet reduced fasting insulin levels by 10 per cent, independent of the BMI of the women in the study.

Additional evidence for adverse effects of high GL foods comes from a series of second meal studies, where the insulinaemic effects of a standard lunch are observed after a low- or high-GL breakfast. Glucose and insulin responses are significantly greater when the same lunch is fed after a high-GI breakfast (Liljeberg, Akerberg and Bjorck 1999). This phenomenon is likely also caused by the postprandial increase in FFA levels as a result of increased release of the counter-regulatory hormones cortisol and glucagon. The FFA would contribute to a transient insulin resistance.

Overall, a low-GL diet has been associated with significant decreased risk of heart disease. Liu *et al.* (2000) found a clear two-fold reduction in CAD risk in women who ate a lower GL diet, comparing lowest to highest tertiles of the population.

5.3.8 WATER-SOLUBLE NON-STARCH POLYSACCHARIDES (FIBRE)

Dietary fibre is an important element in contributing to the low GL of foods, but some types of dietary fibre, such as the soluble non-starch polysaccharides (NSP) may have their own metabolic properties that may help improve insulin sensitivity. The addition of guar gum to the diet can decrease (improve) fasting blood glucose levels and improve insulin sensitivity in both type 2 diabetics and otherwise healthy subjects (Landin *et al.* 1992; Tagliaferro *et al.* 1985). Stahl and Berger (1990) found that eight weeks' supplementation with either 15g/d of guar gum or 30g/d of wheat bran reduced postprandial insulin in diabetic subjects, but only the guar gum lowered total and LDL cholesterol and triglycerides.

Soluble NSPs are significantly better at improving serum lipids than is insoluble fibre. The putative mechanism of metabolic benefit is that gut bacteria digest soluble NSPs, yielding high levels of propionic acid, which are systemically reabsorbed by the large intestine. The propionic acid is taken up by liver cells, where it slows the activity of the hepatic enzyme 3-hydroxy-3-methylglutaryl-coenzyme A (HMG CoA) reductase, instrumental in endogenous cholesterol synthesis (Bueld, Bannenberg and Netter 1996).

While guar gum has been used in most clinical trials, all common beans, other pulses and vegetables like turnip, swede and okra contain large amounts of soluble NSP, and all have extremely low GLs. Furthermore, a therapeutic dose of 10g of soluble NSP is easily achievable with the daily consumption of one or two servings of these foods.

In individuals intolerant to increased dietary pulse consumption, supplementation with the probiotic bacteria *Propionibacterium freudenreichii* may provide a novel avenue for increasing propionic acid production. Supplementation with these bacteria has been shown to increase colonic levels of propionic acid dramatically without a change in dietary fibre intake (Bougle *et al.* 2002). Studies need to be conducted to see if this increase improves lipid parameters.

5.3.9 PALEOLITHIC DIET

One popular diet recommendation for combating metabolic syndrome is the Paleolithic or Paleo diet, whose goal is to take nutrition back to a diet resembling the human diet more than 10,000 years ago. This diet is rich in lean protein and low GL vegetables and fruits; it includes no grains or legumes. While the goal of decreasing GL is laudable, the idea that a modern human could approximate a Paleolithic diet is ludicrous. Civilisation has given us grains and legumes but also every variety of fruit and vegetable commercially available today. Any fruit or vegetable bought or even grown today bears little resemblance to its ancestor of 10,000 years ago (or even several hundred years ago) due to selective breeding in order to create varieties that are higher in yield, calorie/macronutrient content and lower in fibre (McGee 2004).

The same may be said of available animal-derived foods. Domesticating animals increased the fat content approximately ten-fold over that of their pre-domesticated wild ancestors, and the total amount of fat in the diet also plays an important role in the development of insulin insensitivity.

There are several other differences between the Paleolithic and modern lifestyle that would make the reversion at least highly improbable:

- periods of weeks or months of low food availability
- extremely high levels of physical exercise in foraging and hunting
- exposure to the elements with no heating nor air conditioning, and little shelter.

Each of these factors would contribute significantly to the overall metabolic effects of living a Paleolithic lifestyle – the diet is not sufficient in itself. But eating a lower GL-diet is a laudable dietary goal.

6. Specific functional nutrient deficiencies and metabolic syndrome

6.1 Magnesium

Low intake of magnesium (Mg) can contribute to an increased risk of metabolic syndrome, whereas adequate dietary/supplemental intake is associated with reduced risk (Belin and He 2007). Low dietary Mg is also related to the development of type 2 diabetes, characterised by intracellular and extracellular Mg depletion. Reduced intracellular Mg concentrations result in metabolic changes including impaired post-receptor insulin action and worsening of insulin resistance in diabetic patients. Indeed, Mg deficiency has been proposed as a possible underlying common mechanism of the 'insulin resistance' of different metabolic conditions (Barbagallo and Dominguez 2007).

Studies have shown that daily Mg administration increases intracellular Mg concentrations and contributes to improved insulin-mediated glucose uptake. In hypertensive patients Mg administration may be useful in decreasing arterial blood pressure. The benefits deriving from daily Mg supplementation in diabetic and hypertensive patients are further supported by epidemiological studies showing that high daily Mg intake is predictive of a lower incidence of diabetes and hypertension (Paolisso and Barbagallo 1997).

Levels of Mg appear to be directly associated with insulin sensitivity. Humphries, Kushner and Falkner (1999) showed that the lowest levels of Mg were associated with the highest degrees of insulin resistance. Lefébvre, Paolisso and Scheen (1994) concluded that, 'Insulin secretion requires magnesium: magnesium deficiency results in impaired insulin secretion, while magnesium replacement restores insulin secretion.'

Barbagallo *et al.* (2007) observe that *in vitro* and *in vivo* studies have demonstrated that insulin may modulate the shift of Mg from extracellular to intracellular space. Adequate levels of intracellular Mg concentration are essential for the function of the enzyme pyruvate dehydrogenase and the entry of acetyl-CoA into the Citric Acid Cycle, which is a limiting step for oxidative glucose metabolism. Not surprisingly, Paolisso *et al.* (1992) found that Mg repletion restored oxidative glucose metabolism in hypertensive patients. Mg is also necessary for the efficient function of d6D, and deficiency can limit production of long-chain PUFAs, decrease membrane fluidity, and increase insulin resistance.

While levels significantly higher than the RDA for Mg may be necessary for Mg repletion in individuals with metabolic syndrome, type 2 diabetes or hypertension, a diet rich in food sources of Mg should be a therapeutic goal as well. Nuts, seeds, dark leafy greens and pulses are excellent dietary sources of Mg.

6.2 Chromium

Chromium (Cr) is believed to enhance insulin receptor activity through a reciprocal relationship. Insulin binds to the cellular insulin receptor, which stimulates the movement of Cr into the cell, where it binds to and activates a peptide molecule known as Apo-LMW. Functional low molecular weight Cr then binds to the intracellular portion of the insulin receptor, enhancing its activity in stimulating cellular absorption of glucose and amino acids (Vincent 2000). Cr has also been shown to improve glucose uptake and metabolism through up-regulating the production of mRNA coding for the insulin receptors (IR), glucose transporter 4 (GLUT4), glycogen synthase (GS) and uncoupling protein-3 (UCP3) in skeletal muscle cells – all essential for proper insulin-mediated oxidative glucose utilisation (Qiao *et al.* 2009).

While there is no RDA for Cr intake, the Estimated Safe and Adequate Daily Dietary Intake is 25–200mcg per day. Despite this, most Western diets fail to achieve this modest intake of dietary Cr (Anderson, Bryden and Polansky 1992).

Low-Cr diets adversely affect glucose, insulin and glucagon metabolism (Anderson *et al.* 1991). Urinary Cr excretion is increased by a high GL diet (Anderson *et al.* 1990). Type 2 diabetics have 33 per cent lower serum Cr and excrete twice as much compared to controls (Morris 1999). However, fasting plasma Cr in healthy patients has an inverse relationship with insulin, but not in diabetics, suggesting poor Cr utilisation by diabetics (Diabetes Education 2004), and suggesting the effective clinical dose in diabetics may be well above the safe and adequate dose.

The form of Cr supplementation may affect its usefulness: 200–1000mcg supplementation of Cr picolinate leads to enhanced metabolic action of insulin and a reduction in some risk factors for CVD, especially in obese patients, whereas the threshold of effectiveness for high-Cr yeast appears to be 1000mcg Cr. A supplement of 400mcg Cr via high-Cr yeast caused no change in HbA1c in type 2 diabetics (Kleefstra *et al.* 2007). However, 9g/day high-Cr yeast led to significant decreases in cholesterol, total blood lipids and insulin, and improved glucose and insulin sensitivity in older men (Offenbacher and Pi-Sunyer 1980). Cr picolinate is better absorbed and has produced significant improvements in glycaemic control (Broadhurst and Domenico 2006). A supplement of 500mcg Cr picolinate given twice daily to type 2 diabetics for four months led to reduced fasting and postprandial glucose, HbA1c and fasting insulin (Anderson *et al.* 1997); whereas 100mcg twice daily had no significant benefit. Similarly, Lydic *et al.* (2006) reports that women with PCOS taking 1000mcg/d of Cr picolinate experienced a 38 per cent mean improvement in glucose disposal.

The addition of biotin to Cr may be more effective still. A supplement of 2mg biotin + 600mcg Cr (as picolinate) in type 2 diabetics reduced:

- the area under the glucose curve
- fructosamine (a short-term marker for glycosylation)
- triglycerides
- triglyceride:HDL cholesterol ratio
- atherogenic index of plasma (AIP) = log (plasma concentration of triglycerides:HDL cholesterol)
- LDL:HDL ratio
- postprandial glucose
- HbA1c
- fasting glucose.

In patients with high cholesterol already on statins, significant reductions in total lipids, LDL and VLDL cholesterol and AIP were achieved by adding biotin and Cr (Albarracin *et al.* 2007; Geohas *et al.* 2007).

Nicotinic acid complexes with Cr to form glucose tolerance factor (GTF), which facilitates insulin binding to its receptor. Urberg and Zemel (1987) found that neither 200mcg Cr picolinate nor 100mg nicotinic acid given alone elicited a response in healthy subjects, whereas 200mcg Cr picolinate given with 100mg nicotinic acid led to a 15 per cent decrease in the area under the glucose curve and 7 per cent decrease in fasting glucose, indicating enhanced insulin action.

6.3 Herbal medicines and phytochemicals

Phytochemicals found within numerous plants have been found to affect insulin secretion, binding and action. This is perhaps unsurprising, since insulin itself is a 'response molecule' that coordinates the body's metabolism with the availability of food. Many of these bioactive plants have long been used as herbs and spices in traditional cuisine: cinnamon, cloves, turmeric and bay leaf, for instance, have demonstrated significant insulin-potentiating action *in vitro*, increasing insulin action by more than 300 per cent (Khan *et al.* 1990). An extract of cinnamon increased glucose metabolism by more than 20 times *in vitro* (Anderson *et al.* 2004).

Despite their longstanding and frequent use as spices and herbs, and also in traditional medicine, reliable research is lacking and clinical trials are few and small. Their potential as adjuvant therapy for improving insulin resistance is promising but alterations in diet and exercise should always be considered the first line therapy.

6.3.1 GARLIC AND ONIONS (*ALLIUM* SPECIES)

In a double-blind placebo-controlled trial examining the potential protective effects of garlic (800mg/d) on thrombosis, Keisewetter *et al.* (1991) found not only a complete disappearance of spontaneous thrombocyte formation but also a decrease in blood viscosity, diastolic blood pressure (of 9.5%) and fasting blood glucose (of 11.6%), and an increase in the microcirculation of the skin (of 47.6%) in otherwise healthy individuals.

Onions show some ability to reduce the glycaemic response to an oral glucose challenge. Varying doses of an onion extract, equivalent to 30–300g, were administered prior to glucose tolerance testing, reducing the glycaemic response in a dose-dependent manner (Sharma, Gupta and Gupta 1977). Effects were similar with both raw and boiled onions, suggesting that the active constituents in onion are stable in cooking, unlike the allicin in garlic.

Onions and garlic are common foodstuffs and regular inclusion in the diet could help improve glucose and insulin metabolism.

6.3.2 CINNAMON

Cinnamon is the best studied of the herbal therapies. Sixty type 2 diabetics were assigned to groups to receive variable doses of cinnamon (1, 3 or 6g/d) or placebo for 40 days. After treatment, all three levels of cinnamon reduced the mean fasting serum glucose (18–29%), triglyceride (23–30%), LDL cholesterol (7–27%), and total cholesterol (12–26%) levels, while no significant changes were noted in the placebo group. The benefits of cinnamon were not dose dependent, suggesting that 1–3g/d may be an adequate dose for most diabetics to notice improvement in glucose and lipids (Khan *et al.* 2003). In another trial, 79 diabetics were given the equivalent of 3g/d of cinnamon powder or placebo for four months. The treated group experienced a 10.3 per cent drop in fasting glucose levels, compared to 3.4 per cent in the placebo group. No significant changes were observed in HbA1c or plasma lipids (Mang *et al.* 2006).

6.3.3 BITTER MELON (*MOMORDICA CHARANTIA*)

This has been used in traditional medicine in India and China for centuries as a bitter tonic. Diabetic patients were treated with 100mL/d of the aqueous extract of bitter melon. The hypoglycaemic effects were found by the authors 'to be cumulative and gradual, unlike those of insulin' (Srivastava *et al.* 1993). One trial concluded that 73 per cent of type 2 diabetics showed improved glucose tolerance when given the fresh juice (Welhinda *et al.* 1986).

6.3.4 GURMAR (*GYMNEMA SYLVESTRE*)

This is a climbing vine that has been used in Ayurvedic medicine for hundreds of years. Studies have demonstrated its capacity to stimulate insulin secretion and lower cholesterol and triglyceride levels.

Two non-randomised controlled clinical trials by the same team of researchers looked at both insulin-dependent (Shanmugasundaram *et al.* 1990) and non-insulin-dependent diabetics (Baskaran *et al.* 1990). Both groups showed improved glycaemic control with chronic use of an ethanol extract of *Gymnema*, compared with those who received conventional treatment alone. Insulin requirements for insulin-dependent diabetics came down significantly, and in the non-insulin-dependent diabetics blood glucose and HbA1c decreased significantly. Conventional drug dosage could be decreased in all participants, and five of the 22 patients were able to discontinue their conventional drug therapy all together. Baskaran *et al.* also found evidence of pancreas beta-cell regeneration, which if confirmed could be of significant importance for future therapy.

6.3.5 FENUGREEK (*TRIGONELLA FOENUM-GRAECUM*)

Fenugreek seeds are approximately 50 per cent fibre and 20 per cent mucilaginous fibre. While some of the metabolic effects of fenugreek seed may be due to the fibre content, its high saponin content is also likely to play a significant role. Fenugreek has been shown to reduce fasting and postprandial blood glucose levels in diabetic patients. In one trial, ten type 2 diabetics were given 25g of whole fenugreek every day for ten days. At the end of the intervention period participants displayed a significantly reduced area under the plasma glucose curve and an increased rate of metabolic clearance. Additionally, the number of insulin receptors on red blood cells increased. Thus, fenugreek may exert its hypoglycaemic effect not just by fibre-induced slowing of glucose absorption but also by acting at the insulin receptor level (Raghuram *et al.* 1994). Sharma *et al.* (1996) found that type 2 diabetics fed 25g defatted fenugreek seed powder per day had significant reductions in total, LDL and VLDL cholesterol and triglyceride levels, but this is a very large dose and may not be practical for most patients.

7. Are drugs better?

In a now famous study, 3234 subjects with impaired glucose tolerance (pre-diabetes) were randomly assigned to receive either a placebo, or the blood glucose-lowering drug metformin (850mg twice daily), or a lifestyle-modification programme with the goals of at least a 7 per cent weight loss and at least 150 minutes of physical activity per week. The average follow-up was 2.8 years. The incidence of diabetes was 11, 7.8 and 4.8 cases per 100 person-years in the placebo, metformin and lifestyle groups, respectively. The lifestyle intervention reduced the incidence of diabetes by 58 per cent and metformin by 31 per cent, as compared with placebo. Clearly, the lifestyle intervention was significantly more effective than metformin, a drug with sometimes serious side-effects (Knowler *et al.* 2002). Diet and exercise should always be considered the first-line therapy for metabolic syndrome and an essential component of any treatment protocol that includes blood sugar-controlling prescriptive agents and/or insulin.

8. Summary of prevention and treatment recommendations

Metabolic syndrome may well be the greatest public health challenge of the twenty-first century. In terms of its contribution to obesity, heart disease, hypertension and diabetes, it may be the largest single contributor to loss of healthy lifespan in industrialised countries. However it is critical to remember that even as these problems are of our own making, so too are their solutions.

This chapter has attempted to show both the immediate and the evolutionary causes of the metabolic imbalances that are created from the diet and lifestyle changes characteristic of modern times. What follows are some simple recommendations that the author uses in clinical practice for both the prevention and treatment of metabolic syndrome.

8.1 Dr Culp's rules for healthy living

1. Eat less – in general, no more than 2500 calories/day.

2. Exercise daily – brisk walking is fine, but it needs to be a daily occurrence and needs to last at least 20 minutes.

3. Take your time to eat – the same meal eaten slower produces a lower glycaemic response and less insulin secretion.

4. Vegetables, pulses and whole fruits are essential to a healthy diet – apart from potatoes, they all have a lower GL than any grain. Allow yourself an occasional serving of potatoes.

5. Eat more fish – one serving a day is ideal – especially fatty, sustainable fish like salmon, trout, mackerel or herring.

6. Eat at least one serving of a pulse each day – common beans, lentils, split peas and hummus, for example, are extremely low GL, filling, and promote healthy intestinal bacteria.

7. Limit grains to one serving per meal or less (for example, 150g of cooked grain or one slice of bread). All grains have a relatively high GL. Diets without any grain consumption typically have the lowest GL.

8. Use whole fruit as your typical dessert – avoid dried fruit and fruit juice – they are too concentrated a source of sugar, especially fructose – it takes a long time and a lot of effort to eat five apples, but only seconds to drink the juice of five apples.

9. Reduce the consumption of domesticated red meat and poultry to no more than one serving per day.

10. Drink 1–2 glasses of wine every day (preferably red) – beer is OK occasionally – but no more than 1–2 alcoholic drinks per day – moderation is key.

11. Drink more water – most people should drink 1–2 litres per day.

12. Avoid milk – it is high in sugar (lactose).

13. Use olive oil as your main added fat – avoid the excessive use of high omega-6 vegetable oils.

14. Eat nuts and seeds in small amounts daily – all nuts are healthy but the walnut is higher in omega-3 fats.

15. And finally: enjoy life, share your food and laugh often.

References

Albanes, D., Jones, D.Y., Schatzkin, A., Micozzi, M.S. and Taylor, P.R. (1988) 'Adult stature and risk of cancer.' *Cancer Research 48*, 6, 1658–1662.

Albarracin, C., Fuqua, B., Geohas, J., Juturu, V., Finch, M.R. and Komorowski, J.R. (2007) 'Combination of chromium and biotin improves coronary risk factors in hypercholesterolemic type 2 diabetes mellitus: A placebo-controlled, double-blind randomized clinical trial.' *Journal of the Cardiometabolic Syndrome 2*, 2, 91–97.

Allison, D.B., Gadbury, G., Schwartz, L.G., Murugesan, R. *et al.* 2003) 'A novel soy-based meal replacement formula for weight loss among obese individuals: A randomized controlled clinical trial.' *European Journal of Clinical Nutrition 57*, 4, 514–522.

Anderson, E.J., Lustig, M.E., Boyle, K.E., Woodlief, T.L. *et al.* (2009) 'Mitochondrial H2O2 emission and cellular redox state link excess fat intake to insulin resistance in both rodents and humans.' *Journal of Clinical Investigation* 2009 Feb 2. pii: 37048. doi:10.1172/JCI37048. [Epub ahead of print]

Anderson, E.J., Yamazaki, H. and Neufer, P.D. (2007) 'Induction of endogenous uncoupling protein 3 suppresses mitochondrial oxidant emission during fatty acid-supported respiration.' *Journal of Biology and Chemistry 282*, 31257–31266.

Anderson, R.A. (1995) 'Chromium, glucose tolerance, diabetes, and lipid metabolism.' *Journal of Advances in Medicine 8*, 37–50.

Anderson, R.A., Broadhurst, C.L., Polansky, M.M., Schmidt, W.F. *et al.* (2004) 'Isolation and characterization of polyphenol type-A polymers from cinnamon with insulin-like biological activity.' *Journal of Agricultural and Food Chemistry 52*, 1, 65–70.

Anderson, R.A., Bryden, N.A., Polansky, M.M. and Reiser, S. (1990) 'Urinary chromium excretion and insulinogenic properties of carbohydrates.' *American Journal of Clinical Nutrition 51*, 5, 864–868.

Anderson, R.A., Bryden, N.A. and Polansky, M.M. (1992) 'Dietary chromium intake. Freely chosen diets, institutional diet, and individual foods.' *Biological Trace Element Research 32*, 117–121.

Anderson, R.A., Cheng, N., Bryden, N.A., Polansky, M.M. *et al.* (1997) 'Elevated intakes of supplemental chromium improve glucose and insulin variables in individuals with type 2 diabetes.' *Diabetes 46*, 11,1786–1791.

Anderson, R.A., Polansky, M.M., Bryden, N.A. and Canary, J.J. (1991) 'Supplemental-chromium effects on glucose, insulin, glucagon, and urinary chromium losses in subjects consuming controlled low-chromium diets.' *American Journal of Clinical Nutrition 54*, 5, 909–916.

Andersson, A., Sjödin, A., Olsson, R. and Vessby, B. (1998) 'Effects of physical exercise on phospholipid fatty acid composition in skeletal muscle.' *American Journal of Physiology 274*, 3, part 1, E432–38.

Appel, L.J., Moore, T.J., Obarzanek, E., Vollmer, W.M. *et al.* (1997) 'A clinical trial of the effects of dietary patterns on blood pressure. DASH Collaborative Research Group.' *New England Journal of Medicine 336*, 16, 1117–1124.

Argmann, C. and Auwerx J. (2006) 'Insulin secretion: SIRT4 gets in on the act.' *Cell 126*, 5, 837–839.

Assumpcao, C.R., Brunini, T.M.C., Matsuura, C., Resende, A.C. and Mendes-Riberio, A.C. (2008) 'Impact of the L-arginine-nitric oxide pathway and oxidative stress on the pathogenesis of the metabolic syndrome.' *Open Biochemistry Journal 2*,108–115.

Attia, N., Tamborlane, W.V., Heptulla, R., Maggs, D. *et al.* (1998) 'The metabolic syndrome and insulin-like growth factor I regulation in adolescent obesity.' *Journal of Clinical Endocrinology and Metabolism 83*, 5, 1467–1471.

Ballor, D.L. and Poehlman, E.T. (1994) 'Exercise-training enhances fat-free mass preservation during diet-induced weight loss: A meta-analytical finding.' *International Journal of Obesity and Related Metabolic Disorders 18*, 1, 35–40.

Bantle, J.P., Raatz, S.K., Thomas, W. and Georgopoulos, A. (2000) 'Effects of dietary fructose on plasma lipids in healthy subjects.' *American Journal of Clinical Nutrition 72*, 1128–1134.

Barbagallo, M. and Dominguez, L.J. (2007) 'Magnesium metabolism in type 2 diabetes mellitus, metabolic syndrome and insulin resistance.' *Archives of Biochemistry and Biophysics 458*, 40–47.

Barbagallo, M., Dominguez, L.J., Galioto, A., Ferlisi, A. *et al.* (2007) 'Role of magnesium in insulin action, diabetes and cardio-metabolic syndrome X.' *Molecular Aspects of Medicine 24*, 1–3, 39–52.

Baroni, S.S., Amelio, M., Sangiorgo, Z., Gaddi, A. and Battino, M. (1999) 'Solid monounsaturated diet lowers LDL unsaturation trait and oxidisability in hypercholesterolemic (type IIb) patients.' *Free Radical Research 30*, 275–285.

Baskaran, K., Ahamath, B.K., Shanmugasundaram, K.R. and Shanmugasundaram, E.R.B. (1990) 'Antidiabetic effect of a leaf extract from Gymnema sylvestre in non-insulin dependent diabetes mellitus patients.' *Journal of Ethnopharmacology 30*, 295–305.

Baur, J.A., Pearson, K.J., Price, N.L., Jamieson, H.A. *et al.* (2006) 'Resveratrol improves health and survival of mice on a high-calorie diet.' *Nature 444*, 7117, 337–342.

Bebakar, W.M., Honour, J.W., Foster, D., Liu, Y.L. and Jacobs, H.S. (1990) 'Regulation of testicular function by insulin and transforming growth factor-beta.' *Steroids 55*, 6, 266–70.

Beck-Nielsen, H., Pedersen, O. and Lindskov, H.O. (1980) 'Impaired cellular insulin binding and insulin sensitivity induced by high-fructose feeding in normal subjects.' *American Journal of Clinical Nutrition 33*, 273–278.

Belin, R.J. and He, K. (2007) 'Magnesium physiology and pathogenic mechanisms that contribute to the development of the metabolic syndrome.' *Magnesium Research 20*, 107–129.

Boden, G. and Shulman, G.I. (2002) 'Free fatty acids in obesity and type 2 diabetes: Defining their role in the development of insulin resistance and beta-cell dysfunction.' *European Journal of Clinical Investigation 32*, 14–23.

Borkman, M., Storlien, L.H., Pan, D.A., Jenkins, A.B., Chisholm, D.J. and Campbell, L.V. (1993) 'The relation between insulin sensitivity and the fatty-acid composition of skeletal-muscle phospholipids.' *New England Journal of Medicine 328*, 4, 238–244.

Bougle, D., Vaghefi-Vaezzadeh, N., Roland, N., Bouvard, G. *et al.* (2002) 'Influence of short-chain fatty acids on iron absorption by proximal colon.' *Scandinavian Journal of Gastroenterology 37*, 9, 1008–1011.

Broadhurst, C.L. and Domenico, P. (2006) 'Clinical studies on chromium picolinate supplementation in diabetes mellitus – a review.' *Diabetes Technology and Therapeutics 6*, 677–687.

Bueld, J.E., Bannenberg, G. and Netter, K.J. (1996) 'Effects of propionic acid and pravastatin on HMG-CoA reductase activity in relation to forestomach lesions in the rat.' *Pharmacology and Toxicology 78*, 4, 229–234.

Cara, J.F. (1994) 'Insulin-like growth factors, insulin-like growth factor binding proteins and ovarian androgen production.' *Hormone Research 42*, 1–2, 49–54.

Civitarese, A.E., Carling, S., Heilbronn, L.K., Hulver, M.H. et al. (2007) 'Calorie restriction increases muscle mitochondrial biogenesis in healthy humans.' *PLoS Medicine 4*, 3, e76.

Clark, D.O. (1997) 'Physical activity efficacy and effectiveness among older adults and minorities.' *Diabetes Care 20*, 1176–1182.

Cleave, T.L. (1974) *The Saccharine Disease.* Bristol: John Wright and Sons.

Cordain, L., Eades, M.R. and Eades, M.D. (2003) 'Hyperinsulinemic diseases of civilization: More than just Syndrome X.' *Comparative Biochemistry and Physiology Part A 136*, 95–112.

Crawford, M.A., Gale, M.M., Woodford, M.H. and Casped N.M. (1970) 'Comparative studies on fatty acid composition of wild and domestic meats.' *International Journal of Biochemistry 1*, 3, 295–300.

Crovetti, R., Porrini, M., Santangelo, A. and Testolin, G. (1998) 'The influence of thermic effect of food on satiety.' *European Journal of Clinical Nutrition 52*, 7, 482–488.

Das, U.N. (1995) 'Essential fatty acid metabolism in patients with essential hypertension, diabetes mellitus and coronary heart disease.' *Prostaglandins, Leukotrienes and Essential Fatty Acids 52*, 6, 387–391.

Dauncey, M.J. and Bingham, S.A. (1983) 'Dependence of 24 h energy expenditure in man on the composition of the nutrient intake.' *British Journal of Nutrition 50*, 1–13.

de Koning, L., Merchant, A.T., Pogue, J., Anand, S.S. et al. (2007) 'Waist circumference and waist-to-hip ratio as predictors of cardiovascular events: Meta-regression analysis of prospective studies.' *European Heart Journal 28*, 7, 850–56.

Del Prato, S., Leonetti, F., Simonson, D.C., Sheehan P., Matsuda, M. and DeFronzo R.A. (1994) 'Effect of sustained physiologic hyperinsulinaemia, and hyperglycaemia on insulin sensitivity and insulin secretion in man.' *Diabetologia 37*, 1025–1035.

Despres, J-P., Lamarche, B., Mauriege, P., Cantin, B. *et al.* (1996) 'Hyperinsulinemia as an independent risk factor for ischemic heart disease.' *New England Journal of Medicine 334*, 952–957.

Diabetes Education (2004) 'A scientific review: The role of chromium in insulin resistance.' *Diabetes Education* suppl. 2–14. No authors listed.

Elliott, P.J. and Jirousek, M. (2008) 'Sirtuins: Novel targets for metabolic disease.' *Current Opinion in Investigational Drugs 9*, 4, 371–378.

Esposito, K., Marfella, R., Ciotola, M., Di Palo, C. *et al.* (2004) 'Effect of a Mediterranean style diet on endothelial dysfunction and markers of vascular inflammation in the metabolic syndrome: A randomized trial.' *Journal of the American Medical Association 292*, 1440–1446.

Flores-Riveros, J.R., McLenithan, J.C., Ezaki, O. and Lane, M.D. (1993) 'Insulin down-regulates expression of the insulin-responsive glucose transporter (GLUT4) gene: Effects on transcription and mRNA turnover.' *Proceedings of the National Academy of Sciences USA 90*, 2, 512–516.

Folsom, A.R., Kushi, L.H., Anderson, K.E., Mink, P.J. *et al.* (2000) 'Associations of general and abdominal obesity with multiple health outcomes in older women: The Iowa Women's Health Study.' *Archives of Internal Medicine 160*, 14, 2117–2128.

Foster-Powell, K. and Miller, J.B. (1995) 'International tables of glycaemic index.' *American Journal of Clinical Nutrition 62*, 871S–890S.

Foster-Powell, K., Holt, S.H.A. and Brand-Miller, J.B. (2002) 'International tables of glycaemic index and glycaemic load values: 2002.' *American Journal of Clinical Nutrition 76*, 5–56.

Frost, G., Leeds, A., Trew, G., Margara, R. and Dornhorst, A. (1998) 'Insulin sensitivity in women at risk of coronary heart disease and the effect of a low glycemic diet.' *Metabolism 47*, 1245–1251.

Fung, T.T., Rexrode, K.M., Mantzoros, C.S., Manson, J.E., Willett, W.C. and Hu, F.B. (2009) 'Mediterranean diet and incidence of and mortality from coronary heart disease and stroke in women.' *Circulation 119*, 8, 1093–1100.

Gaesser, G.A. (1999) 'Thinness and weight loss: Beneficial or detrimental to longevity?' *Medicine and Science in Sports and Exercise 31*, 8, 1118–1128.

Geohas, J., Daly, A., Juturu, V., Finch, M. and Komorowski, J.R. (2007) 'Chromium picolinate and biotin combination reduces atherogenic index of plasma in patients with type 2 diabetes mellitus: A placebo-controlled, double-blinded, randomized clinical trial.' *American Journal of the Medical Sciences 333*, 3, 145–153.

Hallfrisch, J., Reiser, S. and Prather, E.S. (1983) 'Blood lipid distribution of hyperinsulinemic men consuming three levels of fructose.' *American Journal of Clinical Nutrition 37*, 740–748.

Himsworth, H.P. (1936) 'Diabetes mellitus: Its differentiation into insulin-sensitive and insulin insensitive types.' *Lancet 1*, 117–121.

Horrobin, D.F. (1988) 'The roles of essential fatty acids in the development of diabetic neuropathy and other complications of diabetes mellitus.' *Prostaglandins, Leukotrienes and Essential Fatty Acids 31*, 3, 181–197.

Horrobin, D.F. (1997) 'The use of gamma-linolenic acid in diabetic neuropathy.' *Agents and Actions Supplements 37*, 120–144.

Horrobin, D.F., Ells, K.M., Morse-Fisher, N. and Manku, M.S. (1991) 'The effects of evening primrose oil, safflower oil and paraffin on plasma fatty acid levels in humans: Choice of an appropriate placebo for clinical studies on primrose oil.' *Prostaglandins, Leukotrienes and Essential Fatty Acids 42*, 4, 245–249.

Houstis, N., Rosen, E.D. and Lander, E.S. (2006) 'Reactive oxygen species have a causal role in multiple forms of insulin resistance.' *Nature 440*, 944–948.

Hsueh, W.C., Mitchell, B.D., Aburomia, R., Pollin, T. *et al.* (2000) 'Diabetes in the Old Order Amish: Characterization and heritability analysis of the Amish Family Diabetes Study.' *Diabetes Care 23*, 595–601.

Humphries, S., Kushner, H. and Falkner, B. (1999) 'Low dietary magnesium is associated with insulin resistance in a sample of young, nondiabetic Black Americans.' *American Journal of Hypertension 12*, 8/1, 747–756.

Jenkins, D.J., Wolever, T.M., Ocana, A.M., Vuksan, V. *et al.* (1990) 'Metabolic effects of reducing rate of glucose ingestion by single bolus versus continuous sipping.' *Diabetes 39*, 775–781.

Johannsen, D.L., Redman, L.M. and Ravussin, E. (2007) 'The role of physical activity in maintaining a reduced weight.' *Current Atherosclerosis Reports 9*, 6, 463–471.

Kahana, M., Grossman, E., Feinstein, A., Ronnen, M., Cohen, M. and Millet, M.S. (1987) 'Skin tags: A cutaneous marker for diabetes mellitus.' *Acta Dermato-Venereologica 67*, 2, 175–177.

Katagiri, H., Yamada, T. and Oka, Y. (2007) 'Adiposity and cardiovascular disorders: Disturbance of the regulatory system consisting of humoral and neuronal signals.' *Circulation Research 6*, 101, 1, 27–39.

Keisewetter, H., Jung, F., Pindur, G., Jung, E.M., Mrowietz, C. and Wenzel, E. (1991) 'Effect of garlic on thrombocyte aggregation, microcirculation, and other risk factors.' *International Journal of Clinical Pharmacology, Therapy, and Toxicology 29*, 151–155.

Khan, A., Bryden, N.A., Polansky, M.M. and Anderson, R.A. (1990) 'Insulin potentiating factor and chromium content of selected foods and spices.' *Biological Trace Element Research 24*, 3, 183–188.

Khan, A., Safdar, M., Ali Khan, M.M., Khattak, K.N. and Anderson, R.A. (2003) 'Cinnamon improves glucose and lipids of people with type 2 diabetes.' *Diabetes Care 26*, 12, 3215–3218.

Kleefstra, N., Houweling, S.T., Bakker, S.J., Verhoeven, S. *et al.* (2007) 'Chromium treatment has no effect in patients with type 2 diabetes in a Western population: A randomized, double-blind, placebo-controlled trial.' *Diabetes Care 30*, 5, 1092–1096.

Knowler, W.C., Barrett-Connor, E., Fowler, S.E., Hamman, R.F. *et al.* (2002) 'Reduction in the incidence of type II diabetes with lifestyle intervention or metformin.' *New England Journal of Medicine 346*, 393–403.

Koo, M.M., Rohan, T.E., Jain, M., McLaughlin, J.R. and Corey, P.N. (2002) 'A cohort study of dietary fibre intake and menarche.' *Public Health and Nutrition 5*, 2, 353–360.

Lairon, D. (2007) 'Intervention studies on Mediterranean diet and cardiovascular risk.' *Molecular Nutrition and Food Research 51*, 10, 1209–1214.

Lakka, H.M., Laaksonen, D.E., Lakka, T.A., Niskanen, L.K. *et al.* (2002) 'The metabolic syndrome and total and cardiovascular disease mortality in middle-aged men.' *Journal of the American Medical Association 288*, 21, 2709–2716.

Landin, K., Holm, G., Tengborn, L. and Smith, U. (1992) 'Guar gum improves insulin sensitivity, blood lipids, blood pressure, and fibrinolysis in healthy men.' *American Journal of Clinical Nutrition 56*, 6, 1061–1065.

Lefébvre, P.J., Paolisso, G. and Scheen, A.J. (1994) '[Magnesium and glucose metabolism].' *Therapie 49*, 1, 1–7. Article in French.

Leighton, F., Cuevas, A., Guasch, V., Pérez, D.D. *et al.* (1999) 'Plasma polyphenols and antioxidants, oxidative DNA damage, and endothelial function in a diet and wine intervention study in humans.' *Drugs and Experimental Clinical Research 25*, 133–141.

Liljeberg, H.G., Akerberg, A.K. and Bjorck, I.M. (1999) 'Effect of the glycemic index and content of indigestible carbohydrates of cereal-based breakfast meals on glucose tolerance at lunch in healthy subjects.' *American Journal of Clinical Nutrition 69*, 647–655.

Liu, L., Wang, Y., Lam, K.S. and Xu, A. (2008) 'Moderate wine consumption in the prevention of metabolic syndrome and its related medical complications.' *Endocrine, Metabolic and Immune Disorders Drug Targets* 8, 2, 89–98.

Liu, S., Willett, W.C., Stampfer, M.J., Hu, F.B. *et al.* (2000) 'A prospective study of dietary glycemic load, carbohydrate intake, and risk of coronary heart disease in US women.' *American Journal of Clinical Nutrition 71*, 1455–1461.

Ludwig, D.S. (2002) 'The glycemic index: Physiological mechanisms relating to obesity, diabetes, and cardiovascular disease.' *Journal of the American Medical Association 287*, 2414–2423.

Lydic, M.L., McNurlan, M., Bembo, S., Mitchell, L., Komaroff, E. and Gelato, M. (2006) 'Chromium picolinate improves insulin sensitivity in obese subjects with polycystic ovary syndrome.' *Fertility and Sterility 86*, 1, 243–246.

MacLean, P.S., Zheng, D., Jones, J.P., Olson, A.L. and Dohm, G.L. (2002) 'Exercise-induced transcription of the muscle glucose transporter (GLUT 4) gene.' *Biochemical and Biophysical Research Communications 292*, 409–414.

Madigan, C., Ryan, M., Owens, D., Collins, P. *et al.* (2000) 'Dietary unsaturated fatty acids in type 2 diabetes: Higher levels of postprandial lipoprotein on a linoleic acid-rich sunflower oil diet compared with an oleic acid-rich olive oil diet.' *Diabetes Care 23*, 1472–1477.

Malina, R.M. (1990) 'Research in secular trends in auxology.' *Anthropologischer Anzeiger 48*, 3, 209–227.

Mang, B., Wolters, M., Schmitt, B., Kelb, K. *et al.* (2006) 'Effects of a cinnamon extract on plasma glucose, HbA, and serum lipids in diabetes mellitus type 2.' *European Journal of Clinical Investigation 36*, 5, 340–344.

Mann, N.J., Johnson, L.G., Warrick, G.E. and Sinclair, A.J. (1995) 'The arachidonic acid content of the Australian diet is lower than previously estimated.' *Journal of Nutrition 125*, 10, 2528–2535.

Mayes, P.A. (1993) 'Intermediary metabolism of fructose.' *American Journal of Clinical Nutrition 58*, 754S–765S.

McCay, C.M. and Crowell, M.F. (1934) 'Prolonging the Life Span.' *The Scientific Monthly 39*, 5, 405–414.

McClain, P.A. (2002) 'Hexosamines as mediators of nutrient sensing and regulation in diabetes.' *Journal of Diabetes Complications 16*, 72–80.

McGee, H. (2004) *On Food and Cooking: An Encyclopedia of Kitchen Science, History, and Culture.* London: Hodder and Stoughton.

McKeigue, P.M., Shah, B. and Marmot, M.G. (1991) 'Relation of central obesity and insulin resistance with high diabetes prevalence and cardiovascular risk in South Asians.' *Lancet 16*, 337, 8738, 382–6.

McManus, K., Antinoro, L. and Sacks, F. (2001) 'A randomized controlled trial of a moderate-fat, low-energy diet compared with a low-fat, low-energy diet for weight loss in overweight adults.' *International Journal of Obesity and Related Metabolic Disorders 25*, 1503–1511.

Miller, J.C. (1994) 'Importance of glycaemic index in diabetes.' *American Journal of Clinical Nutrition 59*, 747S–752S.

Mittendorfer, B. and Sidossis, L.S. (2001) 'Mechanism for the increase in plasma triacylglycerol concentrations after consumption of short-term, high-carbohydrate diets.' *American Journal of Clinical Nutrition 73*, 892–899.

Morris, B.W., MacNeil, S., Hardisty, C.A., Heller, S., Burgin, C. and Gray, T.A. (1999) 'Chromium homeostasis in patients with type II (NIDDM) diabetes.' *Journal of Trace Elements in Medicine and Biology 13*, 1–2, 57–61.

Offenbacher, E.G. and Pi-Sunyer, F.X. (1980) 'Beneficial effect of chromium-rich yeast on glucose tolerance and blood lipids in elderly patients.' *Diabetes 29*, 919–925.

Orozco, L.J., Buchleitner, A.M., Gimenez-Perez, G., Roqué, I. *et al.* (2008) 'Exercise or exercise and diet for preventing type 2 diabetes mellitus.' *Cochrane Database Systematic Review 16*, 3, 1–46.

Pamuk, E.R., Williamson, D.F., Madans, J., Serdula, M.K., Kleinman, J.C. and Byers, T. (1992) 'Weight loss and mortality in a national cohort of adults, 1971–1987.' *American Journal of Epidemiology 136*, 6, 686–697.

Pan, D.A., Lillioja, S., Milner, M.R., Kriketos, A.D. *et al.* (1995) 'Skeletal muscle membrane lipid composition is related to adiposity and insulin action.' *Journal of Clinical Investigation 96*, 6, 2802–2808.

Paolisso, G. and Barbagallo, M. (1997) 'Hypertension, diabetes mellitus, and insulin resistance: The role of intracellular magnesium.' *American Journal of Hypertension 10*, 346–355.

Paolisso, G., Di Maro, G., Cozzolino, D., Salvatore, T. *et al.* (1992) 'Chronic magnesium administration enhances oxidative glucose metabolism in thiazide treated hypertensive patients.' *American Journal of Hypertension 5*, 10, 681–686.

Park, Y.K. and Yetley, E.A. (1993) 'Intake and food sources of fructose in the United States.' *American Journal of Clinical Nutrition 58*, 737S–747S.

Parr, T. (1997) 'Insulin exposure and aging theory.' *Gerontology 43*, 3, 182–200.

Pereira, M.A., Jacobs, D.R. Jr., Pins, J.J., Raatz, S.K. *et al.* (2002) 'Effect of whole grains on insulin sensitivity in overweight hyperinsulinemic adults.' *American Journal of Clinical Nutrition 75*, 846–855.

Piatti, P.M., Monti, F., Fermo, I., Baruffaldi, L. *et al.* (1994) 'Hypocaloric high-protein diet improves glucose oxidation and spares lean body mass: comparison to hypocaloric high-carbohydrate diet.' *Metabolism 43*, 12, 1481–1487.

Pischon, T., Boeing, H., Hoffmann, K., Bergmann, M. *et al.* (2008) 'General and abdominal adiposity and risk of death in Europe.' *New England Journal of Medicine 359*, 20, 2105–2120.

Pryer, J.A., Nichols, R., Elliott, P., Thakrar, B., Brunner, E. and Marmot, M. (2001) 'Dietary patterns among a national random sample of British adults.' *Journal of Epidemiology and Community Health 55*, 1, 29–37.

Qiao, W., Peng, Z., Wang, Z., Wei, J. and Zhou, A. (2009) 'Chromium improves glucose uptake and metabolism through upregulating the mRNA levels of IR, GLUT4, GS, and UCP3 in skeletal muscle cells.' *Biological Trace Element Research*, 13 March.

Raghuram, T.C., Sharma, R.D., Sivakumar, B. and Sahay, B.K. (1994) 'Effect of fenugreek seeds on intravenous glucose disposition in non-insulin dependent diabetic patients.' *Phytotherapy Research 8*, 2, 83–86.

Reaven, G.M. (1988) 'Role of insulin in human disease.' *Diabetes 37*, 1595–1607.

Reiser, S., Powell, A.S., Scholfield, D.J., Panda, P., Fields, M. and Canary, J.J. (1989) 'Day-long insulin, glucose and fructose responses of hyperinsulinaemic and non-hyperinsulinaemic men adapted to diets containing either fructose or high amylase cornstarch.' *American Journal of Clinical Nutrition 50*, 1008–1014.

Reiser, S., Powell, A.S., Yang, C.Y. and Canary, J.J. (1987) 'An insulinogenic effect of oral fructose in humans during postprandial hyperglycemia.' *American Journal of Clinical Nutrition 45*, 580–587.

Ros, E., Nunez, I., Perez-Heras, A., Serra, M. *et al.* (2004) 'A walnut diet improved endothelial function in hypercholesterolemic subjects: A randomized crossover trial.' *Circulation 109*, 1609–1614.

Ruano, J., López-Miranda, J., de la Torre, R., Delgado-Lista, J. *et al.* (2007) 'Intake of phenol-rich virgin olive oil improves the postprandial prothrombotic profile in hypercholesterolemic patients.' *American Journal of Clinical Nutrition 86*, 2, 341–346.

Ryan, M., McInerney, D., Owens, D., Collins, P. *et al.* (2000) 'Diabetes and the Mediteranean diet: A beneficial effect of oleic acid on insulin sensitivity, adipocyte glucose transport, and endothelium-dependent vasoreactivity.' *Quarterly Journal of Medicine 93*, 85–91.

Salas-Salvadó, J., Fernández-Ballart, J., Ros, E., Martínez-González, M.A. *et al.* (2008) 'Effect of a Mediterranean diet supplemented with nuts on metabolic syndrome status: one-year results of the PREDIMED randomized trial.' *Archives of Internal Medicine 168*, 22, 2449–2458.

Sarkkinen, E., Schwab, U., Niskanen, L., Hannuksela, M. *et al.* (1996) 'The effects of monounsaturated-fat enriched diet and polyunsaturated-fat enriched diet on lipid and glucose metabolism in subjects with impaired glucose tolerance.' *European Journal of Clinical Nutrition 50*, 9, 592–598.

Schafer, F.Q. and Buettner, G.R. (2001) 'Redox environment of the cell as viewed through the redox state of the glutathione disulfide/glutathione couple.' *Free Radical Biology in Medicine 30*, 1191–1212.

Serra-Majem, L., Roman, B. and Estruch, R. (2006) 'Scientific evidence of interventions using the Mediterranean diet: a systematic review.' *Nutrition Reviews 64*, 2, S27–S47.

Shanmugasundaram, E.R.B., Rajeswari, G., Baskaran, K., Kumar, B.R.R., Shanmugasundaram, K.R. and Ahmath, B.K. (1990) 'Use of Gymnema sylvestre leaf extract in the control of blood glucose in insulin-dependent diabetes mellitus.' *Journal of Ethnopharmacology 30*, 281–294.

Sharma, K.K., Gupta, R.K., and Gupta S. (1977) 'Antihyperglycemic effect of onion: Effect on fasting blood sugar and induced hyperglycemia in man.' *Indian Journal of Medical Research 65*, 422–429.

Sharma, R.D., Sarkar, A., Hazra, D.K., Misra, B. *et al.* (1996) 'Hypolipidaemic effect of fenugreek seeds: A chronic study in non-insulin dependent diabetic patients.' *Phytotherapy Research 10*, 4, 332–334.

Shi, T., Wang, F., Stieren, E. and Tong, Q. (2005) 'SIRT3, a mitochondrial sirtuin deacetylase, regulates mitochondrial function and thermogenesis in brown adipocytes.' *Journal of Biological Chemistry 280*, 14, 13560–13567.

Srivastava, Y., Venkatakrishna-Bhatt, H., Verma, Y., Venkaiah, K. and Raval, B.H. (1993) 'Antidiabetic and adaptogenic properties of Momordica charantia extract: An experimental and clinical evaluation.' *Phytotherapy Research 7*, 4, 285–289.

Stahl, M. and Berger, W. (1990) '[Comparison of guar gum, wheat bran and placebo on carbohydrate and lipid metabolism in type II diabetics].' *Schweizerische medizinische Wochenschrift 120*, 12, 402–408. Article in German.

Storlien, L.H., Jenkins, A.B., Chisholm, D.J., Pascoe, W.S., Khouri, S. and Kraegen, E.W. (1991) 'Influence of dietary fat composition on development of insulin resistance in rats. Relationship to muscle triglyceride and omega-3 fatty acids in muscle phospholipid.' *Diabetes 40*, 2, 280–289.

Storlien, L.H., Pan, D.A., Kriketos, A.D., O'Connor, J. *et al.* (1996) 'Skeletal muscle membrane lipids and insulin resistance.' *Lipids 31*, suppl., S261–S265.

Stout, R.W. (1990) 'Insulin and atheroma.' *Diabetes Care 13*, 631–654.

Su, H.C. and Hung, L.M. (2006) 'Resveratrol possesses an insulin-like effect in diabetic rats.' *American Journal of Physiology – Endocrinology and Metabolism 290*, 6, E1339–1346.

Swinburn, B.A. (1993) 'Effect of dietary lipid on insulin action. Clinical studies.' *Annals of the New York Academy of Sciences 683*, 102–109.

Tagliaferro, V., Cassader, M., Bozzo, C., Pisu, E. *et al.* (1985) 'Moderate guar-gum addition to usual diet improves peripheral sensitivity to insulin and lipaemic profile in NIDDM.' *Diabète e Métabolisme 11*, 6, 380–385.

Tanner, J.M. (1973) 'Trend towards earlier menarche in London, Olso, Copenhagen, the Netherlands and Hungary.' *Nature 243*, 5402, 95–96.

Tebbey, P.W., McGowan, K.M., Stephens, J.M., Buttke, T.M. and Pekala, P.H. (1994) 'Arachidonic acid down-regulates the insulin-dependent glucose transporter gene (GLUT4) in 3T3-L1 adipocytes by inhibiting transcription and enhancing mRNA turnover.' *Journal of Biology and Chemistry 269*, 1, 639–644.

Thappa, D.M. (1995) 'Skin tags as markers of diabetes mellitus: An epidemiological study in India.' *Journal of Dermatology 22*, 10, 729–731.

Thiboutot, D.M. (1996) 'An overview of acne and its treatment.' *Cutis 57*, 1 suppl., 8–12.

Thresher, J.S., Podolin, D.A., Wei, Y., Mazzeo, R.S. and Pagliassotti, M.J. (2000) 'Comparison of the effects of sucrose and fructose on insulin action and glucose tolerance.' *American Journal of Physiology – Regulatory, Integrative and Comparative Physiology 279*, 4, R1334–1340.

United States Department of Agriculture (1997) *Results from USDA 1994–96 Continuing Survey of Food Intakes by Individuals.* Available at www.ers.usda.gov/AmberWaves/November05/Findings/USFoodConsumption.htm, accessed on 10 February 2010.

United States Department of Agriculture, Economic Research Service (2002) *Food Consumption (per capita) Data System, Sugars/Sweeteners.* Washington, DC: USDA.

Urberg, M. and Zemel, M.B. (1987) 'Evidence for synergism between chromium and nicotinic acid in the control of glucose tolerance in elderly humans.' *Metabolism 36*, 9, 896–899.

USDA Food Composition (2009) *USDA National Nutrient Database.* Available at www.nal.usda.gov/fnic/foodcomp/search/, accessed on 5 November 2009.

Vincent, J.B. (2000) 'Quest for the molecular mechanism of chromium action and its relationship to diabetes.' *Nutrition Reviews 58*, 67–72.

Walker, K.Z., O'Dea, K., Johnson, L., Sinclair, A.J. *et al.* (1996) 'Body fat distribution and non-insulin-dependent diabetes: comparison of a fiber-rich, high-carbohydrate, low-fat (23%) diet and a 35% fat diet high in monounsaturated fat.' *American Journal of Clinical Nutrition 63*, 2, 254–260.

Welhinda, J., Karunanayake, E.H., Sheriff, M.H.R. and Jayasinghe, K.S.A. (1986) 'Effect of Momordica charantia on the glucose tolerance in maturity onset diabetes.' *Journal of Ethnopharmacology 17*, 277–282.

Wellen, K.E. and Hotamisligil, G.S. (2005) 'Inflammation, stress, and diabetes.' *Journal of Clinical Investigation 115*, 5, 1111–1119.

Willett, W.C., Sacks, F., Trichopoulou, A., Drescher, G. *et al.* (1995) 'Mediterranean diet pyramid: A cultural model for healthy eating.' *American Journal of Clinical Nutrition 6*, 6 suppl., 1402S–1406S.

Winter, Y., Rohrmann, S., Linseisen, J., Lanczik, O. *et al.* (2008) 'Contribution of obesity and abdominal fat mass to risk of stroke and transient ischemic attacks.' *Stroke 39*, 3145–3151.

Wolever, T.M. and Jenkins, D.J. (1986) 'The use of glycaemic index in predicting the blood glucose response to mixed meals.' *American Journal of Clinical Nutrition 43*, 167–172.

Yun A.J. and Doux J.D. (2007) 'Unhappy meal: How our need to detect stress may have shaped our preferences for taste.' *Medical Hypotheses 69*, 4, 746–751.

Yun, A.J., Lee, P.Y., Doux, J.D. (2006) 'Are we eating more than we think? Illegitimate signaling and xenohormesis as participants in the pathogenesis of obesity.' *Medical Hypotheses 67*, 1, 36–40.

Yusuf, S., Hawken, S., Ounpuu, S., Bautista, L. *et al.* (2005) 'Obesity and the risk of myocardial infarction in 27,000 participants from 52 countries: A case-control study.' *Lancet 366*, 1640–1649.

Zambon, D., Sabate, J., Munoz, S., Campero, B. *et al.* (2000) 'Substituting walnuts for monounsaturated fat improves the serum lipid profile of hypercholesterolemic men and women. A randomized crossover trial.' *Annals of Internal Medicine 132*, 538–546.

Zammit, V.A., Waterman, I.J., Topping, D. and McKay, G. (2001) 'Insulin stimulation of hepatic triacylglycerol secretion and the etiology of insulin resistance.' *Journal of Nutrition 131*, 2074–2077.

Zavaroni, I., Sander, S., Scott, S. and Reaven, G.M. (1980) 'Effect of fructose feeding on insulin secretion and insulin action in the rat.' *Metabolism 29*, 970–973.

Zeigler, E. (1967) 'Secular changes in the stature of adults and the secular trend of the modern sugar consumption.' *Zeitschrift für Kinderheilkunde 99*, 2, 146–166.

Chapter 6

COMPROMISED THYROID AND ADRENAL FUNCTION

Jane Nodder

Introduction

Patients with thyroid and adrenal disorders are usually managed in primary care. This chapter aims to help complementary practitioners understand how they can complement such treatment with safe, effective, evidence-informed interventions as part of an integrated team of health professionals. In particular, the chapter considers those areas that are often the most confusing for complementary health practitioners, such as interpreting thyroid blood tests, issues and controversies in the standard approach to diagnosis and management of thyroid disorders and the debate surrounding the concept of adrenal fatigue.

Part 1 The Thyroid Gland

1. Thyroid function

Thyroid disorders, notably hypothyroidism, are amongst the most common medical conditions particularly in women and the elderly (AACE 2002; Canaris *et al.* 2000; Roberts and Ladenson 2004). In the UK the 20 year follow-up of the Whickham Survey (Vanderpump *et al.* 1995) found a mean incidence of 4.1/1000 survivors per year for all causes of hypothyroidism in women, and 0.6/1000 survivors per year in men. The incidence of hyperthyroidism was 0.8/1000 per year for women, and negligible in men (Vanderpump *et al.* 1995). In a large US population study, the prevalence of elevated thyroid stimulating hormone (TSH) levels was 9.5 per cent, and 40 per cent of people taking thyroid medication had abnormal TSH levels (Canaris *et al.* 2000).

1.1 The thyroid gland

The thyroid is an endocrine gland located in the neck, in front of the trachea and above the collar-bones. The gland secretes two main iodothyronine hormones: tetra-iodothyronine, more commonly called thyroxine (T4), and tri-iodothyronine, (T3).

T4 is made in the follicular cells of the thyroid from tyrosine (amino acid) and four iodine molecules. It is highly lipophilic, binds easily to serum proteins and is the precursor to the active thyroid hormone, T3. T3 is made by detaching one iodine molecule from the T4 molecule. T3 is about ten times more physiologically active than T4 and carries out 90 per cent of thyroid function (Nussey and Whitehead 2001).

1.1.1 SYNTHESIS OF THYROID HORMONES

The synthesis of the iodothyronines requires iodine from the diet (Kelly 2000). Adolescents and adults need around 150µg/day of iodine (Delange 1998), with a standard diet supplying approximately 400–500µg/day, of which the thyroid takes up some 60–80µg/day (Kelly 2000). If the dietary intake of iodine is consistently low, hypothyroidism may develop (Delange 1998). There is no suggested role for iodine in the peripheral metabolism of thyroid tissues (Kelly 2000).

To synthesise thyroid hormones, iodine (in the form of iodide) is drawn from the blood into thyroid follicular cells, where it is activated into a reactive form (iodination) by the iron and selenium-dependent enzyme, thyroid peroxidase (Doerge and Sheehan 2002; Köhrle 2005; Zimmerman and Köhrle 2002). Reactive iodine associates with the polypeptide thyroglobulin (a protein-rich tyrosine residue) to form units of three (tri) or four (tetra) iodine ions. The enzyme thyroid peroxidase is also required for this coupling function. The protein containing the iodothyronines is then stored as colloid in the follicular cells.

The thyroid produces approximately 80–100µg of T4 a day from the gland itself (Leonard and Köhrle 1996; Nussey and Whitehead 2001). The daily production of T3 is about 30µg, 20 per cent from the thyroid gland and 80 per cent by the removal of an iodine atom (deiodination) from T4 in peripheral tissues, mainly in the liver and kidneys, but also in the anterior pituitary and the nervous system (Kelly 2000; Leonard and Köhrle 1996). This deiodination process requires the selenium-dependent 5'-deiodinase enzymes and healthy kidney and liver function (Arthur and Beckett 1999; Kelly 2000).

Thyroid stimulating hormone (TSH)

Thyroid hormone production is regulated by thyrotropin (otherwise known as thyroid stimulating hormone or TSH), secreted from the anterior pituitary gland. TSH stimulates the synthesis of thyroglobulin, the iodide trap, the coupling reactions in the follicular cells and the release of the iodothyronines into the circulation. Release of TSH from the anterior pituitary is controlled by the tripeptide thyrotropin releasing hormone (TRH), secreted from the hypothalamus through the portal system to the anterior pituitary in response to a negative feedback mechanism, predominantly from T4. The release of TSH is pulsatile and circadian with concentrations being higher at night than during the day (Surks, Goswami and Daniels 2005). Significant annual, biannual and quarterly seasonal rhythms have been observed, with the lowest values for TSH occurring in spring (Maes *et al.* 1997) and the highest values occurring during summer and autumn. However, not all studies have identified these seasonal patterns (Plasqui, Kester and Westerterp 2003). Overall, the degree of seasonal individuality found in plasma hormones is too great to accurately identify population-based reference ranges (Maes *et al.* 1997; Plasqui *et al.* 2003).

TRH is a potent stimulator of prolactin (stimulates growth of mammary tissue and milk production) release from the pituitary (Asa and Ezzat 2002). Hyperprolactinaemia is common in **hypothyroid** women, and can result in oligomenorrhoea or amenorrhoea, since high prolactin levels suppress the luteinising and follicle stimulating hormones (LH and FSH) (Mancini 2008; Serri *et al.* 2003).

Reverse T3 (rT3)

3, 3', 5'-triiodothyronine or reverse T3 (rT3) is an iodothyronine isomer with less than 1 per cent of the activity of T4 (Kelly 2000). A very small amount of rT3 is produced in the thyroid gland itself, but the majority (95%) comes from the deiodination of T4 in the periphery to clear some T4 from the body. Under normal conditions some 45–50 per cent of the daily production of T4 is converted to rT3, although this varies considerably between individuals (Kelly 2000).

The level of rT3 reflects the rate of peripheral conversion of T4 to T3. Although rT3 does bind to T3 receptor sites, potentially blocking the action of T3, it does not stimulate thyroid hormone receptors (Kelly 2000). Since T3 is normally the dominant hormone and rT3 has a higher metabolic clearance rate and a lower serum concentration, rT3 does not normally present a problem. However, the rT3/T3 ratio may increase in circumstances such as:

- pregnancy
- oestrogen therapy
- fasting or severe dieting
- infection
- liver or renal disease
- low selenium, potassium or zinc status
- high cadmium, mercury or lead status
- use of certain medications (e.g. some beta blockers, amiodarone)
- elevation of cortisol, catecholamines and some cytokines (Goichot, Sapin and Schlienger 1998).

Changes in rT3/T3 ratio may be designed to slow down metabolism and aid survival (Kelly 2000). It is therefore probably not appropriate to administer thyroid hormone in these situations (Kelly 2000).

1.1.2 THYROID HORMONE CONCENTRATIONS IN PLASMA

Over 99 per cent of thyroid hormones circulating in the blood are bound to plasma transport proteins, mainly thyronine binding globulin (TBG) (75%), but also transthyretin (20%) and thyroxine binding albumin (5%). T3 has a greater affinity for transthyretin and thyroxine binding albumin over TBG. Less than 1 per cent of circulating iodothyronines are free (non-protein bound) in plasma (0.03–0.05% for T4; 0.3% for T3) (Kelly 2000) and it is these free hormones that enter cells, bind to specific cell nuclear receptors and exert metabolic control (Marshall and Bangert 2004).

A cell needs 5–7 times more T4 to bind to cell nuclear receptors to have a physiological effect compared to T3 (Marshall and Bangert 2004). However, although T3 is a more powerful hormone than T4, it has a shorter half-life (about 24 hours compared to approximately one week for T4) due to its lower affinity for transport proteins.

Total thyroid hormone concentrations in plasma are dependent not only on thyroid function, but also on the concentration of binding proteins (Arem 1999; Marshall and Bangert 2004). As these change, thyroid hormone production is adjusted, i.e. as free hormone is taken up, bound hormone dissociates from its binding protein, to maintain stable free hormone concentrations (Marshall and Bangert 2004). Measuring total hormone concentrations can therefore be misleading since many factors, including pregnancy, medication, selenium status and oestrogen therapy, can affect the concentration of binding proteins.

1.1.3 THYROID HORMONE METABOLISM

About 70 per cent of T4 produced in the thyroid is eventually deiodinated in peripheral tissues to T3 or rT3 (Kelly 2000). Thyroid hormone metabolites are further deiodinated to the biologically inactive hormone T2 (Molina 2006) and are eventually excreted in bile (Marshall and Bangert 2004).

1.1.4 CELLULAR EFFECTS OF THYROID HORMONES

T3 and T4 are associated with similar physiological and metabolic functions at cellular level (Table 6.1).

2. Imbalances in thyroid function

A number of imbalances can arise in thyroid function:

- excessive production of thyroid hormones (hyperthyroidism/thyrotoxicosis)

- underproduction of thyroid hormones (hypothyroid state/myxoedema)
- enlarged thyroid (goitre)
- nodules or lumps in the thyroid (multinodular goitre)
- disturbance of normal thyroid function by drugs, e.g. corticosteroids, lithium carbonate, salicylates, sulphonamides, amiodarone
- cancer.

Table 6.1 Cellular effects of thyroid hormones

Function	Mechanism of action of thyroid hormones
Basal metabolic rate	Increase basal metabolic rate of cells by increasing the number and size of mitochondria, oxygen consumption and nutrient utilisation Influence temperature control
Fat metabolism	Increase breakdown of fat to influence levels of body fat and body weight
Carbohydrate metabolism	Increase all aspects of carbohydrate metabolism
Protein metabolism	Stimulate both protein synthesis and degradation and play an important role in normal growth and development
Cardiovascular system	Potentiate the action of catecholamines on cardiac output Tachycardia is associated with high levels of thyroid hormone
Musculoskeletal system	Direct and indirect effect on bone synthesis and turnover through the release of growth hormone and action of insulin-like growth factor −1 (IGF-1)
Central nervous system	Potentiate the action of catecholamines on the central nervous system Essential for mental development (myelination of nerve fibres, development of neurons, speed of reflexes)

2.1 Hyperthyroidism or thyrotoxicosis

2.1.1 CAUSES AND CONTRIBUTING FACTORS FOR HYPERTHYROIDISM

Affecting about 1 per cent of the adult population, thyrotoxicosis is principally an autoimmune condition in which autoantibodies inappropriately stimulate TSH receptors on thyroid follicle cells, resulting in the over-production of thyroid hormones. Graves' disease is the most common form of thyrotoxicosis, although the condition may also arise as a result of the activity of benign tumours in the thyroid gland. Transient hyperthyroidism can occur in thyroiditis, where inflammation of the thyroid results in the release of excess thyroid hormone. The condition may also involve a genetic component. Hyperthyroidism is more common in young to middle-aged women, although it may occur in adolescents, during pregnancy, at the time of menopause and in those over 50.

2.1.2 SIGNS AND SYMPTOMS OF HYPERTHYROIDISM

The symptoms and signs of thyrotoxicosis are due to thyroid hormone excess and the potentiation of the catecholamines. They include:

- weight loss, but normal or increased appetite (in 90% of cases)
- heat intolerance and sweating
- palpitations
- heart failure, particularly in the elderly
- generalised muscle weakness and tiredness
- vomiting or diarrhoea
- irregular periods and infertility in women
- goitre and difficulty swallowing due to possible swelling in throat
- hyperactivity ('always on the go'), anxiety and agitation
- nervousness and irritability
- eye disease (exophthalmos or thyroid associated ophthalmopathy)
- thick skin lesions, particularly over the shins (pretibial myxoedema).

2.2 Hypothyroidism or myxoedema

Hypothyroidism occurs when the thyroid gland fails to produce sufficient thyroid hormones. Primary hypothyroidism is due to a problem in the actual thyroid gland, often as a result of autoimmune destruction of the gland. Secondary (central) hypothyroidism arises from disorders principally in the pituitary gland (e.g. tumour, effects of surgery or (very rarely) a deficiency in TSH production), and possibly also in the hypothalamus, although pituitary or hypothalamic deficiency account for only a very small percentage of hypothyroid cases (British Thyroid Foundation (BTF) 2006). In such conditions, FT4 will be low (Arem 1999). Mild to moderate hypothyroidism can go undetected for many years, and some standard tests may not pick up milder cases that might respond favourably to treatment.

Hypothyroidism is more common in women, in the elderly, in those with other autoimmune disorders (e.g. type 1 diabetes mellitus, Addison's disease), and in those on medication that can affect thyroid function (Nygaard 2007; Roberts and Ladenson 2004).

2.2.1 CAUSES AND CONTRIBUTING FACTORS FOR HYPOTHYROIDISM

Primary hypothyroidism may be due to:

- *lack of iodine*: Worldwide, low dietary iodine is the leading cause of hypothyroidism. Iodine deficiency increases the number of thyrocytes and their mutation rates leading to the development of highly active autonomous nodules in the thyroid (Delange 1998). Where there is chronic iodine deficiency, an acute increase in iodine intake may lead to the development of iodine-induced hyperthyroidism (IIH) (Delange 1998). High iodine intake can also precipitate autoimmune attacks on the thyroid (Arthur and Beckett 1999) and may be linked to rising levels of thyroiditis and thyroid cancer in some parts of the world (Harach and Williams 1995). Data on current iodine status in the UK is currently lacking, although there are concerns about possible low status amongst some pregnant women (International Council for Control of Iodine Deficiency Disorders 2008).

- *autoimmune hypothyroidism*: Antibodies destroy thyroid follicles and block TSH receptors, preventing the thyroid from releasing normal amounts of thyroid hormones. Thyroid autoantibodies (TPO-Ab) are generally detectable in the blood. Hashimoto's thyroiditis is the commonest form of autoimmune hypothyroidism (Marshall and Bangert 2004; Roberts and Ladenson 2004).

- *side-effects of drug therapy*: See Table 6.4.

- *thyroidectomy*: Surgical removal of thyroid.

- *congenital hypothyroidism (CHT)*: A condition in which the thyroid gland fails to develop properly or does not produce adequate thyroid hormones. This condition can produce *cretinism* in the newborn. In the UK babies are screened for CHT at 6–8 days of age (Marshall and Bangert 2004).

- *enzyme defects* in the thyroid.

- *thyroiditis*: Inflammation of the thyroid gland.

2.2.2 SIGNS AND SYMPTOMS OF HYPOTHYROIDISM

Signs and symptoms of low thyroid function can be very mild and develop slowly. They usually relate to an overall 'slowing down' of body functions and may be present before levels of thyroid hormone drop below normal. Subclinical (mild) hypothyroidism should be monitored because of the potential risks associated with the condition, including progression to overt hypothyroidism, possible cardiovascular effects, hyperlipidaemia and neuropsychiatric effects (Gharib *et al.* 2005).

The following signs and symptoms seem to be the most reliable indicators of low thyroid function that practitioners should be alert to (Lindsay and Toft 1997; Nygaard 2007):

- Fatigue, particularly on waking, that improves during the day.

- Weight gain, possibly linked to changes in the production of cortisol and in sleep patterns that can affect appetite and carbohydrate metabolism (Stimson *et al.* 2007).

- Changes in mental health including mood swings, depression, impaired mental processing, memory and concentration. Mental health symptoms can develop with only small decreases in the amount of available thyroid hormone and may be worse with seasonal changes that affect circulating thyroid hormone levels (Bunevicius and Prange 2000; Esposito, Prange and Golden 1997).

- Sensitivity to cold and reduced sweating.

- Possible rise in levels of total and LDL cholesterol and triglycerides. Levels of thyroid hormones and lipids are inversely related – when thyroid hormones are in short supply, lipid levels tend to rise, *potentially* increasing the risk for cardiovascular conditions (Osman, Gammage and Franklyn 2001; Pirich, Mullner and Sinzinger 2000). Thyroid hormone regulates the clearance of LDL cholesterol (Roberts and Ladenson 2004).

- Painful constipation accompanied by abdominal bloating and relieved by diarrhoea with cramping. Depleted thyroid function reduces the normal muscular activity of the bowel.

- Muscle cramps and weakness, pain in the calves, thighs and upper arms, rheumatoid pain in joints and carpal tunnel syndrome (Krupsky 1987).

- Neurological symptoms, e.g. prolonged Achilles tendon reflex time.

- Easy bruising or evidence of blood clotting defects.

Individuals may also experience the following:

- Menstrual disturbances, including amenorrhoea or heavy, irregular or prolonged menstrual periods and pre-menstrual syndrome (PMS). Even minimal thyroid dysfunction may result in menstrual disturbances (Stoffer 1982).

- Absence of sweating and dryness of skin and hair.

- Impotence, low libido or fertility problems with an increased risk of miscarriage in younger women, or exaggerated menopausal symptoms in older women. Such symptoms may be linked to disruption in DHEA production and imbalances between testosterone and oestrogen (Redmond 2004). They may also be linked to chronic thyroiditis (American Association of Clinical Endocrinologists (AACE) 2002).

- Swelling of the thyroid gland in the neck (goitre), deep or hoarse voice.

3. Diagnosis of thyroid function problems

A combination of laboratory tests, medical history and current clinical signs and symptoms is required for the correct diagnosis of hypothyroid conditions (Downing 2000).

Box 6.1 Clinical practice points – Thyroid hormone function

- T3 is about 10x more physiologically active than T4 and carries out 90% of thyroid function.

- Hypothyroidism is more common in women, in the elderly, in those on medication that can affect thyroid function or with other autoimmune disorders.

- Signs and symptoms of hypothyroidism can be very mild and may be present before levels of thyroid hormone drop below normal.

- Key signs and symptoms of hypothyroidism include: fatigue, weight gain, changes in mood and mental health, sensitivity to cold and reduced sweating, menstrual disturbances and constipation.

- Subclinical (mild) hypothyroidism should be monitored.

3.1 Blood tests for thyroid dysfunction

Thyroid stimulating hormone (TSH)

Measuring thyroid stimulating hormone (TSH) in the blood is the 'gold standard' in the initial screening for thyroid disease (Dayan 2001). TSH is highly sensitive to changes in thyroid hormone levels and levels may be raised or lowered long before clinical signs and symptoms of a thyroid condition become apparent, or before levels of thyroid hormones fall outside the 'normal' range (Arem 1999). In unselected populations, measurement of serum TSH has a sensitivity of 89–95 per cent and specificity of 90–96 per cent for thyroid dysfunction, compared to cases confirmed by clinical examination and other tests (De los Santos, Starich and Mazzaferri 1989).

Normal TSH is in the approximate range of 0.3–5mU/L in most laboratories, although there is no universal agreement as to the precise level of TSH which delineates hypothyroidism. In the UK the typical reference range for TSH is 0.4–4.5mU/L. High TSH levels are an indicator of hypothyroidism; abnormally low levels indicate hyperthyroidism/thyrotoxicosis. However, even with highly sensitive TSH assays, results from the TSH test should be correlated with clinical evaluation of symptoms in diagnosing thyroid conditions (Baisier, Hertoghe and Eeckhaut 2000; Beastall and Thomson 1997).

TSH is inhibited by glucocorticoids, dopamine and somatostatin (Marshall and Bangert 2004) – this may be relevant to the thyroid hormone disturbance that occurs in non-thyroidal illness. In patients taking thyroid hormone replacement, TSH levels under 0.2mU/L are associated with osteoporosis and an increased risk of atrial fibrillation (Sawin *et al.* 1994).

Free T4 (FT4)

TSH is frequently measured along with free T4 (FT4) (Krunzel 2001) to give a more satisfactory measure of thyroid function (Dayan 2001). FT4 levels may be affected by severe, chronic liver or kidney disease, some drugs (e.g. heparin), acute illness (e.g. AIDS, hepatitis) and extreme changes in the concentration of binding proteins (Dayan 2001).

The normal range for FT4 is 9–25pmol/L. Levels are high in hyperthyroidism and low in hypothyroidism.

Free T3 (FT3)

Plasma FT3 alone may be too non-specific to be clinically useful as a routine diagnostic test. Concentrations change in fasting, in acute and chronic non-thyroidal disease (e.g. liver, kidney disease, etc.) and with age. FT3 concentrations are also dependent on protein binding status – as the concentration of carrier proteins changes, TT3 levels also change to keep FT3 levels constant (Marshall and Bangert 2004). The concentration of the carrier protein can change in many conditions, including during pregnancy and the administration of oestrogen therapy e.g. oral contraceptive pill (OCP), hormone replacement therapy (HRT).

FT3 is a useful test where an individual clearly appears hyperthyroid but their FT4 test is normal. Levels of FT3 are almost always raised in hyperthyroidism (due to increased peripheral formation from T4) and can become abnormal earlier than FT4, and return to normal later than FT4. Levels of FT3 may be normal in hypothyroidism. Low levels of T3 are frequently associated with depression (Sher 2000).

Normal values for FT3 are generally about 3.5–7.8pmol/L.

Total T4 and T3 (free plus bound)

The total T4 (TT4) and total T3 (TT3) levels can be measured, but are of little use alone since more than 99 per cent of these hormones is bound and the test does not therefore indicate how much free hormone is present. TT4 and TT3 levels are also affected by some medication and other clinical conditions.

Reverse T3

The normal range in adult serum for rT3 is 0.22–0.46nmol/L, although a range of values have been reported (Franklyn and Shephard 2000).

Thyroid antibodies

Thyroid peroxidase antibodies (TPO-Ab) are the main antibody indicators of possible thyroid disease and their appearance usually precedes the development of thyroid disorders (Dayan 2001). Factors that have been considered as triggers for TPO-Ab include infection, genetics, stress, sex hormone status and iodide levels in the thyroid (Bhattacharyya and Wiles 2000). Measurement of TPO-Ab can be very useful when evaluating possible subclinical hypothyroidism, as the presence of antibodies predicts a greater risk for hypothyroidism (4.3% per year compare to 2.1% for those with no antibodies present) (Surks *et al.* 2004). Clinicians may also use this test when deciding whether to treat a patient with subclinical hypothyroidism (McDermott and Ridgeway 2001).

Thyrotrophin releasing hormone (TRH)

TRH is infrequently used as a measure of thyroid function, although measurement may be helpful when the level of TSH is borderline low or high, or pituitary or hypothalamic disease is suspected (BTF 2006).

3.1.1 INTERPRETATION OF THYROID BLOOD TESTS

Interpreting blood tests for thyroid function can be a confusing subject for complementary practitioners. The following section is designed to help practitioners understand test results so that their recommendations for patients with signs and symptoms of possible thyroid disorders can be safe and effective.

In the UK typical serum reference ranges for thyroid hormones in adults are:

TSH – 0.4–4.5mU/L*	TT4 – 60–160nmol/L
FT4 – 9.0–25pmol/L	TT3 – 1.2–2.6nmol/L
FT3 – 3.5–7.8pmol/L	RT3 – 0.22–0.46 nmol/L

*There is ongoing debate about the upper limit of the reference range for serum TSH due to concerns about the risks of patients who are subclinically hypothyroid going on to develop primary hypothyroidism. Some authors have argued in favour of reducing the upper limit to 2.5mU/L (Wartofsky and Dickey 2005), while others have argued to retain the upper limit at 4.5mU/L (Surks *et al.* 2005). The upper limit of 4.5mU/L is the current guideline from the BTF (BTF 2006). The AACE use 0.3–3.0mU/L as an optimal range with a level of 2.0mU/L being of concern for subclinical hypothyroidism (Gharib *et al.* 2005; Wartofsky and Dickey 2005).

Key profiles in blood tests for thyroid function

In clinical practice there are six key profiles (Table 6.2) that may arise from the main thyroid function tests (Dayan 2001).

Table 6.2 Possible profiles from thyroid blood tests

Low TSH (almost undetectable) with **elevated FT3 or FT4**, presence of TSH-receptor antibodies and frequently thyroid peroxidase autoantibodies (TPO-Ab)	Indicative of primary hyperthyroidism
	Individuals with an overactive thyroid can also have normal FT4 levels, with elevated FT3 (Arem 1999)
Low TSH, normal FT3 or FT4 (Gharib *et al.* 2005)	Indicative of subclinical primary hyperthyroidism, e.g. in the elderly or excessive thyroxine ingestion
	Low serum TSH (especially if reduced but >0.1mU/L) may also reflect other non-thyroidal systemic illness or drug therapy
	Complete suppression of TSH (<0.1 mU/L) warrants treatment for hyperthyroidism
	See section 4.2 regarding levels of TSH in patients who are taking replacement thyroid hormone
Low, normal or slightly elevated TSH, low FT3 or FT4	Possible pituitary disease (secondary hypothyroidism) (Beckett and Toft 2003; Wardle, Fraser and Squire 2001; Waise and Belchetz 2000), recent treatment for hyperthyroidism or other non-thyroid illness. Refer to endocrinologist
	Thyroxine therapy should not be started in patients with cortisol deficiency as it may lead to an Addisonian crisis if no preceding glucocorticoid treatment (Murray, Jayarajasingh and Perros 2001). It is important to rule out Addison's disease if clinical symptoms of hypothyroidism worsen after starting thyroid hormone replacement (Murray, Jayarajasingh and Perros 2001)
	TSH may remain suppressed for up to a year in individuals recently treated for hyperthyroidism even where there is low FT4 or FT3 status (Dayan 2001)
Raised TSH (greater than 10mU/L), **low FT3 or FT4.** Possible presence of thyroid antibodies	Characteristic of overt primary hypothyroidism (Klee and Hay 1997; Weetman 1997)
	FT4 may also be low in individuals who have been treated for hyperthyroidism (Dayan 2001)
	Levels of FT3 may be normal due to increased peripheral formation from T4 (Marshall and Bangert 2004)

continued

Table 6.2 Possible profiles from thyroid blood tests *cont.*

Raised TSH, normal FT3 or FT4. Possible presence of positive anti-TPO antibodies	Characteristic of subclinical hypothyroidism. Symptoms are frequently either absent or clinically subtle and non-specific (Owen and Lazarus 2003)
	In individuals taking regular thyroxine, an increase in TSH concentration may indicate thyroxine malabsorption (Choe and Hays 1995) or interference with the assay (Ward *et al.* 1997)
	Changes in thyroid function have also been reported in acute psychiatric illness, although these rarely last longer than 14 days (Dayan 2001)
Normal or raised TSH, raised free FT3 or FT4	Rare profile. May indicate thyroid hormone resistance or a TSH-secreting pituitary tumour, interference with test procedure, presence of antibodies, amiodarone therapy, intermittent excessive thyroxine intake or excessive intake preceding the test sample

Source: Adapted from Dayan 2001

3.2 Radioactive iodine uptake (RIU)

Measuring radioactive iodine uptake is an expensive and inconvenient test that may be used in the differential diagnosis of transient hyperthyroidism (e.g. postpartum).

3.3 Urine hormone assays for thyroid function

Urine hormone assays assess thyroid status by measuring tissue exposure to non-protein-bound thyroid hormones over a 24-hour period. Baisier *et al.* (2000) suggested a useful correlation between unconjugated fractions of urinary T3 and T4 and serum unbound hormone concentrations. The same group also suggested that 24-hour urinary excretion of FT3 may be helpful in defining borderline or subclinical hypothyroidism and overall selenium status. Urinary thyroid assessment is not common in the UK and does not replace serum testing in the diagnosis of thyroid conditions.

3.4 Functional tests

3.4.1 BRODA BARNES TEMPERATURE TEST

The Broda Barnes temperature test measures morning basal body temperature and is sometimes used by complementary practitioners to indicate whether further investigation of thyroid function might be advisable (Barnes and Galton 1976).

The normal range for underarm morning basal body temperature is between 36.6°C (97.8°F) and 36.8°C (98.2°F) (Barnes and Galton 1976). If the recorded temperature is consistently below the normal levels, thyroid function should be tested with blood tests.

Box 6.2 Procedure for the Broda Barnes temperature test

1. Shake down a non-mercury basal thermometer* at night.
2. In the morning, before moving place the thermometer under the armpit for 10 minutes and keep still.
3. Note the temperature after ten minutes.
4. Repeat for 6–12 consecutive mornings,** noting the temperature each time.

*If using a digital thermometer, take the temperature three times a day under the tongue. (Note that temperatures taken in the mouth may be affected by low-grade infection.)

**Pre-menopausal women should start to take their temperature on day 2 of their menstrual cycle (i.e. day 2 of bleeding). Men and post-menopausal women may take it at any time of the month.

** Pre-menopausal women should start to take their temperature on day 2 of their menstrual cycle (i.e. day 2 of bleeding). Men and post-menopausal women may take it at any time of the month.

The temperature test is a screening tool only. It should not be used alone to diagnose a thyroid condition – a fall in temperature is not sensitive enough to diagnose or monitor treatment for thyroid conditions (Arem 1999). Only severe hypothyroidism results in low temperature and temperature is affected by many other factors.

Box 6.3 Clinical practice points – Testing for thyroid conditions

- A combination of laboratory tests, medical history and current clinical signs and symptoms is required for the correct diagnosis of thyroid conditions.

- TSH is highly sensitive to changes in thyroid hormone levels, which may be raised or lowered long before clinical signs and symptoms of a thyroid condition become apparent.

- Minor imbalances in thyroid hormones may not be detectable in blood tests (Arem 1999), e.g. FT4 often remains in the normal range until the TSH level exceeds 20 mU/L or even higher.

- A laboratory result represents a range, not an absolute, and the normal range of thyroid function is very broad between individuals. Other valuable tests (e.g. thyroid autoantibodies) and assays may be required alongside the TSH test.

---

4. Conventional treatment approaches for thyroid conditions

It is important for complementary medicine practitioners to understand standard treatment approaches to thyroid conditions as patients frequently have many questions and issues in this area. Key information is given below and further details can be found in the following references: AACE 2002; Gharib *et al.* 2005 and BTF 2006.

4.1 Hyperthyroidism

Hyperthyroidism is commonly treated with medications to manage the overproduction of thyroid hormones or the side-effects of the condition, surgical removal of part of the thyroid gland (now less common) or radioactive iodine treatment.

4.2 Hypothyroidism

Hypothyroid conditions are usually managed with thyroxine (T4) in tablet form as levothyroxine for conversion to T3. The main aim of replacement therapy is to help the patient feel well and to achieve a serum TSH within the reference range (Ladenson *et al.* 2000; Vanderpump and Franklyn 2003). The mean replacement dosage is 1.6μg/kg of body weight per day (AACE 2002), although it can take time to get the dose of levothyroxine right for an individual. Treatment is generally for life (Walsh 2002). A minimum of two months is usually required to restore stability in thyroid function tests after a change in dose (Gow *et al.* 1987). Annual checks of TSH and FT4 are standard, once the correct dose of thyroxine has been identified.

There is debate about the upper limit of the normal reference range for monitoring treatment of hypothyroidism with thyroxine. The current recommendation is that in medicated patients, the dose of thyroxine should be appropriate to achieve a TSH level within the reference range (traditionally 0.5–5.0mU/L) (Biondi *et al* 2002; Walsh 2002) or between 0.5 and 2.0mU/L (Arem 1999).

Side-effects of thyroxine replacement are unusual, although if too much is prescribed, an individual may develop symptoms of overactive thyroid. In a few individuals a rare genetic mutation may result in thyroid hormone resistance at tissue level (Weiss and Refetoff 2000).

4.3 Subclinical (mild) hypothyroidism

Subclinical hypothyroidism (TSH above, and FT4 within, the reference range) should be monitored by repeat testing 3–6 months after the original result (Gharib *et al.* 2005). Treatment approaches for this condition remain controversial (Fatourechi 2001, 2002a, 2002b; Gharib *et al.* 2005; Owen and Lazarus 2003; Surks *et al.* 2004; Vanderpump 2003). See Table 6.3 for current UK guidelines for the treatment of subclinical hypothyroidism.

4.4 Combination treatment

T4 replacement hormone is usually given in isolation of T3. Some researchers assert combination treatment (T4 with T3) offers benefits particularly with regard to brain function and mental health (Bunevicius *et al.* 1999; Canaris *et al.* 2000; Henneman *et al.* 2004; Wartofsky 2004). A small initial study (Bunevicius *et al.* 1999) generated some interest in this approach and although subsequent reviews have not confirmed the initial beneficial effects (Escobar-Morreale *et al.* 2005; Grozinsky-Glasberg *et al.* 2006), this approach is one that patients often research on the Internet and wish to discuss with complementary practitioners. The current position of the British Thyroid Association (BTA) is that combination treatment with T4/T3 is not recommended, since there is insufficient consistent evidence of benefit and some evidence of undesirable and harmful effects for this approach, particularly with regard to cardiovascular function in people over 55 (BTA 2007).

Additionally, in the USA in particular, there is considerable interest in the use of Armour thyroid as an alternative to synthetic thyroid hormones. Armour thyroid is a desiccated natural thyroid extract, usually from porcine sources. It contains both T4 and T3 in a ratio of around 4:1 (T4:T3) compared to 14:1 in the human thyroid.

There have been concerns regarding the stability of Armour thyroid (BTA 2007) and, in the UK, it is not on the British National Formulary, nor is it a licensed therapy for thyroid conditions, although doctors can 'prescribe an unlicensed medicine to meet a special clinical need for a patient, on their own direct personal responsibility' (BTA 2007). Glandular thyroid products available from nutritional supplement companies have usually had most of the thyroid hormone removed.

5. Issues in the standard approach to diagnosis and management of hypothyroidism

5.1 Interpreting thyroid function tests

It is important for the complementary medicine practitioner to appreciate a number of factors that may affect the results of thyroid function tests (Dayan 2001). Diagnosing thyroid conditions based on the results of the TSH blood test alone may not detect all conditions (O'Reilly 2000; Wardle, Fraser and Squire 2001; Weetman 1997). Blood tests do not measure thyroid hormone levels in tissues and minor imbalances in hormones may not be detectable in blood tests (Arem 1999).

Reference ranges do vary from laboratory to laboratory and the clinical definition of 'normal' values for serum TSH – particularly with regard to the upper reference limit – is frequently discussed (see section 3.1.1 in this chapter).

Test results may not be reliable in situations where thyroid status is unstable, e.g. post-hyperthyroidism or thyroiditis, in the early weeks of thyroxine therapy, or with poor compliance with thyroxine therapy (Wright 1994). Results may also be misleading where hypothyroidism is due to pituitary disease (Wardle *et al.* 2001) or other hormone disorders. High cortisol levels, due to stress or the use of synthetic corticosteroids, may normalise TSH levels and mask hypothyroidism (Pizzorno and Ferril 2005, p.645). Free hormones should therefore be tested in addition to TSH levels (Dayan 2001).

Table 6.3 Guidelines for the treatment of subclinical hypothyroidism

Test results	Action
TSH high, FT4 normal	Exclude non-thyroidal illness and drug interactions. Repeat tests after 3–6 months
TSH >10mU/L, FT4 low or normal	Treatment with thyroxine recommended
TSH above reference range but <10mU/L, FT4 normal	Measure TPOAb
	If positive, monitor TSH annually, or in line with any clinical symptoms. Individual patients, who are not pregnant, may be offered a 3-month trial of thyroxine (Weetman 2006). Start thyroxine if TSH rises above 10mU/L
	If TPOAb negative, measure TSH levels approximately every 3 years

Source: Adapted from British Thyroid Foundation 2006

There are many common interactions between drugs and thyroid function (see Table 6.4), whilst stress, caloric restriction, intensive exercise, exposure to toxic metals, issues with T3 receptors, adrenal insufficiency and serious or chronic illness can also affect thyroid hormone (Kelly 2000) and TSH levels (Marshall and Bangert 2004).

Finally, other valuable tests (e.g. thyroid autoantibodies) may not be performed alongside the TSH test, or assays may be prone to interference that can produce clinically misleading results.

Table 6.4 Common drugs that interact with thyroid medications

• Corticosteroids and dopaminergic drugs	• Tricyclic antidepressants, e.g. imipramine
• Oral anticoagulants, e.g. heparin	• Cholesterol-lowering drugs
• Insulin or oral hypoglycaemics	• Antacids containing aluminium hydroxide
• Oestrogen, oral contraceptives	• Lithium carbonate (for bipolar disorder)
• Iron/iron-containing vitamins	• Beta-blockers, amiodarone (anti-arrhythmic containing iodine)
• Salicylates, phenytoin	
• Digitalis	

5.2 Issues with the conversion of T4 to T3

Patients may be told that their symptoms of hypothyroidism are the result of difficulties with the conversion of thyroid hormones (T4 to T3). Two explanations are frequently offered to try to explain such difficulties:

- the patient may be deficient in selenium (see Box 6.6)

- chronically impaired conversion of T4 to T3 leads to reverse T3 dominance (Wilson 1991). Under certain conditions (e.g. fasting or starvation, impairment of 5'-deiodinase function, liver disease, and other situations that raise levels of cortisol) the conversion of T4 to T3 decreases, and the production of rT3 increases (Kelly 2000). This mechanism may be designed to slow down metabolism and aid survival. Where metabolism slows down, rT3 is not eliminated as quickly as usual and levels therefore rise considerably.

Dr E. Denis Wilson proposed that, under significant physical or emotional stress, this process of impaired conversion of T4 to T3 with an increase in rT3 can become 'stuck', leading to chronically low T3 levels and slowed metabolism that can persist even after the stress has passed (Wilson 1991). He described the key symptoms of this situation as very low body temperature, thyroid blood tests in the normal range and a range of symptoms frequently associated with hypothyroidism, including depression (Wilson 1991). He advocated treating the condition with high doses of T3 and adjusting the dose by monitoring basal temperature, as opposed to thyroid testing.

However, the reduction in T4 to T3 conversion that occurs under significant stress is usually only temporary (lasting only for about 1–3 weeks), even if levels of cortisol remain high (Arem 1999). Currently, there appears to be no evidence for chronically impaired conversion of T4 to T3 (Arem 1999). Arem (1999) suggests that the pattern of symptoms Wilson (1991) described may be due to thyroid hormone deficit in the brain, resulting in depression, rather than true hypothyroidism in other organs. T3 therapy must always be monitored by both thyroid function testing *and* clinical assessment to avoid the risk of the patient becoming hyperthyroid (Arem 1999).

5.3 Dissatisfaction with thyroxine therapy

A substantial percentage of patients continue to experience ongoing symptoms such as fatigue, depression and cognitive problems, despite receiving a seemingly adequate dosage of thyroxine (Walsh 2002). These patients frequently report such ongoing symptoms to a complementary practitioner. It may be helpful to suggest that such patients visit their GP to:

- double-check their thyroid hormone status. Mild or subclinical hypothyroidism can be a coincidental finding, with the patient's symptoms actually being due to another condition (e.g. depression, anaemia, iron deficiency, primary hyperparathyroidism), that is resulting in a temporary increase in serum TSH (Walsh 2002)

- discuss the level of thyroxine replacement they are taking as requirements may vary between individuals. Thyroid hormone absorption can be affected by malabsorptive states, age, lack of bioequivalence and the narrow therapeutic range of commercially produced levothyroxine, and drug interactions (AACE 2002).

Box 6.4 Clinical practice points – Treatment of thyroid conditions

- In medicated patients, the dose of thyroxine should be appropriate to achieve a TSH level within the reference range (traditionally 0.5–5.0mU/L).

- Combination treatment with T4/T3 is not recommended by the British Thyroid Foundation since there is insufficient consistent evidence of benefit, and some evidence of undesirable and harmful effects for this approach, particularly with regard to cardiovascular function in people over 55.

- Patients who continue to report symptoms such as fatigue, depression and cognitive problems, despite thyroxine treatment, should be referred back to their GP.

---

6. Thyroid function and other conditions

6.1 Pregnancy

In the first half of pregnancy oestrogen production increases and TBG concentrations rise, leading to an increase in TT4 and TT3 (AACE 2002; BTF 2006). There may also be a fall in serum TSH during the first trimester as human chorionic gonadotropin (hCG) exerts a mild thyrotrophic effect (Glinoer 1997). By the second and third trimesters, serum FT4 and FT3 levels decrease and could fall below the reference range, which is generally set for non-pregnant women, depending on the testing methods used (BTF 2006).

Women with hypothyroidism need more frequent checks in pregnancy, using trimester-related reference ranges, as their thyroxine requirements tend to increase (AACE 2002; BTF 2006). TPO-Ab testing should also be considered as this may predict both post-partum thyroiditis (occurs in approximately 5–10% of women within 2–6 months after delivery or miscarriage) and/or issues with foetal impairment (BTF 2006; Lazarus 2002). Changes in the immune system during and after pregnancy may also influence autoimmune thyroid disease (BTF 2006).

Pregnant women with type 1 diabetes and/or previous, current or family history of thyroid disease or goitre, should have their thyroid function assessed when pregnancy is confirmed, or in antenatal checks, or before conception if possible (BTF 2006).

6.2 Non-thyroidal illness or euthyroid sick syndrome (ESS)

These terms describe abnormalities in thyroid function that occur in patients with severe infection, trauma or illness but that are not due to primary thyroid or pituitary dysfunction. Such patients may have low circulating FT3, and either normal or reduced TSH levels (De Groot 1999). As the situation continues, FT4 levels also start to fall (De Groot 1999). The low T3 or T4 response is seen as protective – e.g. lowers metabolic or cardiac rate in acute conditions (De Groot 1999; Goichot *et al.* 1998) – and such patients are generally not treated with replacement hormones.

6.3 Other related conditions

Thyroid conditions are associated with a range of complications, including increased risk of osteoporosis, atrial fibrillation, dyslipidaemia, abnormal menstruation, miscarriage, subfertility and depression. Autoimmune thyroid disease has also been particularly associated with Down syndrome (Karlsson *et al.* 1998; Rooney and Walsh 1997) and also with coeliac disease (Sategna-Guidetti *et al.* 1998). UK guidelines recommend that all patients presenting with such conditions or symptoms should be assessed for thyroid function status (BTF 2006).

Part 2 The Adrenals

7. Adrenal function

7.1 The adrenal glands

The two adrenal glands are situated in the abdomen, above the kidneys. They consist of an outer cortex and an inner medulla and have a rich blood and nerve supply for optimal function. In total, the adrenals secrete over 50 hormones (see Table 6.5) that help to control:

- energy production, via the conversion of carbohydrate, protein and fat to blood glucose
- fluid and electrolyte balance in cells, interstitial fluid and the blood stream
- fat storage
- sex hormone production, particularly post-menopause in women.

7.2 Functions of cortisol

Cortisol is a particularly important glucocorticoid (steroid) that regulates a wide range of effects in tissues and organs. Cortisol:

- *increases the flow of glucose and promotes glycogen breakdown and gluconeogenesis from fats and proteins* when blood glucose is low. Acts as an insulin antagonist by inhibiting glucose uptake and oxidation
- *breaks down tissue (e.g. muscle, skin and bone)* to release amino acids, some of which may be used to produce more glucose

- *breaks down body fat*

- *is released as an anti-inflammatory agent* in response to infection or injury and auto-immune reactions. However, excess cortisol decreases white blood cell and T-cell production and activity, reducing the ability to respond to infection

- *raises blood pressure by increasing the sensitivity of the vasculature to adrenaline and noradrenaline* – low levels of cortisol can result in widespread vasodilation and pervasive hypotension. Regulates sodium and potassium in heart cells and increases the strength of contraction of the heart muscle

- *limits the effects of aldosterone.* Cortisol may bind to mineralocorticoid receptors because it is molecularly similar to aldosterone and because glucocorticoids circulate in larger amounts than mineralocorticoids. This effect may be partially blocked by the enzyme 11-beta hydroxysteroid dehydrogenase type II, which prevents overstimulation of target tissues for mineralocorticoid by glucocorticoids. Aldosterone and cortisol need to be in balance for good health

- *controls the body's response to stress* by increasing blood glucose, mobilising fats and proteins for secondary energy, modifying heartbeat, blood pressure, brain function and responses in the nervous and immune systems.

7.3 Cortisol production

The amount of cortisol circulating at any particular time is regulated by a negative feedback system involving the hypothalamus, the pituitary and the adrenal glands (the HPA axis) and ACTH. Cortisol levels follow a daily pattern (or circadian rhythm) in which cortisol concentrations are at their lowest between midnight and 4am, rise to a peak between 6am and 8am and fall throughout the rest of the day. This pattern is frequently disrupted in adrenal fatigue. Cortisol is inactivated in the liver to inactive cortisone.

8. Imbalances in adrenal function

Imbalances in adrenal function can be due to:

- *adrenal hyperfunction*, characterised by a chronic increase in the production of cortisol, usually due to Cushing's Syndrome; or adrenal *hypofunction* or *insufficiency*, characterised by a reduction in the production of adrenal hormones, particularly cortisol, due to Addison's disease. See the National Endocrine and Metabolic Diseases Information Service (http://endocrine.niddk.nih.gov/) for descriptions of these conditions

- *adrenal fatigue*, characterised by less acute variations in hormone output.

Table 6.5 The main adrenal hormones

Adrenal cortex (3 zones)		
Zone	*Main hormones*	*Main functions*
Zona glomerulosa	Aldosterone	Mineralocorticoid that regulates sodium, potassium and fluid volume to maintain blood pressure
Zona fasciculata	Cortisol, under the influence of adrenocorticotropic hormone (ACTH)	Glucocorticoid that particularly mobilises and forms glucose from proteins and fats. Also maintains vascular tone to regulate blood pressure (BP)
Zona reticularis	Progesterone, oestrogen precursors and androgens – dehydroepiandrosterone (DHEA), dehydroepiandrosterone sulphate (DHEA(s)) and androstenedione	Sex hormones that support the development of sexual characteristics. DHEA is also involved in the metabolism of protein, carbohydrates and fats, blood sugar control and the regulation of body weight, BP and immune function
Adrenal medulla		
Main hormones	*Main functions*	
Catecholamines – adrenaline and noradrenaline	Non-steroid hormones that help to manage heart rate and BP, gut motility, pupil and airway dilation and the break down of glycogen and fatty acids	
Adrenomedullin	Regulatory peptide required for the vascular, endocrine, kidney and nervous systems and for growth and development	

8.1 Adrenal fatigue

Adrenal fatigue does not constitute an accepted medical diagnosis since the conventional concept of low adrenal function is usually limited to Addison's disease. The term is however used by complementary medicine practitioners to describe 'sub-optimal or low adrenal function, characterised by a poor response to any kind of intermittent or sporadic stressor' (Heim, Ehlert and Hellhammer 2000). The hypothesis behind adrenal fatigue is that the adrenal glands fail to produce a normal quantity of the stress hormones adrenaline, noradrenaline, cortisol and DHEA, leaving an individual less able to cope with stressful situations. A reduction in adrenal function is often accompanied by the appearance of non-specific signs and symptoms, such as aches and pains, fatigue, low mood, nervousness, sleep disturbances and digestive problems. Adrenal fatigue may also be implicated in other chronic conditions such as depression, other mood disorders, chronic fatigue and fibromyalgia. It is therefore very important to ensure that patients presenting with non-specific symptoms are referred to their medical practitioner for further investigation.

8.1.1 STAGES OF ADRENAL FATIGUE

In 1936 Hans Selye started to develop his theory of the General Adaptation Syndrome (GAS) in which he described the body's response to short and long-term stressors (Selye 1979). Selye identified a number of key stages in the stress response (see Table 6.6).

Table 6.6 Adrenal hormone patterns in the different stages of stress

Stage of stress	Pattern of adrenal hormones
Stage I – Acute or alarm stage	Normal 'fight or flight' response to short term stress. Levels of adrenaline, cortisol and DHEA rise and then return to normal once the stressor is removed
Stage II – Resistance/adaptation stage	State of adrenal overstimulation. Cortisol levels continue to rise at the expense of DHEA which initially stays stable (early compensation response), and then starts to fall (late compensation stage)
Stage III – Exhaustion stage	Later phase of the compensation response in which falling levels of DHEA are followed by a subsequent fall in cortisol levels

8.1.2 DEVELOPMENT OF ADRENAL FATIGUE

A number of factors may contribute to the development of the various stages of adrenal fatigue, including:

- genetics and congenital weakness
- poor nutritional status due to an inadequate diet or poor digestion, absorption and/or elimination
- physical stimulants such as alcohol, caffeine, medical or recreational drugs or a high glycaemic load which shift the HPA axis towards sympathetic overactivity, with increases in cortisol, ACTH and noradrenaline (Tentolouris et al. 2003)
- emotional or psychological stress that constantly provokes the production of adrenal hormones in the fight or flight response
- food allergies/intolerances and infections that involve the release of histamine and other pro-inflammatory mediators, resulting in an increase in cortisol as an anti-inflammatory hormone
- presence of toxic chemicals and substances that may also result in allergic reactions. Controlling these reactions with steroid drugs may in itself create further hormone imbalance.

8.1.3 SIGNS AND SYMPTOMS OF ADRENAL FATIGUE

The many possible signs and symptoms of the different stages of adrenal fatigue can affect all systems in the body and many of the symptoms also overlap with those of hypothyroidism. Common signs and symptoms are outlined in Table 6.7.

Table 6.7 Signs and symptoms of adrenal imbalance

• Fatigue	• Poor circulation	• General depression and anxiety
• Decreased tolerance to cold	• Low blood sugar	
	• Hypotension	• Poor exercise tolerance
• Subnormal body temperature	• Joint aches and pains	• Low levels of hydrochloric acid
• Poor response to thyroxine	• Muscle weakness	• Need for excessive sleep
• Tendency to constipation	• Salt cravings	• Lowered resistance to infection
• Skin pigmentation	• Loss of body hair	• Unstable pupillary reflex
• Prolonged or slow Achilles reflex	• Allergies	

8.1.4 EFFECTS OF ADRENAL FATIGUE OVER TIME

The main effect of adrenal fatigue over time is to disrupt the individual's capacity to produce adrenaline, DHEA and cortisol. The initial impact of this disruption is often on energy levels, as cortisol and DHEA are required to keep blood sugar at adequate levels to meet energy needs. Although each individual will have their own pattern (Wilson 2001), a typical daily energy pattern in adrenal fatigue would be:

1. morning fatigue – with particular difficulty waking early in the morning
2. improvement (after midday)
3. afternoon low (2–4pm)
4. improvement (after 6pm)
5. second wind late at night (after 11pm).

Chronically elevated cortisol and catecholamine levels may lead to immunosuppression and decreased cellular immunity (McEwen 1998). High levels of cortisol also affect the consistency of the gastro-intestinal mucosal barrier and reduce the production of white blood cells and antibodies (e.g. SIgA) that help to fight infection and allergic responses (Wilson 2001). Pathogens can therefore establish themselves more easily, affecting the structural integrity of the gut wall, increasing the risk of intestinal permeability and upsetting the balance of beneficial and less beneficial bacteria in the intestine. Treatment of any stress and immune symptoms with drugs (e.g. antidepressants, analgesics, sedatives, antihistamines, bronchial dilators, etc.) can further disrupt adrenal, digestive and liver function. Individuals in this vicious cycle may need a period of recovery to restore adrenal function (Baschetti 2001).

During long-term stress the parasympathetic nervous system will be dominant in an attempt to slow the body down (Tsigos and Chrousos 2002). This may partly account for the mental health symptoms that patients with adrenal fatigue may describe. Symptoms of depression have been linked to a pattern of elevated morning cortisol and decreased DHEA production (Tafet and Smolovich 2004). In animals, sustained stress reduces serotonin turnover and the response of the 5-HT_{1A} receptor system, which is involved in depression and other mental health conditions (van Praag 2004). The production of serotonin is also inhibited by depletion of B vitamins (especially B6 and biotin) and magnesium, nutrients that are also important for the adrenal cascade. Symptoms of low serotonin status may include depression, anxiety, low energy, poor concentration, insomnia and food cravings (Birdsall 1998).

Insulin, cortisol and adrenaline also interact in an immediate and direct feedback system to influence sex hormone production (Hyman 2005, p.357). Elevated adrenaline may depress production of oestradiol in the ovaries, while high cortisol levels decrease the effects of oestrogen centrally as well as peripherally (Hays 2005, p.229). In addition, although sex hormones are primarily produced in the ovaries and testes, some production takes place in the zona reticularis of the adrenal glands, using the precursor pregnenolone. Sex hormones are also produced via the peripheral conversion of DHEA, particularly after menopause or gynaecological surgery. Disruption in adrenal function can lead to disturbances in sex hormone and DHEA production, which may result in symptoms ranging from menstrual and menopausal irregularities in women, to infertility in both sexes (Wilson 2001).

Box 6.5 Clinical practice points – Adrenal fatigue

- The term 'adrenal fatigue' is used by complementary medicine practitioners to describe 'sub-optimal or low adrenal function characterised by a poor response to any kind of intermittent or sporadic stressor'.

- In adrenal fatigue, an individual's daily energy pattern is often characterised by morning fatigue with improvements in energy later in the day.

---

9. Tests for adrenal function

9.1 Blood tests

Blood tests for cortisol are usually requested to investigate the possibility of Cushing's syndrome and Addison's disease. They may also be useful in other circumstances, e.g. to identify sodium and potassium levels, glucose status, elevated blood urea nitrogen (BUN) and thyroid function status. Many factors can affect blood test results. Cortisol levels may be higher in pregnancy, illness, hyperthyroidism and obesity and when taking certain medication, and lower in hypothyroidism and when taking steroid medication.

Cortisol levels can also be tested by a 24-hour urine collection. However, such samples reflect the total amount of cortisol produced in a 24-hour period, making it difficult to evaluate diurnal variation.

9.2 Adrenal stress index test (ASI)

In this non-invasive saliva test, samples are taken at set times over 24 hours to measure levels of free DHEA and cortisol and the ratio between the two hormones; the results are shown against a reference range for normal adrenal function. Levels of DHEA and cortisol indicate an individual's longer term response to stress and are less influenced by the daily output of adrenaline released to cope with short-term stressors. The respective levels of DHEA and cortisol, and the relationship between the two, indicate where an individual is in the stress cycle.

In summary the test measures:

- *morning cortisol levels* (peak circadian activity) – an indication of peak adrenal function

- *noon cortisol levels* – representing adrenal response to the first few hours of the day and indicative of adaptive adrenal gland function

- *afternoon cortisol levels* – postprandial sample indicative of glycaemic control

- *midnight cortisol levels* – lowest circadian activity, indicating baseline adrenal function.

10. Links between thyroid function and adrenal fatigue

Both too much and too little cortisol can affect thyroid function. A certain level of cortisol is required for the peripheral conversion of T4 to T3 in the liver and kidneys and, in adrenal fatigue, supplies of cortisol may be depleted (Pizzorno and Ferril 2005, p.645). Individuals may therefore produce sufficient T4 but be functionally deficient in thyroid hormone (Pizzorno and Ferril 2005, p.644).

Elevated levels of cortisol suppress the release of TSH and blunt the response of TSH to TRH (Kelly 2000). Where inflammation is present, cytokines can bind to thyroid peroxidase, thyroglobulin and TSH receptors, reducing the production of T4, inhibiting the conversion of T4 to T3 and again increasing the production of rT3 at the expense of T3 (Pizzorno and Ferril 2005, p.645; Vantyghem, Ghularn and Hober 1998). The stress response also results in an increase in levels of lipo-protein lipase and free fatty acids (FFAs), and FFAs may displace thyroid hormone from its carrier (Pizzorno and Ferril 2005, p.645). Elevated cortisol levels suppress immune function and may be linked to conditions such as thyroiditis and Graves' disease, due to a possible increase in the production of thyroid antibodies (Arem 1999).

Adrenaline and thyroid hormones are cardiac irritants (Carvalho-Bianco *et al.* 2004). When adrenaline is chronically elevated, T4 output may fall to reduce the negative effects on the cardiovascular system. This may lead to modest elevation in TSH with symptoms of hypothyroidism. Adding thyroxine does not improve the situation as the requirement is to balance adrenal function. High levels of adrenaline also inhibit the function of T3 at receptor level (Hays 2005, p.229).

11. Nutritional support for the modulation of thyroid and adrenal function

11.1 Overall nutritional approach

When addressing imbalances in both thyroid and adrenal function through nutritional approaches, it is usually necessary to support both glands through one overall dietary protocol, tailored to the needs of each individual.

The main aims of the nutritional management of thyroid and adrenal function are to:

- provide adequate precursors for the production, transport, conversion and tissue receptor uptake of thyroid and adrenal hormones

- support the immune system to reduce the potential for the development of autoimmune conditions

- support hepatic and intestinal detoxification and elimination.

As a general guideline, the diet should be nutritionally dense and based on complex carbohydrates, organic lean meat, poultry, fish, eggs and plant sources of protein, low-fat dairy produce, vegetables and some fruit. It should also contain sources of essential fatty acids and in particular omega-3 fats, from e.g. oily fish, nuts and seeds, to support receptor sites and the production of adrenal hormones (Delarue *et al.* 2003). Where appropriate, specific nutritional guidelines should be considered to deal with particular imbalances that may have developed as a result of adrenal stress or poor thyroid function, e.g. gut dysbiosis, intestinal permeability ('leaky gut') or other inflammatory conditions (see relevant chapters).

Blood sugar management is central to the nutritional protocol. Many people with low thyroid function feel particularly unwell first thing in the morning when blood sugar levels are usually at their lowest point. A state of low blood sugar promotes the production of adrenal hormones, in particular cortisol, to increase the supply of glucose to cells. Eating regular meals (combining fat, protein and complex carbohydrates), with two or three quality snacks of protein with complex carbohydrate should help to maintain blood sugar control and sustain energy levels.

Guidance for portion sizes will vary depending on the situation with regard to weight control. The hyperthyroid patient will have higher metabolic demands and calorie requirements than most hypothyroid patients. They may also require extra protein with severe weight loss, and a higher dietary intake of calcium and phosphorous to protect against the increased risk of osteoporosis (Ajjan and Weetman 2007; Biondi *et al.* 2005).

As well as emphasising foods to include in the diet, it is also important to reduce or eliminate foods that may be promoting immune reactions, and stimulants such as sugar, refined carbohydrates, chocolate, tobacco, alcohol, tea and coffee which may disrupt blood sugar control (see Table 6.8).

Table 6.8 Dietary guidelines for supporting thyroid and adrenal function

Build the diet around whole grains, plant proteins, lightly cooked and raw vegetables, organic, lean meat, fish and poultry, low-fat dairy produce and some fruit.
Include a wide variety of food – add a new food every week or few days.
Eat carbohydrates, fats and proteins at every meal, and protein and carbohydrate at every snack.
For sources of omega-6 and omega-3 fatty acids, include 1–2 tbsp of mixed nuts and seeds (e.g. almonds, walnuts, brazil nuts, pecans, linseed (flaxseeds), hemp, pumpkin, sesame and sunflower seeds), or nut or seed oil, daily; or 2–4 x 140g portions of fresh oily fish per week (depending on age and gender). Avoid tuna, swordfish and marlin because of pollution levels.
Include whole grains (brown rice, barley, oats, quinoa, buckwheat, whole wheat, millet, rye) as sources of complex carbohydrates.
Eat plenty of vegetables. With low thyroid function, cook vegetables in the brassica family (cabbage, kale, Brussels sprouts, broccoli, kohlrabi, turnips) before eating (see section 11.2.4).
Add beans, seeds and nuts for sources of plant protein. Limit intake of soya protein to 2–3 portions/week to avoid any possible effects of soy isoflavones on low thyroid function (Rice, Graves and Larson 1995) (see section 11.2.4).
Avoid coffee, cola, alcohol, black tea and chocolate drinks. Guidelines for total daily fluid intake vary from organisation to organisation. In 2009: <ul><li>the Food Standards Agency (FSA) recommended a total intake of 1.2 litres of fluid/day (Food Standards Agency 2009)</li><li>the British Dietetic Association (BDA) and the British Nutrition Foundation (BNF) recommended a total intake of 1.5–2.5 litres of fluid per day (British Dietetic Association 2009; British Nutrition Foundation 2009).</li></ul> It is important to notice that these guidelines cover *total* fluids consumed and not just water. It is useful to monitor urine output and colour to judge hydration status.
Chew thoroughly.
Avoid eating fruit alone or as juice first thing in the morning to help manage blood sugar levels. At other times, eat fruit *before* meals if digestive symptoms (e.g. bloating, flatulence, acid reflux) occur when fruit is eaten after a meal.
Avoid sugar and refined white flour products. Also consider possible intolerance to gluten, lactose or casein in wheat and dairy products.

11.2 Specific dietary actions for thyroid function

11.2.1 NUTRIENTS AND FOODS THAT SUPPORT THYROID HORMONE PRODUCTION AND CONVERSION

To further enhance the building blocks for thyroid hormone production it is important to include dietary sources of:

- *iodine*: The richest food sources of iodine are fish (salmon, sardines), seafood and sea vegetables (e.g. kelp, dulse, nori, arame, wakame, kombu) followed by eggs, milk and milk products, meat and marine iodised salt. Vegetarians, vegans and other population groups who do not regularly consume these products need to pay particular attention to obtaining sufficient iodine from the diet (Davidsson 1999; Remer, Neubert and Manz 1999).

- *iron*: Iron deficiency may reduce the activity of thyroid peroxidase in the production of T4 and the conversion of T4 to T3 (via 5'-deiodinase), and modify the binding of T3 to receptors (Zimmerman and Köhrle 2002). Low iron status may also increase circulating levels of TSH and reduce the efficacy of iodine supplementation (Zimmerman and Köhrle 2002). Hypothyroid females with heavy periods may have a greater risk of low iron levels. Food sources of iron include meat, poultry, fish, nuts and seeds, legumes and pulses, dried fruits, e.g. apricots, whole grains and fortified cereals.

- *zinc*: Human and animal data indicate that zinc is required for selenocysteine-containing proteins such as 5'-deiodinase, conversion of T4 to T3 and the configuration of T3 receptors (Arthur and Beckett 1999; Kralik, Eder and Kirchgessner 1996). With vitamin C and vitamin E, zinc may protect against cadmium toxicity. Animal studies suggest that cadmium may affect pituitary and thyroid hormones (Lafuente, Cano and Esquifino 2003). Useful food sources of zinc include fresh oysters, ginger root, lamb, pecans, almonds, walnuts, brazil nuts, whole wheat, rye, oats and sardines.

- *Tyrosine*: Tyrosine is derived from phenylalanine and found in avocados, pumpkin and sesame seeds, cashew nuts, bananas and dairy products. Although supplementation with tyrosine does not appear to increase the production of thyroid hormones specifically, adequate protein intake is important for overall nutritional status and hormone production (Bland and Jones 2005, p.602). Tyrosine is also required for the production of noradrenaline, adrenaline and dopamine.

- *vitamin A*: Vitamin A as retinol is needed for the uptake of iodine (Hess and Zimmermann 2004; Zimmermann *et al*. 2004). It is also required for T3 to bind to intracellular receptors (Pizzorno and Ferril 2005, p.646). Retinoid and carotenoid status can be disrupted in both hypo- and hyperthyroid states. Low levels of retinol and betacarotene (vitamin A precursor) have been observed in hyperthyroid patients, while both increases *and* decreases in serum levels of betacarotene and retinol have been noted in hypothyroid patients (Aktuna, Buchinger and Langsteger 1993; Goswami and Choudhury 1999).

Vitamin A status seems to be maintained above deficiency levels where the supply of dietary protein is enough for the liver to produce sufficient retinol-binding protein (RBP) and pre-albumin (Aktuna *et al.* 1993). Zinc is also required for the production of RBP (Aktuna *et al.* 1993).

Food sources of vitamin A include cheese, eggs, oily fish (particularly mackerel), milk, fortified vegetable margarine and yoghurt. Food sources of the carotenoids include yellow and orange vegetables and fruits, including squashes, pumpkins, carrots, apricots, melon, papaya, nectarines, peaches, and green (leafy) vegetables such as spinach, kale, and broccoli.

11.2.2 NUTRIENTS AND FOODS FOR SYMPTOMS OF FATIGUE AND LOW ENERGY

B vitamins are important for the production of energy and for mental health, especially:

- *vitamin B2*: from organ meats, almonds, milk, wild rice, mushrooms, egg yolks, green vegetables

- *vitamin B3*: from rice bran, peanuts, liver, turkey, chicken, dairy products, salmon, mackerel, eggs

- *vitamin B6*: from sunflower seeds, tuna, liver, walnuts, salmon, trout, lentils, beans, brown rice and bananas.

11.2.3 FOOD CONTAINING ANTIOXIDANTS

Antioxidant nutrients may be particularly important in hyperthyroid conditions which are characterised by the over-production of free radicals. Sources include:

- *vitamin C*: from peppers, parsley, green leafy vegetables, strawberries, papaya, and citrus fruits

- *vitamin E*: from sunflower seeds, almonds, peanut oil, olive oil, peanuts, and wheat germ.

11.2.4 THYROID FUNCTION AND FOOD – KEY CAUTIONS

Gluten

Coeliac disease in adults has been associated with autoimmune thyroid diseases, and thyroid disorders have been associated with coeliac disease (Sategna-Guidetti *et al.* 1998). Removing gluten from the diet may help to resolve both the coeliac and the thyroid conditions (Sategna-Guidetti *et al.* 2001).

Box 6.6 Selenium and thyroid function

Selenium is required for the iodination and peripheral deiodination of thyroid hormones and for the maintenance of thyroidal glutathione peroxidase (GPx) and thioredoxin reductase (TR) which protect the thyrocytes, and support immune function, during thyroid hormone production (Beckett and Arthur 2005).

Reference ranges

There are no internationally accepted 'normal' reference ranges for selenium due to complexities in defining normal, optimal or suboptimal intakes and status, and limited understanding of the distribution and roles of the various selenoproteins and species of selenium in different human tissues (Rayman 2008; Rayman, Goenaga Infante and Sargent 2008; Thomson 2004). The baseline selenium requirement to avoid Keshan's disease is 19µg/day, corrected for body weight to 21µg/day for men and 16µg/day for women (WHO/FAO/IAEA 1996 cited in Thomson 2004, p.393).

Selenium in the UK

In the UK:

- the reference nutrient intakes (RNIs) for selenium are 75 and 60 µg/day for adult men and women respectively (Rayman 2000). These figures were originally based on the intake required to maximise the activity of GPx in plasma, which occurs at about 95 (range 89–114) µg/L (Rayman 2000) or 40–50µg/day, but have recently been questioned (Rayman 2008; Turker *et al.* 2006)

- the LRNI is 40µg/day (Murray, Pizzorno and Pizzorno 2005; Rayman 2000)

- the average daily dietary intake is estimated at 29–39µg/day, above the threshold for deficiency diseases, about half the RNI and possibly just below the optimum level (40–50µg/day) for maximising blood and plasma GPx activity (Food Standards Agency 2009; Rayman 1997).

Intake of selenium has declined considerably in the UK in the past 25 years (Rayman 1997) particularly as the import, and therefore consumption, of grains grown in the selenium-rich soils of the USA has fallen amongst both animals and humans (Rayman, Goenaga Infante and Sargent 2008). So far, no truly adverse effects have been associated with the decrease in intake and habitual low consumption of selenium in Europe (Elsom *et al.* 2006; Thomson 2004), although this may vary considerably according to geographical location (Rayman, Goenaga Infante and Sargent 2008). Estimates of intakes that are not associated with any adverse health effects suggest that 25–40µg/day of selenium may be adequate, although not necessarily optimal (Thomson 2004).

Selenium and thyroid function

Animal studies have indicated that, in selenium deficiency, the most important aspects of thyroid metabolism may be preserved by a strict hierarchy for the distribution of selenium, both to specific tissues and to different selenoenzymes within a tissue (Arthur and Beckett 1999). Similarly, in humans, deiodinase enzymes rank high in the cellular and tissue-specific hierarchy of selenium distribution among various selenoproteins (Köhrle 2005; Thomson 2004), and appear to be well protected when the supply of selenium is limited (Arthur and Beckett 1999; Zimmermann and Köhrle 2002).

Indeed, maximal activity of deiodinase enzymes may occur at dietary selenium intakes below those needed for maximal GPx activity (Thomson 2004), and 30µg/day, corresponding to a plasma selenium concentration of 0.82µmol/l or 65µg/l, could be adequate for optimal deiodinase activity (Duffield *et al.* 1999; Thomson *et al.* 2005).

Other metabolic adaptations to low selenium intake include a reduction in excretion (Hawkes and Keim 2003, Hawkes *et al.* 2008).

A large intervention study (Rayman *et al.* 2008) found that supplementing up to 300µg/ day of selenium from yeast in euthyroid elderly subjects did not result in a significant difference in thyroid hormone conversion, despite an increase in plasma selenium status. Although baseline plasma selenium in this study was a little higher (average 91µg/L) than in other studies that have shown benefit for selenium supplementation on T4 to T3 conversion (e.g. Arthur *et al.* 1997; Olivieri *et al.* 1995, 1996), the researchers still concluded that there was no indication for increasing selenium intake to benefit thyroid hormone conversion in the elderly in the UK.

Whilst deiodinase activity appears to be protected when selenium supply is limited, it is still important to maintain an appropriate intake of selenium to optimise the expression of thyroidal GPx and protect against the potential development and maintenance of autoimmune thyroid disease (Arthur and Beckett 1999; Bohnet, Broyer and Peters 2005; Gartner, Gasnier and Dietrich 2002; Rayman 2002). The amount of selenium required to optimise this protection is not yet established (Turker et al. 2006; Rayman 2008).

Selenium and hyperthyroidism

In hyperthyroidism levels of plasma selenium and red cell GPx can fall because hyperthyroidism may reduce the half-life of selenoproteins (Arthur and Beckett 1999).

Coexisting selenium and iodine deficiency

Individuals who are *severely* deficient in both selenium and iodine, or who have a goitre, should not supplement selenium without first receiving iodine or thyroid hormone supplementation. Selenium deficiency with iodine deficiency increases plasma T4 through inhibition of the deiodinases. When selenium is replenished, more T4 is rapidly converted to T3; however, without sufficient iodine, the thyroid is unable to increase T4 output in response to the increased T4 metabolism. Selenium supplementation further impaired thyroid function and goitre in children with cretinism, who were deficient in both selenium and iodine (Contempre, Dumont and Ngo 1991; Köhrle 2005; Vanderpas *et al.* 1993).

Food sources of selenium

Brazil nuts are the richest food source of selenium, although the content varies and brazil nuts frequently contain the toxic metals barium and radium (Rayman 2008). In the UK other food sources of selenium are meat, poultry and fish, followed by bread and cereals. Seeds, seafood and eggs also contain some selenium.

Selenium may protect against mercury, cadmium and silver in marine foods by forming inert metal selenide complexes (Rayman 2000; Soldin, O'Mara and Aschner 2008). However, this may also reduce the bioavailability of selenium from these foods (Rayman 2000).

Toxicity

Selenium has a small therapeutic window and so it is important not to overconsume selenium supplements (Rayman 2000).

Soy isoflavones

The isoflavones in soy (principally genistein and daidzein) have been associated with blocking the activity of thyroid peroxidase in the iodination and coupling reactions required for the production of thyroid hormones (Doerge and Chang 2002; Doerge and Sheehan 2002). Soy isoflavones may also interfere with the thyroid-binding protein transthyretin (TTR), possibly altering the overall distribution of thyroid hormones in the body (Green et al. 2005; Radović, Mentrup and Köhrle 2006). Although these anti-thyroid effects have mainly been noted in vitro and in studies with iodine-deficient rats (Doerge and Sheehan 2002), an increase in TSH within the normal range has been reported in adult humans in the absence of iodine deficiency (Ishizuki et al. 1991) and in children with congenital hypothyroidism or autoimmune thyroid disease fed on soya formula (Fort et al. 1990; Jabbar, Larrea and Shaw 1997). Isoflavones have also been shown to inhibit the sulphotransferase enzymes involved in the inactivation and elimination of thyroid hormones and the recovery of iodine in human thyroid tissue (Ebmeier and Anderson 2004).

While the full clinical significance of these effects is still unknown, it would seem prudent to ensure adequate dietary levels of iodine and selenium if consuming soy isoflavones (Bland and Jones 2005), and to consider the particular needs of special population groups, e.g. infants with congenital hypothyroidism, postmenopausal women consuming soy isoflavones and the elderly (Committee on Toxicity (COT) 2003; Doerge and Sheehan 2002). Eating soya products simultaneously with taking thyroid replacement hormone may reduce absorption of such hormones (Bell and Ovalle 2001) making it advisable not to consume soya products within three hours of taking thyroid medication.

Cruciferous vegetables

Cruciferous vegetables such as broccoli, cauliflower, Brussels sprouts, cabbage, kohlrabi and turnips are dietary sources of glucosinolates that are often labelled 'goitrogenic' and associated with disrupted thyroid function. However, there are very few controlled studies on the relationship between glucosinolates and their effect on thyroid function, and it is important for practitioners to understand how these compounds are broken down and metabolised.

Glucosinolates remain intact unless they are hydrolysed by the plant enzyme myrosinase (following chewing or food processing), or by bacterial myrosinase in the colon (Johnson 2002). Myrosinase releases glucose and breakdown products such as isothiocyanates, the specific compounds that are said to interfere with iodine uptake and thyroid function (Shapiro et al. 1998).

Cooking appears to denature the plant myrosinase, thereby reducing the production of isothiocyanates (Conaway et al. 2000; Rouzaud, Young and Duncan 2004; Rungapamestry et al. 2007). Cooking also affects the site of release of breakdown products from glucosinolates. When cruciferous vegetables are eaten raw, breakdown products are released in the upper gastro-intestinal (GI) tract. Following cooking, glucosinolates are hydrolysed in the colon under the action of the resident microflora. Feeding trials in humans have shown that the hydrolysis of glucosinolates and the absorption of isothiocyanates are much reduced after eating cooked, as opposed to raw, cruciferous vegetables (Conaway *et al.* 2000; Rungapamestry *et al.* 2007).

Individuals with thyroid disorders can probably continue to include lightly cooked cruciferous vegetables in their diet to try to obtain some of the important health benefits of the breakdown products of glucosinolates (Halkier and Gershenzon 2006).

11.2.5 NUTRITIONAL SUPPLEMENTS FOR SUPPORTING THYROID FUNCTION – USE AND KEY CAUTIONS

It is always important to maximise dietary changes to improve nutritional status, digestion and elimination in support of thyroid function *before* considering the use of nutritional supplements. The digestive system and liver detoxification must be functioning effectively for nutrients in supplements to be absorbed and metabolised. Even where supplementation is considered, if a patient is being treated with replacement thyroid hormone or monitored for sub-clinical hypothyroidism, any supplement programme must be managed in collaboration with the patient's GP or prescribing medical professional, and in line with the results of regular laboratory tests. It is important to take account of upper safety limits for all nutrients and to be aware that, in combination with thyroxine, individuals may be more sensitive to the effects of supplements.

Iodine

High iodine intake can precipitate autoimmune attacks on the thyroid (Arem 1999), and iodine supplementation is probably not necessary for most people (Delange 1998; Rose, Saboori and Rasooly 1997). Urinary iodine excretion is a good marker of recent dietary intake of iodine (WHO, UNICEF and ICCIDD 2001). Self-test approaches available on the internet are unlikely to be sufficiently accurate.

Iron

Iron deficiency must be identified by a medical professional testing for ferritin levels before any supplementation is provided, as iron supplements may *decrease* absorption of thyroid hormone medication (Campbell, Hasinoff and Stalts 1992). Iron supplements (including multivitamin and mineral and pre-natal formulations) should not be taken within four hours of taking thyroid replacement hormone.

Calcium

Thyroid hormone replacement may increase urinary loss of calcium (Kung and Pun 1991), although thyroid hormone replacement may not necessarily be associated with reduced bone density (Schneider, Barrett-Connor and Morton 1994, 1995). Calcium supplementation for those on long-term thyroid medication has not yet been proven to be either helpful or necessary.

Calcium formulations should not be taken within four hours of taking thyroid replacement hormone (Singh, Singh and Hershman 2000).

Niacin

Supplementing niacin at high doses to manage levels of cholesterol and triglycerides may decrease thyroid hormone levels (O'Brien, Silverberg and Nguyen 1992; Shakir, Kroll and Aprill 1995).

L-carnitine

Supplementation of L-carnitine at 2–4g/day has been shown to improve some symptoms of **hyperthyroidism** (Benvenga, Ruggeri and Russo 2001). Theoretically, therefore, high levels of carnitine could exacerbate symptoms of hypothyroidism.

Commiphora mukul, Gum guggul, Guggulsterones

These compounds may be helpful for patients with low thyroid function who find it difficult to lose weight (Antonio *et al.* 1999). They may also support dyslipidaemia (Singh, Chander and Kapoor 1997). Once again, the action of guggulsterones may potentiate the effect of thyroid replacement hormone (Antonio *et al.* 1999).

Lipoic acid

Lipoic acid may suppress the production of T3 when given in conjunction with T4 therapy (Segermann *et al.* 1991).

Fibre supplements

In vitro investigations suggest that dietary fibre supplements may decrease the bioavailability of thyroid hormone replacement, due to non-specific binding of thyroxine to fibre, particularly in soluble form in the gut, and increased clearance of T4 (Liel, Harman-Boehm and Shany 1996). However, a similar effect was not seen when certain forms of pharmacological fibre supplements (calcium polycarbophil or psyllium hydrophilic mucilloid) were taken along with thyroid replacement hormone (Chiu and Sherman 1998). A good intake of *dietary* fibre is important to support the management of constipation that frequently accompanies hypothyroid conditions.

Flavonoids

Flavonoids found in vegetables, fruits, grains, nuts, wine and tea may interfere with thyroid hormone production and availability, even though epidemiological studies indicate that these naturally occurring compounds generally have beneficial effects on health, due to their role as antioxidants. *In vivo* and *in vitro* studies using synthetic and natural flavonoids indicate that T4 is displaced from the carrier protein transthyretin, resulting in changes in the amount of thyroid hormone available to tissues (Köhrle 1992; Van der Heide, Kastelyn and Schroeder-van de Elst 2003). Synthetic flavonoid derivatives have also been shown to reduce FT4 concentrations in serum and inhibit both the conversion of T4 to FT3 and the clearance of rT3 (Köhrle 1992; Köhrle *et al.* 1988).

Box 6.7 Clinical practice points – Supplementation and thyroid function

- Maximise dietary changes to improve nutritional status, digestion and elimination in support of thyroid function *before* considering the use of dietary supplements.

- If a patient is being treated with replacement thyroid hormone or monitored for sub-clinical hypothyroidism, any supplementation programme *must* be managed in collaboration with the patient's GP or prescribing medical professional, and in line with the results of regular laboratory tests.

- Iron supplements (including multivitamin and mineral and pre-natal formulations) and calcium formulations should not be taken within four hours of taking thyroid replacement hormone.

11.3 Nutritional supplements for adrenal function – use and cautions

It is equally important to maximise dietary changes to improve nutritional status, digestion, detoxification and elimination to support the adrenal glands *before* considering dietary supplements, particularly for individuals in an advanced stage of the stress cycle where digestion and detoxification may be considerably compromised. Any supplement programme should always be managed in collaboration with the patient's medical practitioner. Restoring adrenal function may improve the uptake of thyroid replacement hormone and could result in thyrotoxicity.

Supplements to consider for supporting adrenal function could include:

- *vitamin C*: This is especially concentrated in the adrenal glands where it is required, with magnesium and pantothenic acid (B5) (Lukaski 2000), for production of cortisol and throughout the adrenal cascade. It also appears to act as an antioxidant in the adrenals themselves (Peters *et al.* 2001). Intake of vitamin C should always be increased and decreased with caution, particularly if the patient is on anti-coagulant medication.

- *vitamin E*: This is indirectly essential in key enzymatic reactions in the adrenal cascade. With vitamin C, it also helps to neutralise free radicals produced in the manufacture of adrenal hormones. Food sources of vitamin E include nuts and seeds, almonds, olive oil, green, leafy vegetables, peanuts and whole grains. Mixed tocopherols are the most useful supplement form. Vitamin E should not be supplemented with anti-coagulant medication.

- *B vitamins*: The entire B-complex is needed in small amounts throughout the adrenal cascade. In particular: B5 is used in the conversion of glucose to energy; B3 is required for the production of niacin-dependent coenzymes required in the adrenal cascade; and B6 is a co-factor in many enzymatic pathways (Heap, Peters and Wessely 1999). Useful food sources of B vitamins include whole grains, cereals, brewers' yeast, almonds, miso, liver, milk, fish, sprouts and green leafy vegetables.

- *magnesium*: This is used in many enzyme reactions in the body, in the metabolism of carbohydrates, fats and proteins and with vitamin C and pantothenic acid to support adrenal function (Lukaski 2000). Magnesium is also important for glucose homeostasis (Paolisso and Barbagallo 1997; Rosolova, Mayer and Reaven 1997). Useful food sources of magnesium include brown rice, beans, nuts, seeds and sea vegetables.

- *L-tyrosine, phosphatidyl serine or precursors*: These may reduce high cortisol levels. Supplements should be used in conjunction with test results to ensure that low levels of cortisol (e.g. in the exhaustion phase of stress) are not further reduced. Supplements should be taken at the meal preceding the high point of cortisol production. Note that tyrosine may potentiate thyroid replacement hormone (Van Spronsen, van Rijn and Bekhof 2001).

- *adrenal glandular/adrenal cortical extracts*: These are liquid or powder extracts of the adrenal cortex, usually from bovine adrenal glands. They are described as providing essential constituents for supporting adrenal function; however, their mechanism of action is not well understood. They are not suitable for vegetarians and vegans and should be used only under the supervision of professionals trained in their prescription.

- *DHEA*: Under stress the body produces dehydroepiandrosterone (DHEA) from dehydroepiandrosterone sulphate (DHEA-S) in the zona reticularis of the adrenal cortex and in the liver. Adults with primary or secondary adrenal insufficiency often have low levels of both DHEA and DHEA-S, and levels may also be low in adrenal fatigue (Wilson 2001).

  DHEA is frequently presented as something of a 'wonder hormone' for a wide range of conditions and scenarios linked to ageing and there is increasing public enthusiasm for purchasing DHEA via the internet for self-administration. However, although Arlt *et al.* (1999) did demonstrate that DHEA replacement in women with adrenal insufficiency had some positive effects for depression, anxiety, general wellbeing, cholesterol status and the physical aspects of sexuality, very few clinical trials have been done on the safety of the long-term use of DHEA. In addition, DHEA is a precursor to androgens and many women, particularly those who may be hyperandrogenic, may not benefit from DHEA unless their adrenal fatigue is considerable (Wilson 2001). In the UK, only a qualified medical practitioner may prescribe or administer hormones.

11.4 Herbal medicine

Adaptogenic herbs such as Siberian ginseng (*Eleutherococcus senticosus* or *sinensis*), rhodiola (*Rhodiola rosea*), maca (*Lepidium meyenii*) and products such as liquorice root and ashwaganda (*Withania somnifera*) have been investigated for their role in supporting thyroid and adrenal function. Advice from an appropriately qualified practitioner of herbal medicine may be helpful for some patients.

11.5 Additional support for thyroid and adrenal function

11.5.1 OTHER BIOCHEMICAL IMBALANCES

It is important to consider other possible biochemical balances that may be present when working to balance thyroid and adrenal function, e.g. sex hormone function, essential fatty acid status, presence of gut dysbiosis and/or intestinal permeability, food intolerances, poor absorption and detoxification. Many of these imbalances can be addressed through the nutritional guidelines outlined above and in other chapters of this publication.

11.5.2 EXERCISE

Exercise promotes thyroid function and increases tissue sensitivity to both thyroid hormones and insulin. An exercise programme must be appropriate for the individual, bearing in mind the degree of thyroid and adrenal imbalance. Appropriate activities could include walking, swimming, cycling, yoga, meditation, relaxation, and tai chi. Excessive or intense exercise may place additional stress on adrenal function.

11.5.3 XENOBIOTICS

Toxic metals, pesticides, hormone and antibiotic residues and smoking have all been shown to impact on thyroid function (Pizzorno and Ferril 2005, p.647). Fluoride in tap water and toothpaste, and chlorine in tap water may also interfere with iodine receptors (Jooste *et al.* 1999).

References

Ajjan, R.A. and Weetman, A.P. (2007) 'Medical management of hyperthyroidism.' *European Endocrine Disease.* Available at http://www.touchendocrinology.com/files/article_pdfs/endo_7494, accessed 2 December 2009.

Aktuna, D., Buchinger, W. and Langsteger, W. (1993) 'Beta-carotene, vitamin A and carrier proteins in thyroid diseases.' *Acta Medica Austriaca 20*, 17–20.

American Association of Clinical Endocrinologists (AACE) (2002) 'Medical guidelines for clinical practice for the evaluation and treatment of hyperthyroidism and hypothyroidism.' *Endocrine Practice 8*, 6, 457–469.

Antonio, J., Colker, C.M., Torina, G.C., Shi, Q., Brink, W.D. and Kalman, D. (1999) 'Effects of a standardized guggulsterone phosphate supplement on body composition in overweight adults: A pilot study.' *Current Therapeutic Research Clinical and Experimental 60*, 4, 220–227.

Arem, R. (1999) *The Thyroid Solution.* New York: Ballantine Books.

Arlt, W., Callies, F., van Vlijmen, J.C., Koehler, I. *et al.* (1999) 'Dehydroepiandrosterone replacement in women with adrenal insufficiency.' *New England Journal of Medicine 341*, 14, 1013–1020.

Arthur, J.R. and Beckett, G.J. (1999) 'Thyroid function.' *British Medical Bulletin 55*, 658–668.

Arthur, J.R., Nicol, F., Mitchell, J.H. and Beckett, G.J. (1997) 'Selenium and iodine deficiencies and selenoprotein function.' *Biomedical and Environmental Sciences 10*, 2–3, 129–135.

Asa, S.L. and Ezzat, S. (2002) 'Medical management of pituitary adenomas: structural and ultrastructural changes.' *Pituitary 5*, 2,133–139.

Baisier, W.V., Hertoghe, J. and Eeckhaut, W. (2000) 'Thyroid insufficiency: Is TSH measurement the only tool?' *Journal of Nutrition and Environmental Medicine 10*, 105–115.

Barnes, B.O. and Galton, L. (1976) *Hypothyroidism: The Unsuspected Illness.* New York: Harper Collins.

Baschetti, R. (2001) 'Chronic fatigue syndrome, decreased exercise capacity, and adrenal insufficiency.' *Archives of Internal Medicine 161*, 12, 1558–1559.

Beastall, G.H. and Thomson, J.A. (1997) 'Treating hypothyroidism. Biochemical tests are important in diagnosis.' *British Medical Journal 315*, 7106, 490.

Beckett, G.J. and Toft, A.D. (2003) 'First-line thyroid function tests – TSH alone is not enough.' *Clinical Endocrinology 58*, 20–21.

Beckett, G.J. and Arthur, J.R. (2005) 'Selenium and endocrine systems.' *Journal of Endocrinology 184*, 3, 455–465.

Bell, D.S. and Ovalle, F. (2001) 'Use of soy protein supplement and resultant need for increased dose of levothyroxine.' *Endocrine Practice 3*, 193–194.

Benvenga, S., Ruggeri, R.M. and Russo, A. (2001) 'Usefulness of L-carnitine, a naturally occurring peripheral antagonist of thyroid hormone action, in iatrogenic hyperthyroidism: A randomized, double-blind, placebo-controlled clinical trial.' *Journal of Clinical Endocrinology and Metabolism 86*, 3579–3594.

Bhattacharyya, A. and Wiles P.G. (2000) 'The aetiology and pathology of thyroid diseases.' *Hospital Pharmacist 7*, 1, 6–13.

Biondi, B., Palmieri, E.A., Lombardi, G. and Fazio, S. (2002) 'Effects of subclinical thyroid dysfunction on the heart.' *Annals of Internal Medicine 137*, 11, 904–914.

Biondi, B., Palmieri, E.A., Klain, M., Schlumberger, M., Filetti, S. and Lombardi, G. (2005) 'Subclinical hyperthyroidism: Clinical features and treatment options.' *European Journal of Endocrinology 152*, 1, 1–9.

Birdsall, T.C. (1998) '5-Hydroxytryptophan: A clinically-effective serotonin precursor.' *Alternative Medicine Review 3*, 4, 271–280.

Bland, J.S. and Jones, D.S. (2005) 'Cellular messaging, Part II – Tissue sensitivity and intracellular response.' In D.S. Jones (ed.) *Textbook of Functional Medicine*. Gig Harbour, WA: Institute for Functional Medicine.

Bohnet, H.G., Broyer, P.A. and Peters, N. (2005) 'Incidence of selenium deficiency in thyroid disease.' Paper presented at British Endocrine Societies 24th Joint Meeting 4–6 April, Harrogate, UK. *Endocrine Abstracts 9*, P173.

British Dietetic Association (2009) 'Fluid – Why you need it and how to get enough.' Available at www.bda.uk.com/foodfacts/070606_fluid.pdf, accessed 2 December 2009.

British Nutrition Foundation (2009) 'Liquids.' Available at www.nutrition.org.uk/nutritionscience/nutrients/liquids?start=1, accessed 2 December 2009.

British Thyroid Association (2007) *Armour Thyroid (USP) and combined thyroxine/tri-iodothyronine as Thyroid Hormone Replacement. A Statement from the British Thyroid Association*. February Available at www.british-thyroid-association.org/info-for-patients/Docs/bta_Armour_T4_T3.pdf, accessed 13 March 2010.

British Thyroid Foundation, British Thyroid Association and The Association for Clinical Chemistry (2006) *UK Guidelines for the Use of Thyroid Function Tests*. Available at http://www.british-thyroid-association.org/info-for-patients/Docs/TFT_guideline_final_version_July_2006.pdf, accessed 27 November 2009.

Bunevicius, R. and Prange, A.J. (2000) 'Mental improvement after replacement therapy with thyroxine plus triiodothyronine: Relationship to cause of hypothyroidism.' *International Journal of Neuropsychopharmacology 3*, 2, 167–174.

Bunevicius, R., Kazanavicius, G., Zalinkevicius, R. and Prange, A.J. Jr. (1999) 'Effects of thyroxine as compared with thyroxine plus triiodothyronine in patients with hypothyroidism.' *New England Journal of Medicine 340*, 6, 424–429.

Campbell, N.R., Hasinoff, B.B. and Stalts, H. (1992) 'Ferrous sulphate reduces thyroxine efficacy in patients with hypothyroidism.' Annals of Internal Medicine *17*, 1010–1013.

Canaris, G.J., Manowitz, N.R., Mayor, G. and Ridgway, E.C. (2000) 'The Colorado thyroid disease prevalence study.' *Archives of Internal Medicine 160*, 4, 526–534.

Carvalho-Bianco, S.D., Kim, B.W., Zhang, J.X., Harney, J.W. *et al.* (2004) 'Chronic cardiac-specific thyrotoxicosis increases myocardial beta-adrenergic responsiveness.' *Molecular Endocrinology 18*, 7, 1840–1849.

Chiu, A.C. and Sherman, S.I. (1998) 'Effects of pharmacological fibre supplements on levothyroxine absorption.' *Thyroid 8*, 8, 667–671.

Choe, W. and Hays, M.T. (1995) 'Absorption of oral thyroxine.' *Endocrinologist 5*, 222–228.

Committee on Toxicity of Chemicals in Food, Consumer Products and the Environment (2003) *Phytoestrogens and Health*. London: Food Standards Agency.

Conaway, C.C., Getahun, S.M., Liebes, L.L., Pusateri, D.J. *et al.* (2000) 'Disposition of glucosinolates and sulforaphane in humans after ingestion of steamed and fresh broccoli.' *Nutrition and Cancer 38*, 2, 168–178.

Contempre, B., Dumont, J.E. and Ngo, B. (1991) 'Effect of selenium supplementation in hypothyroid subjects of an iodine and selenium deficient area: the possible danger of indiscriminate supplementation of iodine-deficient subjects with selenium.' *Journal of Clinical Endocrinology and Metabolism 73*, 213–215.

Davidsson, L. (1999) 'Are vegetarians an 'at risk group' for iodine deficiency?' *British Journal of Nutrition 81*, 1, 3–4.

Dayan, C.M. (2001) 'Interpretation of thyroid function tests.' *Lancet 357*, 619–624.

De Groot, L.J. (1999) 'Dangerous dogmas in medicine: The nonthyroidal illness syndrome.' *Journal of Clinical Endocrinology and Metabolism 84*, 1, 151–164.

Delange, F. (1998) 'Risks and benefits of iodine supplementation.' *Lancet 351*, 9107, 923–924.

Delarue, J., Matzinger, O., Binnert, C., Schneiter, P., Chiolero, R. and Tappy, L. (2003) 'Fish oil prevents the adrenal activation elicited by mental stress in healthy men.' *Diabetes and Metabolism 3*, 289–295.

De los Santos, E.T., Starich, G.H. and Mazzaferri, E.L. (1989) 'Sensitivity, specificity, and cost-effectiveness of the sensitive thyrotropin assay in the diagnosis of thyroid disease in ambulatory patients.' *Archives of Internal Medicine 149*, 3, 526–532.

Doerge, D.R. and Chang, H.C. (2002) 'Inactivation of thyroid peroxidase by soy isoflavones, in vitro and in vivo.' *Journal of Chromatography B, Analytical Technologies in the Biomedical and Life Sciences 777*, 1–2, 269–279.

Doerge, D.R. and Sheehan D.M. (2002) 'Goitrogenic and estrogenic activity of soy isoflavones.' *Environmental Health Perspectives 110*, suppl. 3, 349–353.

Downing, J. (2000) 'Hypothyroidism: Treating the patient not the laboratory.' *Journal of Nutritional and Environmental Medicine 10*, 101–103.

Duffield, A.J., Thomson, C.D., Hill, K.E. and Williams, S. (1999) 'An estimation of selenium requirements for New Zealanders.' *American Journal of Clinical Nutrition 70*, 896–903.

Ebmeier, C.C. and Anderson, R.J. (2004) 'Human thyroid phenol sulfotransferase enzymes 1A1 and 1A3: Activities in normal and diseased thyroid glands, and inhibition by thyroid hormones and phytoestrogens.' *Journal of Clinical Endocrinology and Metabolism 89*, 11, 5597–5605.

Elsom, R., Sanderson, P., Hesketh, J.E., Jackson, M.J. *et al.* (2006) 'Functional markers of selenium status: UK Food Standards Agency workshop report.' *British Journal of Nutrition 96*, 5, 980–984.

Escobar-Morreale, H.F., Botella-Carretero, J.I., Escobar del Rey, F. and Morreale de Escobar, G. (2005) 'Treatment of hypothyroidism with combinations of levothyroxine plus liothyronine.' *Journal of Clinical Endocrinology and Metabolism 90*, 8, 4946–4954.

Esposito, S., Prange, A.J. Jr. and Golden, R.N. (1997) 'The thyroid axis and mood disorders: Overview and future prospects.' *Psychopharmacology Bulletin 33*, 2, 205–217.

Fatourechi, V. (2001) 'Subclinical thyroid disease.' *Mayo Clinic Proceedings 76*, 4, 413–416.

Fatourechi V. (2002a) 'Subclinical hypothyroidism: How should it be managed?' *Treatments in Endocrinology 1*, 4, 211–216.

Fatourechi V. (2002b) 'Mild thyroid failure [subclinical hypothyroidism]: To treat or not to treat?' *Comprehensive Therapy 28*, 2, 134–139.

Food Standards Agency (FSA) (2009) '8 Tips for Eating Well.' Available at www.eatwell.gov.uk/healthydiet/eighttipssection/8tips/, accessed 2 December 2009.

Fort, P., Moses, N., Fasano, M., Goldberg, T. and Lifshitz, F. (1990) 'Breast and soy-formula feedings in early infancy and the prevalence of autoimmune thyroid disease in children.' *Journal of the American College of Nutrition 9*, 2, 164–167.

Franklyn, J. and Shephard, M. (2000) *Evaluation of Thyroid Function in Health and Disease*. Available at http://www.thyroidmanager.org/Chapter6/6-frame.htm, accessed 12 February 2010.

Gartner, R., Gasnier, B.C. and Dietrich, J.W. (2002) 'Selenium supplementation in patients with autoimmune thyroiditis decreases thyroid peroxidase antibodies concentrations.' *Journal of Clinical Endocrinology and Metabolism 87*, 1687–1691.

Gharib, H., Tuttle, R.M., Baskin, H.J., Fish, L.H., Singer, P.A. and McDermott, M.T. (2005) 'Subclinical thyroid dysfunction: A joint statement on management from the American Association of Clinical Endocrinologists, the American Thyroid Association, and the Endocrine Society.' *Journal of Clinical Endocrinology and Metabolism 90*, 1, 581–585.

Glinoer, D. (1997) 'The regulation of thyroid function in pregnancy: Pathways of endocrine adaptation from physiology to pathology.' *Endocrine Reviews 18*, 3, 404–433.

Goichot, B., Sapin, R. and Schlienger, J.L. (1998) 'Euthyroid sick syndrome: Recent physiopathologic findings.' *Revue de Medicine Interne 19*, 9, 640–648.

Goswami, U.C. and Choudhury, S. (1999) 'The status of retinoids in women suffering from hyper- and hypothyroidism: Interrelationship between vitamin A, beta-carotene and thyroid hormones.' *International Journal of Vitamin Nutrition Research 69*, 2, 132–135.

Gow, S.M., Caldwell, G., Toft, A.D., Seth, J., *et al.* (1987) 'Relationship between pituitary and other target organ responsiveness in hypothyroid patients receiving thyroxine replacement.' *Journal of Clinical Endocrinology and Metabolism 64*, 2, 364–370.

Green, N.S., Foss, T.R. and Kelly, J.W. (2005) 'Genistein, a natural product from soy, is a potent inhibitor of transthyretin amyloidosis.' *Proceedings of the National Academy of Sciences of the USA 102*, 41, 14545–14550.

Grozinsky-Glasberg, S., Fraser, A., Nahshoni, E., Weizman, A. and Leibovici, L. (2006) 'Thyroxine-triiodothyronine combination therapy versus thyroxine monotherapy for clinical hypothyroidism: Meta-analysis of randomized controlled trials.' *Journal of Clinical Endocrinology and Metabolism 91*, 7, 2592–2599.

Halkier, B.A. and Gershenzon, J. (2006) 'Biology and biochemistry of glucosinolates.' *Annual Review of Plant Biology 57*, 303–333.

Harach, H.R. and Williams, E.D. (1995) 'Thyroid cancer and thyroiditis in the goitrous region of Salta, Argentina, before and after iodine prophylaxis.' *Clinical Endocrinology 43*, 6, 701–706.

Hawkes, W.C. and Keim, N.L. (2003) 'Dietary selenium intake modulates thyroid hormone and energy metabolism in men.' *Journal of Nutrition 133*, 11, 3443–3448.

Hawkes, W.C., Richter, B.D., Alkan, Z., Souza, E.C. *et al.* (2008) 'Response of selenium status indicators to supplementation of healthy North American men with high-selenium yeast.' *Biological Trace Element Research 122*, 2, 107–121.

Hays, B. (2005) 'Female hormones: The dance of the hormones, part 1.' In D.S. Jones and S. Quinn (eds) *Textbook of Functional Medicine*. Gig Harbour, WA: Institute for Functional Medicine.

Heap, L.C., Peters, T.J. and Wessely, S. (1999) 'Vitamin B status in patients with chronic fatigue syndrome.' *Journal of the Royal Society of Medicine 4*, 183–185.

Heim, C., Ehlert, U. and Hellhammer, D.H. (2000) 'The potential role of hypocortisolism in the pathophysiology of stress-related bodily disorders.' *Psychoneuroendocrinology 25*, 1, 1–35.

Henneman, G., Doctor, R., Visser, T.J. and Postema, P.T. (2004) 'Thyroxine plus low-dose slow release triiodothyronine replacement in hypothyroidism – proof of principle.' *Thyroid 14*, 4, 271–275.

Hess, S.Y. and Zimmermann, M.B. (2004) 'The effect of micronutrient deficiencies on iodine nutrition and thyroid metabolism.' *International Journal for Vitamin and Nutrition Research 74*, 103–115.

Hyman, M. (2005) 'Clinical approaches to environmental inputs.' In D.S. Jones and S. Quinn (eds) *Textbook of Functional Medicine*. Gig Harbour, WA: Institute for Functional Medicine.

International Council for Control of Iodine Deficiency Disorders (2008) *IDD Newsletter 29*, 3, 9.

Ishizuki, Y., Hirooka, Y., Murata, Y. and Togashi, K. (1991) 'The effects on the thyroid gland of soybeans administered experimentally in healthy subjects.' *Nippon Naibunpi Gakkai Zasshi 67*, 5, 622–629.

Jabbar, M.A., Larrea, J. and Shaw, R.A. (1997) 'Abnormal thyroid function tests in infants with congenital hypothyroidism: The influence of soy-based formula.' *Journal of the American College of Nutrition 16*, 3, 280–282.

Johnson, I.T. (2002) 'Glucosinolates: Bioavailability and importance to health.' *International Journal of Vitamin Nutrition Research 72*, 1, 26–31.

Jooste, P.L., Weight, M.J., Kriek, J.A. and Louw, A.J. (1999) 'Endemic goitre in the absence of iodine deficiency in schoolchildren of the Northern Cape Province of South Africa.' *European Journal of Clinical Nutrition 53*, 1, 8–12.

Karlsson, B., Gustafsson, J., Hedov, G., Ivarsson, S.A. and Annerén, G. (1998) 'Thyroid dysfunction in Down's syndrome: Relation to age and thyroid autoimmunity.' *Archives of Disease in Childhood 79*, 3, 242–245.

Kelly, G. (2000) 'Peripheral metabolism of thyroid hormones: A review.' *Alternative Medicine Review 5*, 4, 306–333.

Klee, G.G. and Hay, I.D. (1997) 'Biochemical testing of thyroid function.' *Endocrinology and Metabolism Clinics of North America 26*, 4, 763–775.

Köhrle J. (1992) 'The trace components – selenium and flavonoids – affect iodothyronine deiodinases, thyroid hormone transport and TSH regulation.' *Acta Med Austriaca 19*, suppl. 1, 13–17.

Köhrle, J (2005) 'Selenium and the control of thyroid hormone metabolism.' *Thyroid 15*, 8, 841–853.

Köhrle, J., Spanka, M., Irmscher, K. and Hesch, R.D. (1988) 'Flavonoid effects on transport, metabolism and action of thyroid hormones.' *Progress in Clinical and Biological Research 280*, 323–340.

Kralik, A., Eder, K. and Kirchgessner, M. (1996) 'Influence of zinc and selenium deficiency on parameters relating to thyroid hormone metabolism.' *Hormone and Metabolic Research 5*, 223–226.

Krunzel, T.A. (2001) 'Thyroid function testing: Dealing with interpretation difficulties.' *Journal of Naturopathic Medicine 1*, 1–9.

Krupsky, M. (1987) 'Musculoskeletal symptoms as a presenting sign of long-standing hypothyroidism.' *Israeli Journal of Medical Sciences 23*, 1110–1113.

Kung, A.W.C. and Pun, K.K. (1991) 'Bone mineral density in premenopausal women receiving long-term physiological doses of levothyroxine.' *Journal of the American Medical Association 265*, 2688–2691.

Ladenson, P.W., Singer, P.A., Ain, K.B., Bagchi, N. *et al.* (2000) 'American Thyroid Association guidelines for detection of thyroid dysfunction.' *Archives of Internal Medicine 160*, 11, 1573–1575.

Lafuente, A., Cano, P. and Esquifino, A.I. (2003) 'Are cadmium effects on plasma gonadotropins, prolactin, ACTH, GH and TSH levels, dose-dependent?' *Biometals 16*, 2, 243–250.

Lazarus, J.H. (2002) 'Epidemiology and prevention of thyroid disease in pregnancy.' *Thyroid 12*, 10, 861–865.

Leonard, J.L. and Köhrle, J. (1996) 'Intracellular Pathways of Iodothyronine Metabolism.' In L.E. Braverman and R.D. Utiger (eds) *Werner and Ingbar's The Thyroid: A Fundamental and Clinical Text*, 7th edn. Philadelphia: Lippincott-Raven.

Liel, Y., Harman-Boehm, I. and Shany, S. (1996) 'Evidence for a clinically important adverse effect of fiber-enriched diet on the bioavailability of levothyroxine in adult hypothyroid patients.' *Journal of Clinical Endocrinology and Metabolism 81*, 857–859.

Lindsay, R.S. and Toft, A.D. (1997) 'Hypothyroidism.' *Lancet 349*, 9049, 413–417.

Lukaski, H.C. (2000) 'Magnesium, zinc, and chromium nutriture and physical activity.' *American Journal of Clinical Nutrition 2*, suppl., 585S–593S.

Maes, M., Mommen, K., Hendrickx, D., Peeters, D. *et al.* (1997) 'Components of biological variation, including seasonality, in blood concentrations of TSH, TT3, FT4, PRL, cortisol and testosterone in healthy volunteers.' *Clinical Endocrinology 46*, 587–598.

Mancini, T. (2008) 'Hyperprolactinaemia and prolactinomas.' *Endocrinology and Metabolism Clinics of North America 37*, 67.

Marshall, W.J. and Bangert, S.K. (2004) *Clinical Chemistry*, 5th edn. London: Elsevier Health Sciences.

McDermott, M.T. and Ridgway, E.C. (2001) 'Subclinical hypothyroidism is mild thyroid failure and should be treated.' *Journal of Clinical Endocrinology and Metabolism 86*, 10, 4585–4590.

McEwen, B.S. (1998) 'Protective and damaging effects of stress mediators.' *New England Journal of Medicine 338*, 3, 171–179.

Molina, P.E. (2006) *Endocrine Physiology.* Lange Physiology Series. New York: McGraw-Hill.

Murray, J.S., Jayarajasingh, R. and Perros, P. (2001) 'Lesson of the week: Deterioration of symptoms after start of thyroid hormone replacement.' *British Medical Journal 323*, 7308, 332–333.

Murray, M., Pizzorno, J. and Pizzorno, L. (2005) *The Encyclopaedia of Healing Foods.* London: Time Warner Books.

Nussey, S.S. and Whitehead, S.A. (2001) *Endocrinology: An Integrated Approach.* London: Taylor and Francis.

Nygaard, B. (2007) *Hypothyroidism (Primary).* British Medical Journal Clinical Evidence. Available at www.ncbi.nlm.nih.gov/pubmed/19450344, accessed on 13 March 2010.

O'Brien, T., Silverberg, J.D. and Nguyen, T.T. (1992) 'Nicotinic acid-induced toxicity associated with cytopenia and decreased levels of thyroxine-binding globulin.' *Mayo Clinic Proceedings 67*, 465–468.

Olivieri, O., Girelli, D., Azzini, M., Stanzial, A.M. *et al.* (1995) 'Low selenium status in the elderly influences thyroid hormones.' *Clinical Science (London) 89*, 6, 637–642.

Olivieri, O., Girelli, D., Stanzial, A.M., Rossi, L., Bassi, A. and Corrocher, R. (1996) 'Selenium, zinc, and thyroid hormones in healthy subjects: Low T3/T4 ratio in the elderly is related to impaired selenium status.' *Biological Trace Element Research 51*, 1, 31–41.

O'Reilly, D.S. (2000) 'Thyroid function tests – time for re-assessment.' *British Medical Journal 320*, 7245, 1332–1334.

Osman, F., Gammage, M.D. and Franklyn, J.A. (2001) 'Thyroid disease and its treatment: Short-term and long-term cardiovascular consequences.' *Current Opinion in Pharmacology 1*, 6, 626–631.

Owen, P.J. and Lazarus, J.H. (2003) 'Subclinical hypothyroidism: The case for treatment.' *Trends in Endocrinology and Metabolism 14*, 6, 257–261.

Paolisso, G. and Barbagallo, M. (1997) 'Hypertension, diabetes mellitus, and insulin resistance: The role of intracellular magnesium.' *American Journal of Hypertension 10*, 3, 346–355.

Peters, E.M., Anderson, R., Nieman, D.C., Fickl, H. and Jogessar, V. (2001) 'Vitamin C supplementation attenuates the increases in circulating cortisol, adrenaline and anti-inflammatory polypeptides following ultramarathon running.' *International Journal of Sports Medicine 7*, 537–543.

Pirich, C., Mullner, M. and Sinzinger, H. (2000) 'Prevalence and relevance of thyroid dysfunction in 1922 cholesterol screening participants.' *Journal of Clinical Epidemiology 53*, 6, 623–629.

Pizzorno, L. and Ferril, F. (2005) 'Thyroid.' In D.S. Jones and S. Quinn (eds) *Textbook of Functional Medicine.* Gig Harbour, WA: Institute for Functional Medicine.

Plasqui, G., Kester, A.D. and Westerterp, K.R. (2003) 'Seasonal variation in sleeping metabolic rate, thyroid activity, and leptin.' *American Journal of Physiology – Endocrinology and Metabolism 285*, 2, E338–343.

Radović, B., Mentrup, B. and Köhrle, J. (2006) 'Genistein and other soya isoflavones are potent ligands for transthyretin in serum and cerebrospinal fluid.' *British Journal of Nutrition 95*, 6, 1171–1176.

Rayman, M.P. (1997) 'Dietary selenium: Time to act.' *British Medical Journal 14*, 7078, 387–388.

Rayman, M.P. (2000) 'The importance of selenium to human health.' *Lancet 356*, 233–241.

Rayman, M.P. (2002) 'The argument for increasing selenium intake.' *Proceedings of the Nutrition Society 61*, 203–215.

Rayman, M.P. (2008) 'Food-chain selenium and human health: emphasis on intake.' *British Journal of Nutrition 100*, 254–268.

Rayman, M.P., Goenaga Infante, H. and Sargent, M. (2008) 'Food-chain selenium and human health: Spotlight on speciation.' *British Journal of Nutrition 100*, 238–253.

Rayman, M.P., Thompson, A.J., Bekaert, B., Catterick, J. *et al.* (2008) 'Randomized controlled trial of the effect of selenium supplementation on thyroid function in the elderly in the United Kingdom.' *American Journal of Clinical Nutrition 87*, 2, 370–378.

Redmond, G.P. (2004) 'Thyroid dysfunction and women's reproductive health.' *Thyroid 14*, suppl. 1, S5–15.

Remer, T., Neubert, A. and Manz, F. (1999) 'Increased risk of iodine deficiency with vegetarian nutrition.' *British Journal of Nutrition 81*, 1, 45–49.

Rice, M., Graves, A. and Larson, E. (1995) 'Estrogen replacement therapy and cognition: Role of phytoestrogens (abstract).' *Gerontologist 35*, suppl. 1, 169.

Roberts, C.G. and Ladenson, P.W. (2004) 'Hypothyroidism.' *Lancet 363*, 9411, 793–803.

Rooney, S. and Walsh, E. (1997) 'Prevalence of abnormal thyroid function tests in a Down's syndrome population.' *Irish Journal of Medical Science 166*, 2, 80–82.

Rose, N.R., Saboori, A.M., Rasooly, L. and Burek, C.L. (1997) 'The role of iodine in autoimmune thyroiditis.' *Critical Reviews in Immunology 17*, 5–6, 511–517.

Rosolova, H., Mayer, O. Jr. and Reaven, G.J. (1997) 'Effect of variations in plasma magnesium concentration on resistance to insulin-mediated glucose disposal in nondiabetic subjects.' *Journal of Clinical Endocrinology and Metabolism 82*, 11, 3783–3785.

Rouzaud, G., Young, S.A. and Duncan, A.J. (2004) 'Hydrolysis of glucosinolates to isothiocyanates after ingestion of raw or microwaved cabbage by human volunteers.' *Cancer Epidemiology, Biomarkers and Prevention 13*, 1, 125–131.

Rungapamestry, V., Duncan, A.J., Fuller, Z. and Ratcliffe, B. (2007) 'Effect of cooking brassica vegetables on the subsequent hydrolysis and metabolic fate of glucosinolates.' *Proceedings of the Nutrition Society 66*, 1, 69–81.

Sategna-Guidetti, C., Bruno, M., Mazza, E., Carlino, A. *et al.* (1998) 'Autoimmune thyroid diseases and coeliac disease.' *European Journal of Gastroenterology and Hepatology 10*, 11, 927–931.

Sategna-Guidetti, C., Volta, U., Ciacci, C., Usai, P. *et al.* (2001) 'Prevalence of thyroid disorders in untreated adult celiac disease patients and effect of gluten withdrawal: An Italian multicenter study.' *American Journal of Gastroenterology 96*, 3, 751–757.

Sawin, C.T., Geller, A., Wolf, P.A., Belanger, A.J. *et al.* (1994) 'Low serum thyrotropin concentrations as a risk factor for atrial fibrillation in older persons.' *New England Journal of Medicine 331*, 19, 1249–1252.

Schneider, D.L., Barrett-Connor, E.L. and Morton, D.J. (1994) 'Thyroid hormone use and bone mineral density in elderly women. Effects of estrogen.' Journal of the American Medical Association *271*, 16, 1245–1249.

Schneider, D.L., Barrett-Connor, E.L. and Morton, D.J. (1995) 'Thyroid hormone use and bone mineral density in elderly men.' *Archives of Internal Medicine 155*, 18, 2005–2007.

Segermann, J., Hotze, A., Ulrich, H. and Rao, G.S. (1991) 'Effect of alpha-lipoic acid on the peripheral conversion of thyroxine to triiodothyronine and on serum lipid-, protein- and glucose levels.' *Arzneimittelforschung 41*, 12, 1294–1298.

Selye, H. (1979) 'Stress and the reduction of distress.' *Journal of the South Carolina Medical Association 75*, 11, 562–566.

Serri, O., Chik, C.L., Ur, E. and Ezzat, S. (2003) 'Diagnosis and management of hyperprolactinaemia.' *Canadian Medical Association Journal 169*, 6, 575–581.

Shakir, K.M.M., Kroll, S. and Aprill, B.S. (1995) 'Nicotinic acid decreases serum thyroid hormone levels while maintaining a euthyroid state.' Mayo Clinic Proceedings 70, 556–558.

Shapiro, T.A., Fahey, J.W., Wade, K.L., Stephenson, K.K. and Talalay, P. (1998) 'Human metabolism and excretion of cancer chemoprotective glucosinolates and isothiocyanates of cruciferous vegetables.' *Cancer Epidemiology Biomarkers and Prevention 7*, 12, 1091–1100.

Sher, L. (2000) 'The role of brain thyroid hormones in the mechanisms of seasonal changes in mood and behaviour.' *Medical Hypotheses 55*, 1, 56–59.

Singh, K., Chander, R. and Kapoor, N.K. (1997) 'Guggulsterone, a potent hypolipidaemic, prevents oxidation of low density lipoprotein.' *Phytotherapy Research 11*, 291–294.

Singh, N., Singh, P.N. and Hershman, J.M. (2000) 'Effect of calcium carbonate on the absorption of levothyroxine.' Journal of the American Medical Association *283*, 2822–2825.

Soldin, O.P., O'Mara, D.M. and Aschner, M. (2008) 'Thyroid hormones and methylmercury toxicity.' *Biological Trace Element Research 126*, 1–3, 1–12.

Stimson, R.H., Johnstone, A.M., Homer, N.Z., Wake, D.J. *et al.* (2007) 'Dietary macronutrient content alters cortisol metabolism independently of body weight changes in obese men.' *Journal of Clinical Endocrinology and Metabolism 92*, 11, 4480–4484.

Stoffer, C.S. (1982) 'Menstrual disorders and mild thyroid insufficiency.' *Postgraduate Medicine 72*, 75–82.

Surks, M.I., Goswami, G. and Daniels, G.H. (2005) 'The thyrotropin reference range should remain unchanged.' *Journal of Clinical Endocrinology and Metabolism 90*, 9, 5489–5496.

Surks, M.I., Ortiz, E., Daniels, G.H., Sawin, C.T. *et al.* (2004) 'Subclinical thyroid disease: Scientific review and guidelines for diagnosis and management.' *Journal of the American Medical Association 291*, 2, 228–238.

Tafet, G.E. and Smolovich, J. (2004) 'Psychoneuroendocrinological studies on chronic stress and depression.' *Annals of the New York Academy of Sciences 1032*, 276–278.

Tentolouris, N., Tsigos, C., Perea, D., Koukou, E. *et al.* (2003) 'Differential effects of high-fat and high-carbohydrate isoenergetic meals on cardiac autonomic nervous system activity in lean and obese women.' *Metabolism 52*, 11, 1426–1432.

Thomson, C.D. (2004) 'Assessment of requirements for selenium and adequacy of selenium status: A review.' *European Journal of Clinical Nutrition 58*, 391–402.

Thomson, C.D., McLachlan, S.K., Grant, A.M., Paterson, E. and Lillico, A.J. (2005) 'The effect of selenium on thyroid status in a population with marginal selenium and iodine status.' *British Journal of Nutrition. 94*, 6, 962–968.

Tsigos, C. and Chrousos, G.P. (2002) 'Hypothalamic-pituitary-adrenal axis, neuroendocrine factors and stress.' *Journal of psychosomatic research 53*, 4, 865–871.

Turker, O., Kumanlioglu, K., Karapolat, I. and Dogan, I. (2006) 'Selenium treatment in autoimmune thyroiditis: 9-month follow-up with variable doses.' *Journal of Endocrinology 190*, 1, 151–156.

Van der Heide, D., Kastelyn, J. and Schroder-van de Elst, J.P. (2003) 'Flavonoids and thyroid disease.' *Biofactors 19*, 3–4, 113–119.

Vanderpas, J.B., Contempré, B., Duale, N.L., Deckx, H. *et al.* (1993) 'Selenium deficiency mitigates hypothyroxinemia in iodine-deficient subjects.' *American Journal of Clinical Nutrition 57*, 2 suppl., 271S–275S.

Vanderpump, M.P. (2003) 'Subclinical hypothyroidism: The case against treatment.' *Trends in Endocrinology and Metabolism 14*, 6, 262–266.

Vanderpump, M.P. and Franklyn, J.A. (2003) 'Thyroid function tests and hypothyroidism. Restoring serum TSH to reference range should be goal of replacement.' *British Medical Journal 326*, 1086–1087.

Vanderpump, M.P.J., Tunbridge, W.M.G., French, J.M., Appleton, D., Bates, D. and Clark, F. (1995) 'The incidence of thyroid disorders in the community: A twenty-year follow-up of the Whickham survey.' *Clinical Endocrinology 43*, 55–68.

Van Praag, H.M. (2004) 'Can stress cause depression?' *Progress in Neuro-Psychopharmacology and Biological Psychiatry 28*, 5, 891–907.

Van Spronsen, F.J., van Rijn, M. and Bekhof, J. (2001) 'Phenylketonuria: Tyrosine supplementation in phenylalanine-restricted diets.' *American Journal of Clinical Nutrition 73*, 153–157.

Vantyghem, M.C., Ghularn, A. and Hober, C. (1998) 'Urinary cortisol metabolites in the assessment of peripheral thyroid hormone action: Overt and subclinical hypothyroidism.' *Journal of Endocrinological Investigation 21*, 219–225.

Waise, A. and Belchetz, P.E. (2000) 'Lesson of the week: Unsuspected central hypothyroidism.' *British Medical Journal 321*, 7271, 1275–1277.

Walsh, J.P. (2002) 'Dissatisfaction with thyroxine therapy – could the patients be right?' *Current Opinions in Pharmacology 2*, 6, 717–722.

Ward, G., McKinnon, L., Badrick, T. and Hickman, P.E. (1997) 'Heterophilic antibodies remain a problem for the immunoassay laboratory.' *American Journal of Clinical Pathology 108*, 4, 417–421.

Wardle, C.A., Fraser, W.D. and Squire, C.R. (2001) 'Pitfalls in the use of thyrotropin concentration as a first-line thyroid-function test.' *Lancet 357*, 9261, 1013–1014.

Wartofsky, L. (2004) 'Combined levotriiodothyronine and levothyronine therapy for hypothyroidism – are we a step closer to the magic formula?' *Thyroid 14*, 4, 247–248.

Wartofsky, L. and Dickey, R.A. (2005) 'The evidence for a narrower thyrotropin reference range is compelling.' *Journal of Clinical Endocrinology and Metabolism 90*, 9, 5483–5488.

Weetman, A.P. (1997) 'Hypothyroidism: Screening and subclinical disease.' *British Medical Journal 314*, 1175–1178.

Weetman, A.P. (2006) 'Whose thyroid hormone replacement is it anyway?' *Clinical Endocrinology (Oxford) 64*, 3, 231–233.

Weiss, R.E. and Refetoff, S. (2000) 'Resistance to thyroid hormone.' *Reviews in Endocrine and Metabolic Disorders (United States) 1*, 1–2, 97–108.

WHO/FAO/IAEA (1996) 'Trace Elements in Human Nutrition and Health.' In C.D. Thomson (2004) 'Assessment of requirements for selenium and adequacy of selenium status: A review.' *European Journal of Clinical Nutrition 58*, 391–402.

WHO, UNICEF and ICCIDD (2001) *Assessment of the Iodine Deficiency Disorders and Monitoring their Elimination.* Geneva: WHO. WHO/NHD/01.1. 1–107.

Wilson, E.D. (1991) *Wilson's Syndrome: The Miracle of Feeling Well.* Florida: Cornerstone Publishing.

Wilson, J.L. (2001) *Adrenal Fatigue, the 21st Century Stress Syndrome.* Petaluma, CA: Smart Publications.

Wright, E.C. (1994) 'A lesson in non-compliance.' *Lancet 343*, 8909, 1305.

Zimmermann, M.B. and Köhrle, J. (2002) 'The impact of iron and selenium deficiencies on iodine and thyroid metabolism: biochemistry and relevance to public health.' *Thyroid 12*, 10, 867–878.

Zimmermann, M.B., Wegmueller, R., Zeder, C., Chaouki, N. and Torresani, T. (2004) 'The effects of vitamin A deficiency and vitamin A supplementation on thyroid function in goitrous children.' *Journal of Clinical Endocrinology and Metabolism 89*, 5441–5447.

Additional resources

British Thyroid Foundation

www.btf-thyroid.org

British Thyroid Association

www.british-thyroid-association.org

Chapter *7*

SEX HORMONE IMBALANCES

Kate Neil

1. The environment, hormonal and developmental health

The year 1993 marked a pivotal time in understanding the impact of sex hormone imbalance in disease. In that year BBC *Horizon* televised 'The Assault on the Male', publicising research findings by Sharpe and Skakkebaek that implied a possible 50 per cent decline in human sperm count and a doubling of baby boys born with reproductive abnormalities, including undescended testes and hypospadias (Sharpe and Skakkebaek 1993). They also reported a trebling of testicular cancer rates. The unifying theory was that sertoli cells were under the influence of the predominantly female hormone oestrogen. Sertoli cells are responsible for the descent of the testes before birth, commit to sperm development and are the cells that go awry in testicular cancer. These worrying findings appeared to be happening over a relatively short period of history, suggesting environmental influences. The researchers concluded that the most likely cause for these changes were environmental oestrogens, termed xenoestrogens. Later, this theory was broadened to include environmental hormone manipulators, called endocrine disruptors (Toppari and Skakkebaek 1998).

The research findings of Dr Theo Colborn were also televised as part of this programme. Dr Colborn had come to the realisation that at least 16 top predator species were showing reproductive problems (Colborn, vom Saal and Soto 1993). Shortly after the publication of the book *Our Stolen Future* (Colborn, Dumanoski and Peterson Myers 1996), Deborah Cadbury's book *The Feminization of Nature* was published (Cadbury 1997). Both books described the influence of xenoestrogens on reproduction in different species and suggested that toxic pollutants have the capacity to alter genetic expression, resulting in death or deformities.

Cadbury (1997) reports that researchers found elevated levels of oestrogen in male and female alligators in Lake Apopka in 1991. Male alligators were also found to have levels of testosterone that were three times lower than normal. By six months of age the sex of many male alligators could not be differentiated. These findings continue to be reproduced in other contaminated lakes (Guillette, Edwards and Moore 2007). Cadbury goes on to say that around 25 per cent of turtles appeared to be affected in a similar way, that researchers in Paris were noting 'feminised' eels on the river Seine and that panthers in Florida were exhibiting severe reproductive abnormalities.

In 1962 Rachel Carson (writer, scientist and ecologist) had authored *Silent Spring*, which describes in detail how DDT entered the food chain and accumulates in fatty tissues of animals and humans, with the potential to cause genetic damage and cancer. Agricultural and industrial processes are heavily reliant on synthetic chemicals, many of which have been shown to disrupt thyroid, pituitary, hypothalamic and sex hormones, and which are now collectively described as 'endocrine disruptors' (Newbold *et al.* 2007).

The impact of excess oestrogen on males is profound, as they are relatively unused to significant levels of circulating oestrogen. In contrast, excess oestrogen in women may be less overt but it is increasingly being linked to many health problems, including: breast, uterine and ovarian cancer (International Agency for Research on Cancer (IARC) 1999; Kaaks *et al.* 2005; McArdle and O'Mahony 2008); fibroids; endometriosis; premenstrual syndrome (PMS); obesity; migraines and infertility (Bulun 2009; Ross *et al.* 1986; Wardle and Fox 1989).

In 2005 Professor Bill Ledger from Sheffield University reported that one in seven couples have difficulty conceiving, and that this could rise to one in three couples. However, there are many factors involved in the increased incidence of sub- and infertility; the effect of environmental toxicity is just one. Infertility, more than most health problems, directly threatens human survival.

The rest of this chapter aims to:

- clarify current thinking on how endocrine disruptors exert biological effects
- inform the practitioner of various inter-relationships between oestrogen and other hormones
- demonstrate how important the efficient functioning of all major body processes is to the safe handling of oestrogen
- consider possible assessment and treatment options.

Table 7.1 at the end of this chapter provides a quick reference guide to the function and effects of nutrients and foods on hormone balance; and also the potential impact of environmental chemicals. The reader can refer to this guide whilst reading the chapter.

1.1 Endocrine disruptors

Endocrine disruptors are chemicals with the potential to alter hormone action within the body and to interact and/or interfere with oestrogen or androgen signalling mechanisms (see Box 7.1). The increased incidence of breast cancer and testicular dysgenesis syndrome (low sperm counts, testicular cancer, cryptorchidism and hypospadias) has fuelled the debate over the possibility of endocrine disruptors causing ill health (Sharpe and Irvine 2004).

Box 7.1 Some common endocrine disruptors

Phthalates – used as plasticisers in PVC products, as well as in many cosmetics and toiletries, amongst other things

Organochlorines – used as pesticides; of particular note are DDT and lindane

PAHs (polycyclic aromatic hydrocarbons) – products of burnt or charred foodstuffs/ organic material

PCBs (polychlorinated biphenyls) – primarily used as cooling and insulating fluids

Dioxins – by-products of:

- various industrial processes that involve chlorinated organic compounds (such as bleaching)
- incomplete combustion of materials
- natural processes

Toxic minerals – mercury, cadmium, arsenic, lead

Rather than endocrine disruptors exerting their effects through receptor binding, a mechanism that now appears relatively innocuous, Sharpe and Irvine (2004) report that endocrine disruptors appear to be potent suppressors of oestrogen sulphotransferase and that phthalates appear to depress endogenous testosterone production. Such suppression of oestrogen sulphotransferase could prolong the action of oestrogen, a factor potentially relevant to breast cancer and other oestrogen-mediated diseases.

According to Sharpe and Irvine (2004) it is 'unlikely that endocrine disruptors with weak intrinsic oestrogenic activity can be as important hormonal players in the aetiology of breast cancer as the woman's own potent endogenous oestrogens' (p.448). The researchers also say that 'arguably the most important lesson from the phthalate studies has been the recognition that environmental chemicals with the potential to alter endogenous oestrogen production or metabolism pose a greater risk than do the many weak, receptor-mediated endocrine disruptor agents described in the literature' (p.449).

The aetiological involvement of endocrine disruptors in testicular dysgenesis syndrome is mainly theoretical. Phthalate exposure has reignited interest as a causal factor in this syndrome. Phthalates are prolific in the environment – 2 million tons are produced each year worldwide (Okamoto *et al.* 2004).

Sharpe and Irvine (2004) report that:

- human exposure to phthalates is higher than has been presumed and women of reproductive age have notably higher exposure, even though the levels are considerably lower than those used in animal studies

- animal research has shown that certain phthalates, when administered in pregnancy, induce a syndrome that resembles testicular dysgenesis in male offspring

- endometriosis in women, shorter gestation periods in pregnant women and reduced sperm quality have all been significantly related to certain phthalate metabolites.

A recent study in Mexico also indicates that phthalate exposure in the third trimester of pregnancy may cause a two to four-fold increased risk of premature delivery (Meeker *et al.* 2009).

In a large US study women were shown to have mostly higher concentrations of phthalate metabolites in their urine than men; and in some cases children (aged 6–11) had the highest concentrations of all (Centers for Disease Control and Prevention 2005). Animal data (albeit from small studies) indicates that phthalates can cross the placenta and pass into breast milk, thereby passing onto the developing foetus and newborn via the mother (Dorey 2003).

Breast tissue is a potential storage site for lipophilic chemicals and a possible route of transfer from mother to baby during breast feeding. Sharpe and Irvine (2004) explain that transfer can also occur from mother to foetus *in utero*.

Oily fish are also potent absorbers of endocrine-disrupting chemicals, including the toxic metal mercury (see Chapter 4). This has led to sufficient concern over oily fish intake that the UK government has produced guidelines on restricting intake in pregnancy, for infants and children. It is unclear, however, whether the benefit of limiting the intake of oily fish outweighs the risk. Research data continues to accumulate on the vital importance of the omega-3 fatty acids for foetal and infant development (Helland *et al.* 2008; Hibbeln *et al.* 2007). Most fish oils available in supplement form today are considered 'purified' from endocrine-disrupting chemicals and may be a viable alternative to consuming more than recommended amounts of oily fish, while incomplete and contradictory data prevails. Fish is a good source of protein and it is important to ensure adequate intake of other good sources of protein when limiting fish.

1.2 Obesogens

In an emerging hypothesis, Newbold *et al.* (2007) propose that exposures to environmental chemicals, both *in utero* and during early development, may play a role in the development of obesity later in life. An increasing number of studies report that exposure to chemicals during critical periods of differentiation, at low environmentally relevant doses, alters developmental programming, potentially resulting in obesity.

Fat cells are storage sites for lipophilic pollutants. Weight loss and yo-yo dieting are common phenomena in modern times and can initiate the release of such chemicals into circulation. Energy production may also be reduced as a result of the impact of such pollutants on enzymes involved in the conversion of fuels into energy (Lord and Bralley 2008), making weight loss harder to achieve. Hormones, neural pathways and neurotransmitters appear to frequently malfunction in obese individuals (Baillie-Hamilton 2002).

Proving cause and effect on health and disease in terms of diet, toxic exposures and lifestyle is fraught with difficulty, as human beings are complex organisms living in an even more complex environment.

2. Conceptual frameworks for viewing hormonal health

2.1 Systems biology

A new scientific discipline has been emerging over the past decade or more, in the form of 'systems biology'. This new science promises exciting new possibilities for the future, where it should increasingly become possible to develop mathematical and computational techniques to model biochemical interactions and understand them as networks. This should lead to more useful scientific data and further opportunities for personalised healthcare.

Hormones do not work in isolation and the imbalance of one hormone can impact on another (Hays 2005). Complex interactions between the hormonal, neuronal and immune systems are becoming increasingly better understood.

Box 7.2 Systems biology

The goal of systems biology is to fundamentally transform the practice of medicine, and researchers from the Institute for Systems Biology in Seattle have taken the leadership role in catalysing this transformation. They are developing new tools and techniques, and pursuing research that will usher in a new era of predictive, preventive and personalised medicine. (Jones, Hofmann and Quinn 2009, p.A11)

2.2 Allostasis

Many readers will be familiar with the principles of homeostasis where, after a challenge, the body returns to balance. The concept of allostasis has been emerging over the last forty years and, as seen in Chapter 1, proposes that the body does not necessarily return to balance but achieves stability through adaptation and change. For example, blood pressure may reset at a higher point in response to ongoing challenge.

Neurotransmitters and glucocorticoids are the primary mediators of the stress response and in the short term play a protective role. 'Over longer time intervals, they exact a cost (allostatic load) that can accelerate disease processes' (McEwen 2000, p.108). Allostasis is the price the body has to pay for either doing its job less efficiently or simply being overwhelmed by too many challenges.

When allostasis is prolonged, chronic mental and physical disease may result (McEwen and Seeman 1999).

2.3 Resilience theory

Resilience is a name for a set of processes showing that small things can make a big difference. It is about what we can do as opposed to what we can't do. According to Rutter (1999, p.135):

> therapeutic actions need to focus on steps that may be taken in order to reduce negative chain reactions and ... protection may also lie in fostering positive chain reactions. Resilience theory helps individuals to work towards better outcomes and ... therapists across disciplines to plan therapeutic programmes that support positive chain reactions.

In developmental science, individual resilience also 'refers to the processes of, capacity for, or patterns of positive adaptation during or following exposure to adverse experiences that have the potential to disrupt or destroy the successful function or development of the person' (Masten and Obradovic 2008, p.9).

2.4 Moving towards 'ease'

Dis-ease literally means 'moving away from ease'. By supporting the body's major functional processes (of digestion, absorption, elimination, detoxification, transport, mitochondrial function, defence, hormonal and neuronal cellular communication) it becomes much harder for disease to occur. A functional approach works with the 'purpose and design' of the human body and towards restoring normal function, thus aiding a state of 'ease'.

Whether a client presents with a diagnosed sex hormone problem, arthritis, depression, Alzheimer's disease, eczema or an autistic spectrum disorder, the functional practitioner will systematically explore the client's personal and family history to help identify the factors that are most likely to have contributed to a breach of integrity in the body's major functional processes.

Most functional processes are genetically driven and we cannot change our genes. However, in many instances changes to diet, toxin exposure and lifestyle can alter the way our genes are expressed. Functional medicine medical practitioner Dr Leo Galland (1997) coined the concept of 'patient-centred diagnosis' to describe the personalised quality of the functional approach.

Increasingly, nutritional therapists employ a functional approach to underpin their treatment strategies. Sex hormone imbalances are integral to many chronic illnesses and are well suited to functional laboratory assessment to inform, guide and monitor treatment protocols that support the body towards a state of 'ease'.

3. Sex hormones

The sex hormones oestrogen, progesterone and testosterone belong to the steroid hormone group, which also includes dehydroepiandrosterone (DHEA), corticosteroids and aldosterone. According to J.S. Bland (1998), steroid hormones influence cellular physiology in many ways, acting as facilitators of gene expression in coordinating neuro-endocrine and metabolic systems, separately and together, to achieve repair and rebalancing of physiology.

3.1 Synthesis of steroid hormones

Approximately 80 per cent of the sterol cholesterol is made in the body from acetate, mainly derived from acetyl co-enzyme A, a pivotal metabolite in the biochemical pathway that converts fuels into energy.

Cholesterol is not an essential dietary nutrient – it is found naturally only in animal produce and the body can make all it requires; vegans, for example, rely entirely on endogenous synthesis of cholesterol. However, ingestion of cholesterol acts to reduce the amount of cholesterol that the body needs to make *de novo*.

Cholesterol plays a strategic role in the interaction of the steroid hormones, as can be seen from Figure 7.1, and is integral to the structure of all cell membranes in the body. The integrity of cell membranes is vital for, amongst other things, hormone function, neurotransmission and nutrient transport.

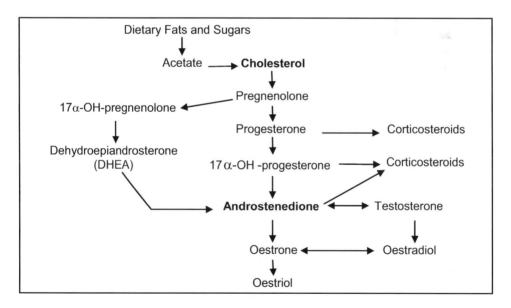

Figure 7.1 Synthesis of steroid hormones

3.2 Oestrogen – not just one hormone

The three major forms of oestrogen are oestrone, oestradiol and oestriol. As can be seen from Figure 7.1, oestrone is metabolised from androstenedione, and oestradiol from testosterone. Oestrone and oestradiol are inter-convertible.

Oestrone is considered to be the most potent form of oestrogen, in that it can undergo biotransformation to form the potentially damaging 4-OHE1 (4-hydroxyoestrone) and 16α-OHE1 (16α-hydroxyoestrone) oestrogen metabolites. Conversion to 2-OHE1 (2-hydroxyoestrone) metabolites is considered a potentially 'safer' biotransformation.

3.3 Oestrogen dominance

The concept of oestrogen dominance, a term first coined by Lee (1993, p.42), describes a state when there is either an excess of oestrogen, or a normal level of oestrogen with a relative deficiency of progesterone. Since that time, data suggests that very small amounts of oestrogen appear to have large effects in the body (Hays 2005) and, according to Caulfield *et al.* (1998), the body views oestrogen as a potential toxin, unlike DHEA and progesterone.

Elevated levels of 4-OHE1 and 16α-OHE1 oestrogen metabolites are increasingly associated with disease risk, including hormone-dependent cancers (Bolton and Thatcher 2008), other oestrogen-mediated diseases and autoimmune disorders such as systemic lupus erythematosus (SLE) and rheumatoid arthritis (RA) (Weidler *et al.* 2004).

4. Functional processes involved in the safe management of oestrogen and other hormones

The following functional discussion focuses heavily on the role of detoxification. To achieve a greater depth of understanding it could be read in conjunction with Chapter 3.

In practice therapists often find that detoxification support is a frontline strategy for supporting hormonal balance. Rather than focusing too much on the amount of circulating hormone, the practitioner needs to focus on the safe handling and removal of hormones and their metabolites.

4.1 Detoxification (digestion and absorption)

Supporting efficient digestion and absorption underpins many nutritional strategies. Reference to the importance of digestive health will not be independently discussed here, as it is covered in depth in Chapter 2, but will be referred to contextually throughout this chapter.

Adequate detoxification is a fundamental process in the 'safe' handling of oestrogen. Toxins, whether generated within the body or that enter the body from the environment, are prepared for elimination using phase I and phase II detoxification pathways. Toxins are rendered water-soluble for elimination mainly in bile or urine.

After a toxin has been processed by phase I enzymes, intermediate metabolites are produced, many of which are more toxic than the original compound. Reactive oxygen species (ROS), such as the superoxide and peroxyl anions, are also generated as part of phase I detoxification. The toxic metabolites are then passed to phase II detoxifiers for elimination.

The function of both phases of detoxification is under considerable genetic control, resulting in wide variance among the human population. It is now possible to assess for specific genetic weaknesses in detoxification processes, thus providing the practitioner with an enhanced ability to personalise treatment strategies.

4.2 Phase I detoxification of sex hormones

Phase I detoxification relies on the cytochrome P450 (CYP) enzyme system, which disposes of oestrogen by forming 2-OH, 4-OH and 16α-OH metabolites, as well as ROS. The balance of oestrogen metabolites has potential in predicting oestrogen-driven hormone-related cancers (Bland *et al.* 1999; Bolton and Thatcher 2008).

4.2.1 NUTRIENTS REQUIRED TO SUPPORT PHASE I DETOXIFICATION

Haem is incorporated into CYP enzymes. The synthesis of haem is dependent on **succinic acid**, the amino acid **glycine** and **iron**. Iron is part of the haem molecule and is released during phase 1 detoxification, participating in the generation of reactive oxygen species (ROS). Toxins and nutrient deficiencies can reduce the synthesis of haem.

Adequate **antioxidant** support is needed to reduce oxidative stress, implicated in the pathology of most chronic degenerative disorders (see Chapter 9). In addition, **B vitamins**, **magnesium** and **lipoic acid** are required for the synthesis of succinic acid. The synthesis of all enzymes, including CYP enzymes, is dependent on adequate dietary **protein**. **Vitamin B6** and **zinc** are important nutrients for the manufacture of enzymes used in the process.

4.2.2 ENZYMES INVOLVED IN PHASE I DETOXIFICATION

CYP1A1

CYP1A1 is responsible for the breakdown of oestradiol into the catechol oestrogen, 2-hydroxyoestradiol. Two common gene polymorphisms have been shown to increase the activity of this enzyme, leading to increased accumulation of metabolites expected to be carcinogenic (de Jong *et al.* 2002). However, Masson *et al.* (2005) reported that a meta-analysis of 17 studies plus more recent studies could not confirm a causal link between increased breast cancer risk and CYP1A1 variants. 2-OH oestrogen metabolites are generally considered 'safer'; however, the safety of 2-OH oestrogen metabolites is critically dependent on the addition of methyl groups to form 2-methoxyoestrogens. Phase II detoxification will include a discussion on the methylation of oestrogens.

Hays (2005) reports that glucosinolates such as indole-3-carbinol (I3C) found in the brassica vegetables (cabbage, kale, broccoli, Brussels sprouts, cauliflower) can upregulate the activity of CYP1A1, thereby increasing the levels of the precursor for 2-methoxyestrone and providing a powerfully protective anti-oestrogen.

CYP2C subfamily and CYP3A4

The CYP2C subfamily of enzymes and CYP3A4 convert oestrogen to 16-αOH metabolites. Gregory *et al.* (2000) reported wide variations in the ratio of 2-OH oestrogens to 16α-OH oestrogens in groups with a higher breast cancer risk e.g. oral contraceptive pill (OCP) users.

A high level of 16α-OHE1 generally represents a non-beneficial shift in oestrogen metabolism with increased risk of lupus, breast cancer and other oestrogen-dependent diseases (Weidler *et al.* 2004). Obesity, low thyroid function and pesticide exposure are all associated with higher levels of this metabolite. However, in post-menopausal South Asian women this metabolite is associated with increased protection from osteopaenia (Sung *et al.* 1997)

Omega-3 fatty acids (Hyman 2005) flaxseed lignans, cruciferous vegetables (Bonnesen *et al.* 1999), exercise and normalising body weight all help minimise the influence of 16α-OHE1 and are associated with increased production of the 'safer' 2-OHE1. Hyman (2005) reported that eicosaepentaenoic acid (EPA) has been shown to increase C-2 hydroxylation and decrease C-16α hydroxylation in breast cancer cells, whereas diets high in saturated fat have the opposite effect.

CYP1B1

Human CYP1B1 is a major enzyme for carcinogenic oestrogen metabolism, forming 4-OH oestrogen metabolites. CYP1B1 is known to be expressed at a high frequency in various human cancers, but not in normal tissues (Tan *et al.* 2007). CYP1B1 has been found to be present in cancers of the bladder, brain, breast, colon, connective tissue, kidney, liver, lung, lymph node, oesophagus, ovaries, skin, small intestine, stomach, testicles and uterus (Tan *et al.* 2007).

According to Hays (2005) CYP1B1 can be up- and down-regulated by many drugs and down-regulated by avoidance of polycyclic aromatic hydrocarbons (PAHs). Tan *et al.* (2007) also report that CYP1B1 plays an important role in the metabolism of various anti-cancer drugs.

The 4-hydroxylated metabolites have been described as the 'oestrogen on fire', due to their ability to be rapidly converted to DNA-damaging quinones.

4.2.3 ENZYME MODIFIERS

Salvestrols and CYP1B1

Tan *et al.* (2007) report that CYP1B1 may act as a tumour-specific rescue enzyme. If CYP1B1 is provided with natural agents (termed salvestrols) in the diet, a stream of chemical agents should be unleashed within the cancer cells that are deadly to themselves. In this context Tan *et al.* (2007) suggest that CYP1B1 may be acting as a 'Trojan horse', as it appears that this enzyme provides cancer cells with the seeds of their own destruction.

Well-conducted clinical trials are needed to evaluate the efficacy of salvestrols as a cancer preventative and therapeutic strategy. Anecdotal data is mixed regarding its use as a therapeutic agent in the management of cancer. Salvestrol products are commercially available.

> Salvestrols belong to a group of phytochemicals called phytoalexins, which are produced by plants as a result of a direct challenge by pathogenic bacteria. Resveratrol was the first Salvestrol identified and, since its discovery, more beneficial natural molecules have been identified with even greater potency than resveratrol. (Tan *et al.* 2007, p.44)

Resveratrol is found in red grapes and red wine and may be one of the health-protective factors associated with moderate intake of red wine. Many fruits and vegetables should provide the active compounds in salvestrols; good sources are tangerines, strawberries and cranberries. These compounds have been part of the human diet and eaten safely for millions of years.

Tan *et al.* (2007) report that initial screening by researchers for these compounds in fruit and vegetables only yielded a result when (according to unpublished studies) organic produce was used. This has led to the observation that modern agricultural techniques have probably depleted the levels of salvestrols in the modern diet, which may help to partially explain the rise of cancer in humans.

Because many agrochemicals are used for general crop protection, the plants are no longer challenged by diseases and so the production of salvestrols is not induced in sprayed plants, leading to only low levels being found in non-organic produce. Salvestrols generally have a bitter taste and there is an ever-increasing demand for sweeter-tasting fruits and vegetables to pander to the modern palate. Given the 'no added sugar' drive by the government, food manufacturers have been forced to remove bitter agents in fruit juices in order to accommodate this and still maintain palatability.

4.2.4 PHTHALATES AND 4-HYDROXYLATION (4-OH)

As outlined previously, phthalates are among the most ubiquitous synthetic chemicals in the environment. Due to their chemical nature they are widely distributed in the atmosphere and hydrosphere and, as such, we are all exposed to them.

Okamoto *et al.* (2004) reported that, once phthalate esters are hydroxylated at the ring 4-position, the resulting compounds exhibit unequivocal binding affinity for human oestrogen receptors (OR). The researchers state that phthalate esters are potentially oestrogenic but results from many investigators remain inconsistent. Phthalate esters (without this hydroxylation) have a very weak OR-binding affinity.

4.2.5 TESTING FOR PHASE 1 DETOXIFICATION OF HORMONES

Saliva tests that measure the 'free' hormone have increasingly played a role in understanding the balance of oestrogen, progesterone, testosterone, DHEA and cortisol. As indicated previously, a little oestrogen can be harmful but a saliva test that measures the amount of oestrogen available to target tissues will not provide information on the balance of oestrogen metabolites, which in many instances may be what the practitioner really needs to know.

Saliva hormone testing can still be a useful adjunct to testing for oestrogen metabolites. It is possible to identify oestrogen dominance through saliva testing. However, this does not confirm whether the more helpful 2-MeOE metabolites are being formed. It may be, for example, that an individual has an excess of oestrogen but is of a favourable genotype and has the available nutrient resources to form more 2-MeOE metabolites.

Other reasons for using a single sample (or a comprehensive eleven-sample) saliva hormone assay include confirmation of oestrogen deficiency and/or progesterone dominance/deficiency, as these, like oestrogen dominance, can underpin many chronic hormone-related conditions in menstruating and post-menopausal women.

It is now possible, through simple urine testing, to assess levels of 2-OHE1, 4-OHE1 and 16α-OHE1 oestrogen metabolites, the ratio between metabolites and, as importantly, the ratios of 2-OHE1 oestrone to 2-MeOE (2-methoxyoestrone, the metabolite that occurs following phase II methylation) and of 4-OHE1 oestrone to 4-MeOE, thus providing practitioners with further opportunities to target personalised nutrition support in the prevention and management of oestrogen-driven diseases.

Imbalances in the level of sex hormones are associated with many conditions, including: infertility, irregular bleeding, fibroids (Okolo 2008), endometriosis, polycystic ovarian syndrome (PCOS), obesity (Cleary and Grossmann 2009), cardiovascular disease (Oqita, Node and Kitakaze 2003), hormone-related cancers (IARC 1999; Kaaks *et al.* 2005; McArdle and O'Mahony 2008), migraines, osteoporosis (Lerner 2006) and depression (Douma *et al.* 2005). Combining a saliva assay with an assessment for oestrogen metabolites provides a more comprehensive appraisal of sex hormone status to inform treatment options.

All three oestrogen metabolites (2-OHE1, 4-OHE1 and 16α-OHE1) created through phase I require quick conjugation with a phase II detoxifier to limit the potential tissue damage caused by these reactive metabolites. Methylation, sulphation, glutathione conjugation and glucuronidation are the principal phase II oestrogen detoxification mechanisms (Hays 2005).

4.3 Phase II detoxification of sex hormones

4.3.1 TRANSMETHYLATION AND TRANS-SULPHURATION

Methylation, sulphation and glutathione conjugation are vital for the safe handling of oestrogen. Glutathione is generated in the body via trans-sulphuration. Clayton (2008) states that methyl donors are reported to be 'the only 'micronutrient' group that, if deficient, is directly carcinogenic' (p.4).

2-OH, 4-OH and 16α-OH oestrogens are methylated as part of the detoxification process. Unmethylated oestrogen metabolites are potentially damaging and injurious to DNA, particularly 4-OHE1 and 16α-OHE1 (Bolton and Thatcher 2008). Prior to elimination these metabolites are conjugated with glutathione, a phase II detoxifier. The essential amino acid methionine is the precursor for the production of S-adenosylmethionine (SAMe), the major methyl donor in the body, and is also required for the synthesis of glutathione (see Figure 7.2). Oestrogen bound to sulphate is inactive; sulphated oestrogen acts as a store for oestrogen as well as being a detoxification outcome (Hays 2005).

4.3.1A METHYLATION

Methylation involves transfer of a methyl group (CH_3) from one compound to another. Methyl donors include methionine, SAMe, choline, betaine (tri-methylglycine), vitamin B12 and folate (Park *et al.* 2008). Transmethylation probably occurs in every cell in the body and involves a series of enzyme reactions that result in a methylated product X-CH_3 (see Figure 7.2) and S-adenosylhomocysteine (SAH), which is then hydrolysed to homocysteine and adenosine. SAMe is required for a number of methylation reactions involving hormones and neurotransmission. For example, methylation is required for the conversion of serotonin to melatonin (Fournier *et al.* 2002) and noradrenaline to adrenaline (Miller 2008).

Undermethylation and high homocysteine are both increasingly associated with many chronic illnesses (Clayton 2008). The production of SAMe can be inhibited due to a lack of vitamin B12, magnesium and methionine. If B12 is deficient then the body can have difficulty using folate. As can be seen from Figure 7.2, dietary dihydrofolate (DHF) is converted to its active form tetrahydrofolate (THF). THF is then converted to either N5, N10 methylene THF or N5, N10 methenyl THF. Both these forms of THF can be metabolised for purine formation. However N5, N10 methylene THF can also be converted by the enzyme methylene THF reductase (MTHFR) to N5 methyl THF.

Homocysteine can be converted back to methionine using betaine (see Figure 7.2). However the formation of betaine (tri-methyl glycine) requires methyl donors and glycine. SAMe is only available on prescription in the UK and is an expensive supplement. Betaine is a relatively cheap source of supplemental methyl groups. Although supplementing betaine would help provide essential methyl groups for important reactions, it does not resolve a methyl trap problem. Non-medical nutrition practitioners should look to support vitamin B12, folate, methionine and magnesium

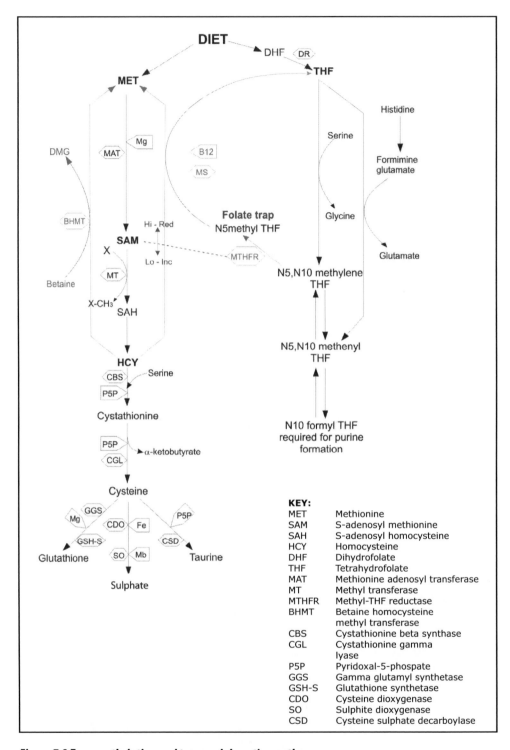

Figure 7.2 Transmethylation and trans-sulphuration pathway

Box 7.3 The methyl trap hypothesis

Vitamin B12, a cofactor for the enzyme methionine synthase, converts homocysteine to methionine (see Figure 7.2). If B12 is deficient this reaction is inhibited, potentially leading to poor methionine status, poor production of SAMe and high homocysteine. This would be compounded by a diet deficient in methionine and low in magnesium. In B12 deficiency folate can also become trapped at N5 methyl THF, because the conversion from N5, N10 methylene THF to N5 methyl THF is not bidirectional (see Figure 7.2).

The trapping of folate is further compounded by a low level of SAMe as, in normal circumstances, SAMe would reduce the activity of MTHFR, diverting more N5, N10 methylene THF towards purine synthesis. Therefore the speed of conversion to N5 methyl THF is increased when SAMe is low, contributing to the trapping of folate. Folate is trapped at N5 methyl THF, as without B12 it cannot be reconverted to THF. Normally the methyl group from N5 methyl THF would be donated to B12 to form methylcobalamin to aid the conversion of homocysteine to methionine. Trapping folate is known as the methyl trap hypothesis (Lieberman, Marks and Smith 2009). Methionine synthase is the only mammalian reaction known to require both B12 and folate.

status to encourage endogenous production of SAMe and, if necessary, communicate with a nutritionally-orientated medical practitioner to prescribe SAMe. Both under- and over-methylation are implicated in cancer, therefore supplementing methyl donors should be considered with care and their use is best supported by laboratory data.

Every tissue in the body utilises the methionine cycle and is therefore able to synthesise adenosylmethionine, employ it for transmethylation, hydrolyse adenosylhomocysteine and remethylate homocysteine (Finkelstein 1998). The liver has a unique isoenzyme, methionine adenosyl transferase (MAT), which enables excess methionine to be used for the continued synthesis of SAMe (Finkelstein 1998).

4.3.1B TRANS-SULPHURATION

Trans-sulphuration occurs only in the liver, kidney, small intestine and pancreas and provides the means of breaking down homocysteine to cysteine. This part of the pathway is called trans-sulphuration because the molecules in this pathway contain a 'thiol' (a double sulphur group).

Homocysteine

Homocysteine is an important intermediate metabolite in the methionine pathway and leads to the production of the major antioxidants and/or detoxifiers: cysteine, glutathione, sulphate and taurine. Too low a level could indicate poor production of these vital compounds and too high a level could indicate a block in converting homocysteine to these compounds.

Vitamin B6, as pyridoxal-5-phosphate (P5P), is used as a cofactor for the enzymes converting homocysteine to cysteine. Along the way, α-ketobutyrate is produced and, if high, is an indication that there is high flux from methionine through to glutathione. Cysteine also requires P5P to convert to taurine; magnesium to convert to glutathione; and molybdenum, iron and B2 to convert to sulphate.

Genetic polymorphisms in MTHFR and cystathionine β-synthase are not uncommon and can lead to raised homocysteine and reduced endogenous production of cysteine, glutathione, taurine and sulphate.

It is worth noting that excessive homocysteine can auto-oxidise and react with ROS, thus increasing requirements for phase I detoxification support. Sufficient magnesium, B12 and folate are needed to sustain adequate reaction rates of SAMe formation and homocysteine remethylation in order to minimise metabolic oxidative stress. Low taurine can allow oxidative activity to go unchecked (Bralley and Lord 2001).

Although a raised homocysteine level has been recognised as an independent risk factor for the development of vascular disease, more recently a relationship between high homocysteine and neurodegenerative diseases, particularly Alzheimer's disease, has been demonstrated (Brosnan *et al.* 2004). Data remains sparse in context of hormone-related cancers and other reproductive problems, including PCOS. However it should be clear from the above discussion and what follows that adequate methylation, glutathione conjugation and sulphation, as well as taurine status, are important players in sex hormone balance.

Glutathione (a tripeptide formed from cysteine, glycine and glutamate) is necessary for the detoxification of the quinones produced from the metabolism of oestrogens during phase I detoxification. 4-quinone oestrogen is highly reactive and can damage DNA (Bland 2004). Antioxidant nutrients may also help reduce the formation of quinones from oestrogens (Hyman 2005).

4.3.2 SUPPORTING METHYLATION AND TRANS-SULPHURATION

The dietary essential amino acid methionine and the essential nutrients, vitamins B12, B6, folate and magnesium, are key nutrients for successful methylation and trans-sulphuration. Betaine is also required but is not considered an essential nutrient; it is found in seafood, spinach, wheat germ and bran. The non-essential nutrient choline is intimately involved in methylation as it is a precursor for the production of betaine. Eggs, liver, wheat germ and soybeans are very good sources of choline. B12, folate and vitamin B2 are used to convert choline to betaine.

Green leafy vegetables and liver are excellent sources of folate. Animal produce is the best source of vitamin B12, as there is, to date, no convincing evidence that seaweed-derived similes of B12 are utilised by the body. Vegans should consider supplemental B12. Meat, liver, wheat and corn are good sources of vitamin B6.

Milk and liver provide good levels of vitamin B2; liver, red meat, eggs, wholegrain, dark green vegetables, beans, lentils, nuts and seeds are good sources of iron; and beans, lentils and peas are the best sources of molybdenum. B2, iron and molybdenum are essential for converting cysteine to sulphate.

Good food sources of sulphur include eggs, brazil nuts, onions, garlic, leeks, cabbage, kale, broccoli and other cruciferous vegetables. Relatively little dietary sulphur is absorbed. Most sulphate in the body is derived from endogenous release from methionine and cysteine.

Supplementary sources of sulphur should be used with care as excess sulphur can be converted to hydrogen sulphide by sulphate-reducing bacteria in the gut. This can contribute to the gut's inflammatory load. Epsom salt baths are used therapeutically as they are a source of sulphur and magnesium, both of which are reported to be absorbed through the skin (Waring 2004).

Adequate dietary protein to supply the essential amino acid methionine is fundamental for methylation and sulphation. Vegans especially need to ensure that they have an adequate mix of plant proteins in their diet, as legumes, nuts and pulses are relatively low in methionine. In the absence of adequate methionine, the non-essential amino acid cysteine becomes conditionally essential for the formation of glutathione and sulphate.

Frequently, digestive processes require support to aid digestion and absorb nutrients. Hypochlorhydria and poor digestive enzyme function can lead to poor uptake of dietary nutrients across the gut membrane. Even supplemental nutrients can be poorly absorbed if the gut membrane is too porous. At a fundamental level, hormone balance is dependent on nutrient absorption.

4.3.3 KEY LABORATORY TESTS FOR TRANSMETHYLATION AND TRANS-SULPHURATION

Fasting plasma homocysteine is a useful biomarker for methylation, glutathione and sulphation capacity, all vital processes for the detoxification of oestrogen. Interestingly, low homocysteine may indicate a functional need for glutathione, taurine and sulphate. According to Lord and Fitzgerald (2006) any condition that increases oxidative stress generally increases functional demand for glutathione synthesis. They report that as homocysteine is drawn into glutathione production plasma homocysteine levels can fall, leading to a critically depleted glutathione status. Homocysteine evaluation should be interpreted in the context of the individual's overall presentation. Urine or blood amino acids and organic acids are useful functional assessments to help the practitioner evaluate nutritional support for methylation, glutathione and sulphate status.

Organic acids analysis provides functional assessment for folate (formimino-glutamate), B12 (methylmalonate) and B6 (kynurenate and xanthurenate). Amino acid testing will provide direct values for methionine, cystathionine and cysteine (amongst others). It will also measure the three amino acids that form glutathione (cysteine, glycine and glutamate). In addition, sarcosine is measured, which, when elevated, is a further indication that B12 and/or folate are required.

Red blood cell folate, serum B12 and functional B6 assessment are also alternative and valuable assessments, alongside plasma homocysteine, that can provide a good insight into methylation and sulphation reactions, at a cost that will be more affordable for many individuals.

Screening for a genetic polymorphism may also be helpful, particularly when the family or personal history suggests this may be relevant. Combining genetic screening with functional assessment enables the practitioner to better advise clients regarding short- and long-term requirements for nutritional support. In future years genetic diagnostics will increasingly facilitate the provision of personalised support by the practitioner. The ethics of genetic screening is outside the context of this chapter.

A detoxification challenge (requiring both a urine and saliva sample) is another alternative assessment that can provide valuable insights into both phase I and phase II detoxification capacity, enabling the practitioner to design a personalised programme to support these pathways. Caffeine is used to challenge phase I, while aspirin and paracetamol are used to challenge phase II pathways.

4.3.4 GLUCURONIDATION

Glucuronide is the only phase II detoxifier derived from glucose and acts as a major alternative pathway for the elimination of toxins such as bilirubin, steroid and thyroid hormones, bile acids and xenobiotics. Glucuronidation is the major excretory pathway for oestrogens. The enzymes that control the glucuronidation pathway are under considerable genetic influence.

Oestrogens are conjugated with glucuronide and then pass via bile into the gut for elimination in the stool. Oestrogen can be recycled via the entero-hepatic circulation; this process is enhanced by imbalanced gut flora that can produce excessive amounts of the enzyme β-glucuronidase. This enzyme de-conjugates oestrogens from glucuronide, facilitating the reabsorption of oestrogens. The freed oestrogen is sulphated by gut mucosal cells and in this form is reabsorbed and released into the circulation.

4.3.5 SUPPORTING GLUCURONIDATION: THE IMPORTANCE OF DIGESTIVE HEALTH

Certain foods and nutrients have been shown, via different mechanisms, to positively influence glucuronidation. These include: garlic, onion, carrot, broccoli and Brussels sprouts, garden cress; flavonoids, including luteolin; fibre; and oleic acid, of which olive oil is a good source. Although Kirk *et al.* (2001) caution the use of flavonoids, due to their potential to inhibit sulphotransferase activity (see later discussion in this chapter), thus leading to excess free oestrone, they suggest that the overall protection conferred by flavonoids is due to their ability to up-regulate glucuronidation, the major route for oestrogen disposal.

4.4 Transport and binding of oestrogen

Most steroid hormones are fat-soluble and as such need to be transported on protein carriers/binders, otherwise they would stick to blood vessel walls and form globules. They have access to all living cells and are able to penetrate membranes without the need of a trans-membrane carrier. When they are produced, they have to be circulated from the site of generation to all tissues in order to influence target tissues, such as breast, uterus, brain, bone and prostate. In the bound form, steroid hormones are inactive. The physiology and clinical consequences of steroid hormones is determined by the balance between the bound and unbound forms.

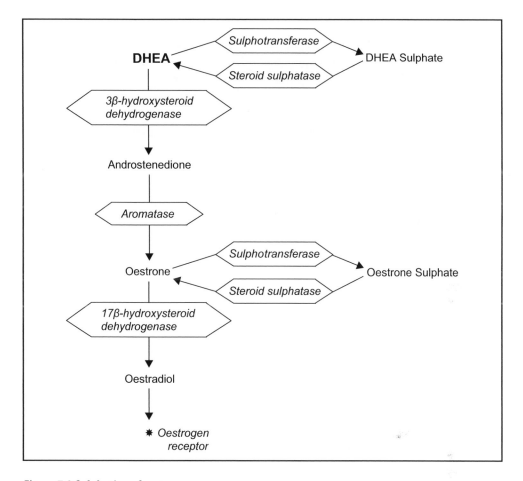

Figure 7.3 Sulphation of oestrone

4.4.1 SEX HORMONE BINDING GLOBULIN (SHBG)

The interaction between hormones is largely mediated by binding globulins. Sex hormone binding globulin (SHBG) is an important regulator of oestrogen balance. Therapies that affect SHBG levels should be undertaken with caution if the release or binding of free oestrogen or testosterone is not the intended outcome (Hays 2005).

According to Hays (2005) a high level of SHBG suggests oestrogen dominance and a low level of SHBG indicates an increased testosterone to oestrogen ratio. She reports that low SHBG is seen in hirsutism, acne vulgaris and PCOS, and may also be seen in hypothyroidism and obesity. Raised levels are associated with oestrogen dominance, low progesterone, pregnancy and oestrogen-replacement therapy.

The level of SHBG declines post-menopause. This may be a protective mechanism, enabling oestrogen to function at target tissues for longer. Although testosterone also declines post-menopause, it is high relative to oestrogen. It can be seen from Figure 7.3 that androstenedione, a metabolite of testosterone, is converted to oestradiol; this can occur in peripheral tissues, such as bone, without increasing blood oestrogen levels. According to Hays (2005) testosterone would be available to stimulate bone building as well as increasing the ability of oestrogen to inhibit bone breakdown.

High levels of insulin down-regulate the production of SHBG. Selva *et al.* (2007) report on new research indicating that excess sugar consumption may have a more significant impact on the production of SHBG than insulin *per se*. Excess sugar can be converted into fats in the liver. The researchers discovered that increased production of fat reduced the amount of SHBG in the blood, leading to excess free testosterone and oestrogen in circulation. This is associated with an increased risk of acne, infertility, polycystic ovarian syndrome (PCOS) and uterine cancer in overweight women. Improving insulin sensitivity and reducing circulating levels of insulin have been shown to benefit women with PCOS (Nestler 1996). Low glycaemic index/load food choices, meals that have an overall low glycaemic load, stress management and exercise are all indicated.

Longcope *et al.* (2000) found that low-protein diets in elderly men might increase SHBG, decreasing the bioactivity of testosterone and thus resulting in decreased sexual function, muscle mass and possibly contributing to loss of bone density. The mechanisms by which a low-protein diet exerts this effect are unclear; although a low-protein intake leads to lower insulin levels, potentially enabling SHBG levels to rise.

Xenoestrogens have been shown to displace testosterone and oestradiol from SHBG, potentially altering the androgen to oestrogen balance in humans. Dechaud *et al.* (1999) propose that binding with SHBG may transport some contaminant xenoestrogens into the plasma and have an impact on their bioavailability to cell tissues. Four xenoestrogens, used as surfactants in many commercial products, and bisphenol A (widely used in plastics) were identified by the researchers as potent binders to SHBG. Further investigation is needed to identify whether these chemicals could reach high enough levels in the blood to cause harm.

Hodgert Jury, Zacharewski and Hammond (2000) found that the xenoestrogens and phytoestrogens they tested bound to SHBG with a much lower affinity than our own sex hormones. They suggested that the most physiologically relevant situations would be when SHBG levels are high and endogenous sex hormone production is low, such as in women taking oral contraceptives and pre-pubertal children.

Phytoestrogens, particularly isoflavones and lignans, have been reported to stimulate the synthesis of SHBG (Low *et al.* 2007; Pino *et al.* 2000) but as yet clinical trials have not borne out the findings from cell culture data. Several short term studies have shown increased urinary excretion of phytoestrogens following increased intake of flax or soy over a 4–12 week period, and only one study noted a significant rise in SHBG. The sample sizes were small, so data should be interpreted cautiously and the association remained weak at the time of the research (Tham, Gardner and Haskell 1998).

Testing SHBG levels

Assessment of SHBG status is currently used to determine the amount of free testosterone, providing key information for diagnosing hormonal problems, and is also a screening tool for those at risk of type 2 diabetes and cardiovascular disease. Hays (2005) indicates that SHBG can be used as a marker for the total amount of oestrogen and testosterone traversing the liver and can also help in estimating the total oestrogen burden in the presence of normal testosterone levels.

Selva *et al.* (2007) discovered that low levels of SHBG in the blood indicate that the liver is functioning suboptimally, due to an inappropriate diet or an inherent problem with the liver. As a result, the researchers reported that SHBG can be used as a biomarker of liver function well before symptoms of hormonal imbalance arise and as a means of monitoring the effectiveness of dietary interventions and pharmaceutical strategies targeted towards improving the metabolic function of the liver.

Clearly, identifying the level of SHBG is fundamental, as treatment strategies will differ for raising or lowering the level of this binder.

4.4.2 CORTISOL BINDING GLOBULIN (CBG)

The stress hormone cortisol and the sex hormone progesterone are transported on a specialised carrier, cortisol binding globulin (CBG). It has a higher affinity for cortisol than progesterone and is capable of binding only one molecule of either cortisol or progesterone at a time.

Cortisol is a catabolic hormone and an excess is tantamount to physiological stress at target tissues, leading to breakdown of bone and muscle. As CBG has a higher affinity for cortisol than progesterone, it will preferentially bind cortisol, which then gives a feedback message to the hypothalamus to produce more cortisol.

As can be seen from Figure 7.1 progesterone is the precursor for corticosteroid hormones and diverting progesterone to corticosteroids can give rise to low progesterone availability, thus forcing the body to use the androgen pathway via DHEA.

Women with PCOS and postmenopausal women utilise the androgen pathway for continued production of oestrogen, hence the increased propensity to facial hair growth, scalp hair loss and acne.

4.4.3 BIO-IDENTICAL HORMONE THERAPY

The use of bio-identical (otherwise known as 'natural') progesterone can potentially displace cortisol from CBG through the principle of 'mass action', leading to an excess level of free-circulating cortisol, which would also be seen by target tissues as stress.

DHEA supplementation can cause a surge of oestrogen or testosterone through displacement on SHBG. Natural hormones are prescription-only medicines in the UK. Natural hormones can have a role to play and should be used with caution and in conjunction with a medical practitioner who is competent in their use. A nutritional programme should underpin the use of natural hormones, as the 'hormone' approach alone, whether natural or synthetic, is somewhat a 'band-aid' strategy and does not attempt to address why the balance of hormones is disrupted.

As well as the hormone tests previously described, tests for levels of stress hormones, thyroid function, and insulin (among other useful biomarkers) can be used to assist in the development of an appropriate personalised nutritional programme.

4.4.4 BINDING OF OESTROGEN WITH SULPHATE

Sulphate, like SHBG, is another compound in the body that potentially protects against too much free oestrogen (see Figure 7.3).

Sulphated oestrone acts as a store of oestrogen and in this form can be eliminated from the body via bile or urine as part of the phase II detoxification process. Sulphatase enzymes can convert sulphated oestrone back into its free unbound state of oestrone. Sulphotransferase enzymes convert free oestrone into oestrone sulphate. The activity of these enzymes is important in terms of how much free oestrogen is made available to hormone-sensitive tissues.

A major source of oestradiol in post-menopausal breast tumours is thought to be the steroid sulphates (see Figure 7.3). Although most epidemiological data suggests protective effects of dietary flavonoids on breast tissue, Waring and colleagues from the University of Birmingham (UK) suggest caution, as they have shown certain flavonoids to exert powerful inhibiting effects on the sulphotransferase enzymes (see Figure 7.3) that convert free oestrone to oestrone sulphate. Inhibition of sulphotransferase would lead to increased levels of free oestrogen. However, as previously discussed in this chapter, flavonoids have been shown to upregulate glucuronidation, the major pathway for oestrogen detoxification.

Compounds in celery (luteolin), onions (quercetin) and particularly genistein in soy were found by the researchers to be the most potent inhibitors of the flavonoids tested for their effect on sulphotransferases. The researchers suggest that the paradox may be explained by the fact that sulphotransferases are involved in activating pro-carcinogens found in overcooked meats, which have also been implicated in the aetiology of breast cancer (Kirk *et al.* 2001).

In practice, limiting exposure to endocrine disruptors and overcooked meats that might influence the expression of sulphotransferase should be considered first. The fact that flavonoids upregulate glucuronidation would seem to outweigh their potential impact on sulphotransferase activity.

4.5 Cholesterol transport

Women from menarche onwards have higher high density lipoprotein (HDL) levels than men. Triglycerides come down as HDL goes up, providing cardiovascular protection through oestrogen. Oestrogens suppress the liver enzyme hepatic lipase, responsible for consuming HDL. This enzyme has been shown to be much lower in women, providing a mechanism for higher HDL (Berk-Planken *et al.* 2003). Oestrogen failure is linked to increase in low density lipoprotein (LDL), change in distribution of body fat and increased iron stores, all associated risks for cardiovascular disease.

5. Immune system health (defence)

The onset and perpetuation of autoimmune disease, according to Bland (2007), appears to be significantly influenced by the balance of sex hormones. Women are more commonly affected by autoimmune disease, with a predominance of between 5 and 10 to 1 over men, depending on the autoimmune disorder.

Bland (2007) goes on to report that the sera of patients with systemic lupus erythematosus (SLE) and the synovial fluid of patients with rheumatoid arthritis (RA) show elevated levels of hydroxylated oestrogens. Metabolites of 16α-OHE1 can stimulate the proliferation of cells in synovial tissue (Cappellino *et al.* 2008; Cutolo *et al.* 2004). As previously discussed, 4-OHE1 is metabolised to the DNA-injurious quinones. The DNA adducts formed may be seen as 'foreign' by the immune system in individuals with specific genetic uniqueness and trigger an inflammatory response (Khan *et al.* 2009).

In conversion of oestrone to the hydroxylated forms, the inflammatory cytokines TNF-α, IL-1 and IL-6 are released. 4- and 16-hydroxylated metabolites increase the production of NFkB-mediated gene expression of inflammatory cytokines. Many plant compounds may inhibit or modulate the expression of NFkB, including soy isoflavones and curcumin (turmeric) (Kunnumakkara and Aggarwal 2008; Singh and Khar 2006).

6. Communication

Steroid hormones are freed from their binders and can easily float through a cell membrane. If they encounter and subsequently bind to an accessible receptor, they form an activated complex that migrates into the cell nucleus and binds with accessible DNA. This results in the formation of specific RNA, enabling the hormone to function. If an appropriate receptor is lacking in the cell, the hormone will simply float out of the cell.

The concentration of a hormone, its affinity to a receptor, the number of receptor sites already occupied and the duration of binding at a receptor site all determine the activity of a hormone at a target cell.

A substance that competes with a hormone for binding is described as an *agonist* if the response of the cell is the same as, or mimics the action of the hormone. A substance that competes with a hormone for binding to a receptor is referred to as an *antagonist* if it blocks or inhibits the response of the cell to the action of the hormone.

6.1 Phytoestrogens

Phytoestrogens, along with oestrogen medication (whether or not it is bio-identical) and xenoestrogens, can compete with the body's own endogenous oestrogen for binding to oestrogen receptor sites on cell surfaces, although all are less potent than endogenous oestrogen. Numerous studies have shown that all the main isoflavonoids bind to oestrogen receptors and exert weak oestrogenic activity.

Post-menopause, oestrogen declines to approximately 40 per cent of pre-menopausal production. Phytoestrogens are thought to act as oestrogen agonists by filling the available receptor sites, potentially conferring oestrogenic benefits at this time.

Genistein and, more particularly, coumestrol have been shown *in vitro* to inhibit the conversion of oestrone to 17-beta oestradiol, a form of oestrogen that is highly stimulating to breast and uterine tissue (Cheeke 1989; Makela *et al.* 1994). However, although there are numerous studies on phytoestrogens, many of the studies are fraught with confounding factors, differences in study design and methodology, giving rise to contradictory and inconclusive data. Various types of soy products with differing chemical composition have been used, further complicating interpretation of the data.

It is worthy of mention that dietary phytoestrogens are acted on by gut bacteria and converted into other compounds that exert weak oestrogenic effects at receptor sites. It has been proposed that the metabolism of genistein and daidzein by gut bacteria may vary considerably from one individual to another, which may help explain inconsistencies in results from clinical trials (Atkinson, Frankenfeld and Lampe 2005; Matthies *et al.* 2008).

Trock *et al.* (2006) report that a meta-analysis showed a small reduction in risk of breast cancer with high versus low intake of soy; the correlation was stronger among pre-menopausal women than amongst post-menopausal women.

Much of the evidence of a role for soy phytoestrogens in bone health has been conducted in animals; any human studies have generally been of short duration. Recent data, however, from a long-term study suggest protective effects on bone in menopausal women, but more data will be required to evaluate the impact of consumption on fracture rates (Cassidy 2003).

The influence of phytoestrogens on hormonal balance remains controversial and often contradictory. In practice, including dietary phytoestrogens in a food plan appears advisable. If using soy, then encourage inclusion of some fermented sources of soy such as miso, tempeh, natto and soy sauce, as they appear to confer many health benefits. The pros and cons of soy are outside the context of this chapter.

Soy is a significant source of dietary amines and, as discussed later, oestrogen excess may inhibit the breakdown of amines. Gut flora support may be indicated prior to the inclusion of phytoestrogens, in order to facilitate appropriate conversion to active metabolites. In the case of soy, one small study showed no difference in isoflavone absorption from soy milk or miso, so long as the intestinal microflora is capable of hydrolysing the isoflavone glucosides (Maskarinec *et al.* 2008).

6.2 Oestrogen and tryptophan metabolism

Oestrogen metabolites have been shown to impair the function of enzymes that convert the essential amino acid tryptophan to NAD (from vitamin B3) (Bender and Totoe

1984). Overt vitamin B3 deficiency is a cause of depression. The oral contraceptive pill (OCP) has been known to affect tryptophan metabolism since the late 1960s (Salih, Zein and Bayoumi 1986). Depressed mood, irritability and emotional instability are frequently reported in OCP users. The metabolite xanthurenic acid, an indicator of low functional B6, has been found in higher levels in OCP users (Smit Veninga 1984).

Tryptophan is the precursor for serotonin, a neurotransmitter involved in mood and appetite control, and for melatonin, a sleep-regulating hormone and powerful antioxidant. The breakdown of tryptophan is stimulated by stress hormones and inflammation. Under these circumstances the production of serotonin is lowered, due to the exhaustion of co-factor nutrients like vitamin B6.

6.3 Oestrogen and monoamine oxidase

Oestrogens suppress monoamine oxidase enzymes (MAOs), giving a feeling of wellbeing. However, if MAO enzymes are too inactive, amine levels can become too high, causing headaches, migraines, high blood pressure or feelings of mania (Grant 1994). Zinc, vitamin B6 and magnesium are needed to break down amines and sulphur is needed to inactivate them.

Amines, found in a diverse range of foods, are also formed by bacterial metabolism of free amino acids in the large bowel. Reduction of amine load by supporting gut health, nutrient status and reduced intake of high amine foods should be considered in individuals presenting with migraines, high blood pressure and depression.

Aged cheeses, raspberries, yeast extract, bananas, chicken liver, red plums, wines (especially red), avocados, beer, aubergines (eggplant), other fermented beverages, soy, tomatoes, vinegar and pickles are particularly potent sources of amines (Joneja 2003).

7. Mitochondrial function – oxidative stress

Oxidative injury can occur through metabolic processes and from exogenous sources, including toxic metals, industrial pollutants and drugs, as well as nutrient deficiencies. The largest endogenous source of reactive oxygen species (ROS) is from mitochondrial respiration converting fuels into energy.

Haem is also incorporated into electron transport proteins (see earlier discussion on phase I detoxification) and so deficiency of haem would disrupt the final stages of converting fuels into energy.

The cumulative damage from ROS is one of the strongest theories of ageing and determinants of maximum lifespan – now called the 'free radical-mitochondrial theory of ageing' (Harman 1972). About 5 per cent of oxygen is converted to ROS even under the most favourable conditions.

Support for phase I detoxification is key in managing ROS. Generation of ROS eventually 'wins' the ageing war. Dietary antioxidants help but some ROS escape control – we all age eventually.

Table 7.1 Sex hormone balancing at a glance

Nutrient/Compounds	Function	Effect	Comment
Antioxidants A, C, E, Zn, Se, CoQ10, lipoic acid, carotenoids, flavonoids, taurine, tryptophan, tyrosine, methionine, cysteine and glutathione	Protect cholesterol from oxidation Generally protect cells from oxidation	Reduce formation of DNA-damaging quinones	Flavonoids particularly from soy, celery and onions may inhibit sulphotransferase enzymes though overall considered protective
B1, B2, B3, B5, biotin, Mg, tryptophan, glycine, cysteine, serine, alanine, lysine, leucine	Conversion of fats and sugars to acetate needed to synthesise cholesterol		Supplementation particularly with amino acids is best supported by clinical testing
Protein	Hormone transport, storage, enzyme and receptor function, detoxification Improve insulin function	Prevent high levels of SHBG decreasing available testosterone	Too much protein can be acidic and is best balanced with alkaline vegetables and fruit to limit acid effect
Reduce sugar	Prevent lowering of SHBG leading to elevated testosterone and oestrogens	Reduce cholesterol synthesis Reduce small dense cholesterol	This applies to added sugar, excessive intake of fruit and fruit juice, confectionery, cakes, biscuits, buns etc and refined cereals products Aim for 2–3 portions of whole fruit daily and 6–7 portions of vegetables each the size of a medium apple Vegetables and wholegrain are generally slow-releasing and give low glycaemic effect Combining with meals containing protein and fat helps slow sugar effect and reduce glycaemic load
Fibre	Helps eliminate cholesterol and oestrogen preventing recirculation		Soluble fibres from oats and rice and vegetables most effective

Nutrient/Compounds	Function	Effect	Comment
Balance fat intake	Fish oils improve insulin, sex hormone, brain, immune, cardiovascular, joint and skin health	Reduce cholesterol synthesis EPA shown to increase C-2 hydroxylation and decrease 16α hydroxylation in breast cancer cells	Limit saturated fats and aim to achieve a balance of omega-6 and 3 fats, 3:1 in favour of omega 6 Avoid trans fats and those labelled hydrogenated Avoid using omega-3 and 6 fats at high temperatures Olive oil, butter, palm and coconut oil safer for cooking
Phytoestrogens and soy	Potentially increase SHBG	Potentially act as oestrogen agonists and antagonists	Data conflicting: fermented sources of soy, such as natto, tempeh, miso, soy sauce are considered preferable Soy, like other goitrogens, may inhibit thyroid function – cooking reduces this effect Healthy gut flora required for proper use
Zinc, B6, Mg	Promote reproduction, neurotransmission and immunity on several levels	Balance with copper Help break down amines	Supplementation best supported by clinical testing
Sulphur-containing foods/glucosinolates Eggs, brazil nuts, garlic, onions, leeks, chives, broccoli, Brussels sprouts, cabbage, cauliflower, kale	Support phase II sulphur detoxification pathway Support gastric hormone function, thyroid, oestrogen and DHEA, fat digestion, gut membrane health	Upregulate CY 1A1 increasing 2-methoxyestrone, a powerful protective anti-oestrogen Supplementation with I3C shown to be helpful for women suffering with SLE	Caution: see above re: goitrogenic effect of soy (brassica family high in goitrogens) Excess sulphur in the gut can convert to hydrogen sulphide giving rise to unpleasant flatulence and damage to gut membranes Epsom salt baths are a way of improving sulphur and magnesium status that bypasses the gut

continued

Table 7.1 Sex hormone balancing at a glance *cont.*

Nutrient/Compounds	Function	Effect	Comment
B12, folate, B6, Mb, Mg, choline, methionine, betaine (seafood, spinach, wheatgerm and bran)	Support methylation, glutathione and sulphuration detoxification pathways	COMT enzyme helps break down amines	Overmethylation can also be problematic and support for methylation is best considered on the basis of testing
Avoid overcooked meats, charred and BBQ food	Tax sulphotransferase activity	Increase need for antioxidants	Best avoided with cancer Otherwise enjoy occasionally, eat with uncharred vegetables and fruit and take antioxidants
Salvestrols Strawberries, tangerines, cranberries, red grapes, red wine, olive oil	Activate CYP1B1 to unleash chemical agents thought to be 'deadly' to cancer cells		Even organic produce can be cultivated to give a sweeter taste Supplementing salvestrols should be considered Alcohol depletes many nutrients including folic acid Clinical trials need to be conducted
Organic produce	Higher salvestrol content	Reduced exposure to endocrine disruptors	Cost may be an issue Many people overeat so eating less and purchasing better quality is a consideration
Garlic, onions, carrot, broccoli, Brussels sprouts, garden cress, flavonoids, oleic acid (olive oil)	Support glucuronidation major pathway for oestrogen detoxification		See cautions re: goitrogens and flavonoids Good gut flora required for action of β-glucuronidase to aid efficient elimination of oestrogen

Nutrient/Compounds	Function	Effect	Comment
Amine-containing foods Aged cheeses, raspberries, yeast extract, bananas, chicken liver, red plums, wines (especially red), avocados, beer, aubergine (eggplant), other fermented beverages, tomatoes, vinegar and pickles	Potent sources of amines that can trigger headaches, migraine, high blood pressure and feelings of mania	High oestrogen can suppress activity of enzymes that break down amines in these foods	Those on MAO medication should restrict intake of these amines Reactions to amines are not allergies and reducing total load can be helpful and then increase to identify tolerance level without giving rise to symptoms
Limit exposure to endocrine disruptors including Toxic metals, plasticisers in PVC products including building and furnishing materials, floorings, furniture, food packaging, toys, clothing, car interiors, cables, medical equipment, lubricating oils, fixatives, adhesives, paints, sealants, surface coatings, insecticides, detergents, printing inks, car-care products, soaps, shampoos, hand lotion, nail polish, cosmetics and perfumes	Prevent displacement of testosterone and oestrogen from SHBG Compete with essential metal binders potentially disrupting zinc to copper balance PCBs and PAHs potent suppressors of oestrogen sulphotransferase	4-hydroxylated phthalate esters unequivocal binding affinities for oestrogen receptors Disrupt oestrogen and potentially androgen receptor binding Tax phase I and II sulphation, methylation and glutathione detoxification May disrupt hormones, neural pathways and neurotransmitters involved in appetite regulation and may contribute to the obesity epidemic	Oily fish are potent absorbers of endocrine disrupting chemicals Controversial re: risk/benefit of reducing oily fish intake as reduces n-3 fatty acid intake. Most fish oil supplements are purified Avoid exposure in pregnancy and breastfeeding
Oral contraceptive pill	Depletes many nutrients including folic acid, B6, zinc and magnesium Disrupts gut flora	Known to affect tryptophan metabolism potentially leading to B3 depletion	Modern OCPs have lower oestrogen dose Vitamin B6 can be helpful

continued

Table 7.1 Sex hormone balancing at a glance *cont.*

Nutrient/Compounds	Function	Effect	Comment
Water	All cellular reactions occur in a medium of water	Supports detoxification	Aim for 6–8 250ml glasses of filtered or bottled water daily Avoid drinking too much water Glass bottles are better than plastic bottles Avoid regularly drinking direct from plastic bottles as they may contain endocrine-disrupting chemicals Fruit and vegetables are a good source of 'natural' water
Exercise and stress management	Improve insulin sensitivity Reduce cortisol output	Weight management	Slow weight loss recommended and avoidance of yo-yo dieting Fat cells are storage sites for toxic metals and slow release is recommended combined with reducing exposure to toxins and a healthy supportive diet to mop up toxins for elimination

8. Conclusion

In conclusion it should be clear from the discussion that scientific data is often incomplete and contradictory and that making clinical decisions based on the data is fraught with difficulty. The use of laboratory evaluation is instrumental in aiding the practitioner in both making informed treatment decisions and monitoring the effectiveness of their interventions. Thus the practitioner is better able to use the scientific data as a guide to informing and justifying their decisions for individual clients based on a functional model.

The art of making clinical decisions in a world of scientific uncertainty is a reality for all healthcare practitioners.

References

Atkinson, C., Frankenfeld, C.L. and Lampe, J.W. (2005) 'Gut bacterial metabolism of the soy isoflavone daidzein: Exploring the relevance to human health.' *Experimental Biology and Medicine 230*, 155–170.

Baillie-Hamilton, P. (2002) 'Chemical toxins: A hypothesis to explain the global obesity epidemic.' *Journal of Alternative and Complementary Medicine 8*, 185–192.

Bender, D.A. and Totoe, L. (1984) 'Inhibition of tryptophan metabolism by oestrogens in the rat: A factor in the aetiology of pellagra.' *British Journal of Nutrition 51*, 219–224.

Berk-Planken, I.I.L, Hoogerbrugge, N., Stolk, R.P., Bootsma, A.H. *et al.* (2003) 'Atorvastatin dose-dependently decreases hepatic lipase activity in type 2 diabetes. Effect of sex and the LIPC promoter variant.' *Diabetes Care 26*, 2, 427–432.

Bland, J.S. (1998) *Improving Genetic Expression in the Prevention of the Diseases of Aging.* Gig Harbour, WA: HealthComm International Inc, p8.

Bland, J.S. (2004) *Nutrigenomic Modulation of Inflammatory Disorders: Arthralgias, Coronary Artery Disease, PMS and Menopause-Associated Inflammation.* Gig Harbour, WA: Metagenics Inc.

Bland, J. (2007) 'Estrogen Metabolism and Detoxification Pathways Associated with Autoimmune Diseases with Emphasis on Systemic Lupus Erythematosus.' *Understanding the Origins and Applying Advanced Nutritional Strategies for Autoimmune Diseases.* Gig Harbour, WA: Metagenics Inc.

Bland, J.S., Costarella, L., Levin, B., Liska, D. *et al.* (1999) *Clinical Nutrition: A Functional Approach.* Gig Harbour, WA: Institute for Functional Medicine.

Bolton J.L. and Thatcher, G.R. (2008) 'Potential mechanisms of estrogen quinone carcinogenesis.' *Chemical Research in Toxicology 21*, 1, 93–101.

Bonnesen, C., Stephensen, P.U., Andersen, O., Sørensen, H. and Vang, O. (1999) 'Modulation of cytochrome P-450 and glutathione S-transferase isoform expression in vivo by intact and degraded indolyl glucosinolates.' *Nutrition and Cancer 33*, 2, 178–187.

Bralley, J. and Lord, R. (2001) *Laboratory Evaluations in Molecular Medicine*, 1st edn. Atlanta, GA: IAMM.

Brosnan, J., Jacobs, R.L., Stead, L.M. and Brosnan, M.E. (2004) 'Methylation demand: A key determinant of homocysteine metabolism.' *Acta Biochimica Polonica 51*, 2, 405–413.

Bulun, S.E. (2009) 'Endometriosis.' *New England Journal of Medicine 360*, 3, 268–279.

Cadbury, D. (1997) *The Feminization of Nature.* Toronto: Penguin Books.

Capellino, S. Montagna, P., Villaggio, B. Soldano, S. Straub, R.H. and Cutolo, M. (2008) 'Hydroxylated estrogen metabolites influence the proliferation of cultured human monocytes: Possible role in synovial tissue hyperplasia.' *Clinical and Experimental Rheumatology 26*, 5, 903–909.

Carson, R. (1962) *Silent Spring*. London: Penguin.

Cassidy, A. (2003) 'Dietary phytoestrogens and bone health.' *Journal of the British Menopause Society 9*, 1, 17–21.

Caulfield, L., Zavaleta, N., Shankar, A.H. and Merialdi, M. (1998) 'Potential contribution of maternal zinc supplementation during pregnancy to maternal and child survival.' *American Journal of Clinical Nutrition 68*, suppl., 499S–508S.

Centers for Disease Control and Prevention (2005) *Third National Report on Human Exposure to Environmental Chemicals*. Atlanta, GA: CDC. Available at www.cdc.gov/exposurereport/pdf/results_06.pdf, accessed 8 November 2009.

Cheeke, P.R. (1989) *Toxicants of Plant Origin IV – Phenolics*. Florida: CRC Press.

Clayton, P, (2008) *Hypomethylation: A Nutritional Disorder with Multiple Consequences*. Cytoplan Technical Information Series, Issue 5.

Cleary, M.P. and Grossmann, M.E. (2009) 'Minireview: Obesity and breast cancer: The estrogen connection.' *Endocrinology 150*, 6, 2537–2542.

Colborn, T., Dumanoski, D. and Peterson Myers, J. (1996) *Our Stolen Future*. New York: Penguin.

Colborn, T., vom Saal, F.S. and Soto, A.M. (1993) 'Developmental effects of endocrine-disrupting chemicals in wildlife and humans.' *Environmental Health Perspectives 101*, 5, 378–384.

Cutolo, M., Villaggio, B., Seriolo, B., Montagna, P. *et al.* (2004) 'Synovial fluid estrogens in rheumatoid arthritis.' *Autoimmunity Reviews 3*, 3, 193–198.

Dechaud, H., Ravard, C., Claustrat, F., Brac de la Perrière, A. and Pugeat, M. (1999) 'Xenoestrogen interaction with human sex hormone-binding globulin (hSHBG).' *Steroids 64*, 5, 328–334.

de Jong, M.M., Nolte, I.M., te Meerman, G.J., van der Graaf, W.T.A. *et al.* (2002) 'Genes other than BRCA1 and BRCA2 involved in breast cancer susceptibility.' *Journal of Medical Genetics 39*, 4, 225–242.

Dorey, C. (2003) *Chemical Legacy – Contamination of the Child*. London: Adobe. Available at www.greenpeace.org/raw/content/international/press/reports/chemical-legacy-contaminatio.pdf, accessed on 24 November 2009.

Douma, S.L., Husband, C., O'Donnell, M.E., Barwin, B.N. and Woodend, A.K. (2005) 'Estrogen-related mood disorders: Reproductive life cycle factors.' *ANS Advances in Nursing Science 28*, 4, 364–375.

Finkelstein, J. (1998) 'The metabolism of homocysteine: Pathways and regulation.' *European Journal of Paediatrics 157*, S40–S44.

Fournier, I., Ploye, F., Cottet-Emard, J.M., Brun, J. and Claustrat, B. (2002) 'Folate deficiency alters melatonin secretion in rats.' *Journal of Nutrition 132*, 9, 2781–2784.

Galland, L. (1997) *The Four Pillars of Healing: How the New Integrated Medicine – The Best of Conventional and Alternative Approaches – Can Cure You*. New York: Random House.

Grant, E. (1994) *Sexual Chemistry: Understanding our Hormones, the Pill and HRT*. London: Cedar.

Gregory, J., Lowe, S., Bates, C.J., Prentice, A. *et al.* (2000) *National Diet and Nutrition Surveys*. London: HMSO.

Guillette, L.J. Jr, Edwards, T.M. and Moore, B.C. (2007) 'Alligators, contaminants and steroid hormones.' *Environmental Science 14*, 6, 331–347.

Harman, D. (1972) 'A biologic clock: The mitochondria?' *Journal of American Geriatric Society 20*, 4, 145–147.

Hays, B. (2005) 'Female Hormones: The Dance of the Hormones, part 1.' In D. Jones (ed.) *The Textbook of Functional Medicine*. Gig Harbour, WA: Institute for Functional Medicine.

Helland, I.B., Smith, L., Blomén, B, Saarem, K., Saugstad, O.D. and Drevon, C.A. (2008) 'Effect of supplementing pregnant and lactating mothers with n-3 very-long-chain fatty acids on children's IQ and body mass index at 7 years of age.' *Pediatrics 122*, 2, 472–479.

Hibbeln, J.R., Davis, J.M., Steer, C., Emmett, P. *et al.* (2007) 'Maternal seafood consumption in pregnancy and neurodevelopmental outcomes in childhood (ALSPAC study, an observational cohort study).' *Lancet 369*, 9561, 578–585.

Hodgert Jury, H., Zacharewski, T.R., and Hammond, G.L. (2000) 'Interactions between human plasma sex hormone binding globulin and xenobiotic ligands.' *Journal of Steroid Biochemistry and Molecular Biology 75*, 2–3, 167–176.

Hyman, M. (2005) 'Clinical Approaches to Environmental Inputs.' In D. Jones (ed.) *The Textbook of Functional Medicine*. Gig Harbour, WA: Institute for Functional Medicine.

International Agency for Research on Cancer (IARC) (1999) 'Post-menopausal oestrogen therapy (group 1).' *Summaries and Evaluations 72*, 399. Available at www.inchem.org/documents/iarc/vol72/vol72-3. html, accessed on 9 November 2009.

Joneja, J. (2003) *Dealing with Food Allergies: A Practical Guide to Detecting Culprit Foods and Eating a Healthy, Enjoyable Diet*. Colorado: Bull Publishing Company.

Jones, D., Hofmann, L. and Quinn, S. (2009) '21st century medicine: A new model for medical education and practice.' Gig Harbour, WA: Institute for Functional Medicine.

Kaaks, R., Rinaldi, S., Key, T.J., Berrino, F. *et al.* (2005) 'Postmenopausal serum androgens, oestrogens and breast cancer risk: The European prospective investigation into cancer and nutrition.' *Endocrine-Related Cancer 12*, 4, 1071–1082.

Khan, W.A., Uddin, M., Khan, M.W.A. and Chabbra, H.S. (2009) 'Catecholoestrogens: Possible role in systemic lupus erythematosus.' *Rheumatology 48*, 11, 1345–1351.

Kirk, C.J., Harris, R.M., Wood, D.M., Waring R.H. and Hughes, P.J. (2001) 'Do dietary phytoestrogens influence susceptibility to hormone-dependent cancer by disrupting the metabolism of endogenous oestrogens?' *Biochemical Society Transactions 29*, 209–216.

Kunnumakkara, A.B. and Aggarwal, B.B. (2008) 'Chemoprevention of GI cancers with dietary agents: Are we there yet?' *AGA Perspectives*, 9–10. Available at www.jivaresearch.org/research/curcumin/GM_02-17-2008.pdf, accessed on 1 February 2010.

Ledger, B. (2005) 'Infertility threatening Europe's population.' *The Medical News*. Available at www.news-medical.net/news/2005/06/21/11224.aspx, accessed on 12 September 2009.

Lee, J. (1993) *Natural Progesterone: The Multiple Roles of a Remarkable Hormone*. Sebastopol, CA: BLL Publishing.

Lerner, U.H. (2006) 'Bone remodelling in post-menopausal osteoporosis.' *Journal of Dental Research 85*, 7, 584–595.

Lieberman, M., Marks, A.D. and Smith, C. (2009) *Marks' Basic Medical Biochemistry: A Clinical Approach*, 3rd edn. Philadelphia; Wolters Kluwer Health.

Longcope, C., Feldman, H.A., McKinlay, J.B. and Araujo, A.B. (2000) 'Diet and sex hormone binding globulin.' *Journal of Clinical Endocrinology and Metabolism 85*, 1, 293–296.

Lord, R.S. and Bralley, J.A. (2008) *Laboratory Evaluations for Integrative and Functional Medicine*. Georgia, USA: Metametrix Institute.

Lord, R. and Fitzgerald, K. (2006) *Significance of Low Plasma Homocysteine*. Metametrix Clinical Laboratory, Dept of Science and Education. Georgia, USA: Metametrix Inc.

Low, Y.-L., Dunning, A.M., Dowsett, M., Folkerd, E. (2007) 'Phytoestrogen exposure is associated with circulating sex hormone levels in postmenopausal women and interact with ESR1 and NR1I2 gene variants.' *Cancer Epidemiology, Biomarkers and Prevention 16,* 1009.

Makela, S., Davis, V.L., Tally, W.C., Korkman, J. *et al.* (1994) 'Dietary estrogens act through estrogen receptor-mediated processes and show no antiestrogenicity in cultured breast cancer cells.' *Environmental Health Perspectives 102,* 6–7, 572–578.

Maskarinec, G., Watts, K., Kagihara, J., Hebshi, S.M. and Franke, A.A. (2008) 'Urinary isoflavonoid excretion is similar after consuming soy milk and miso soup in Japanese-American women.' *British Journal of Nutrition 100,* 2, 424–429.

Masson, L.F., Sharp, L., Cotton, S.C. and Little, J. (2005) 'Cytochrome P-450 1A1 gene polymorphism and risk of breast cancer.' *American Journal of Epidemiology 161,* 10, 901–915.

Masten, A.S. and Obradovic, J. (2008) 'Disaster preparation and recovery: lessons from research on resilience in human development.' *Ecology and Society 13,* 1, 9. Available at www.ecologyandsociety.org/vol13/iss1/art9, accessed 22 March 2010.

Matthies, A., Clavel, T., Gütschow, M., Engst, W. *et al.* (2008) 'Conversion of daidzein and genistein by an anaerobic bacterium newly isolated from the mouse intestine.' *Applied and Environmental Microbiology 74,* 15, 4847–4852.

McArdle, O. and O'Mahony, D. (2008) *Oncology: An Illustrated Colour Text.* Philadelphia: Churchill Livingstone, Elsevier.

McEwen, B.S. (2000) 'Allostasis and allostatic load: Implications for neuropsychopharmacology.' *Neuropsychopharmacology 22,* 108-124.

McEwen, B.S, and Seeman, T. (1999) 'Protective and damaging effects of mediators of stress – Elaborating and testing the concepts of allostasis and allostatic load.' *Annals of the New York Academy of Sciences 896,* 1, 30–47.

Meeker, J., Hu, H., Cantonwine, D.E., Lamadrid-Figueralt, H. *et al.* (2009) 'Urinary phthalate metabolites in relation to preterm birth in Mexico City.' *Environmental Health Perspectives 117,* 10, 1587–1592.

Miller, A.L. (2008) 'The methylation, neurotransmitter and antioxidant connections between folate and depression.' *Alternative Medicine Review 13,* 3, 216–226.

Nestler, J.E. and Jakubowicz, D.J. (1996) 'Decreases in ovarian cytochrome P450c17a activity and serum free testosterone after reduction in insulin secretion in women with polycystic ovary syndrome.' *New England Journal of Medicine 335,* 617–623.

Newbold, R.R., Padilla-Banks, E., Snyder, R.J. Phillips, T.M. and Jefferson, W.N. (2007) 'Developmental exposure to endocrine disruptors and the obesity epidemic.' *Reproductive Toxicology 23,* 3, 290–296.

Okamoto, Y., Okajima, K., Toda, C., Ueda, K. *et al.* (2004) 'Novel estrogenic microsomal metabolites from phthalate ester.' *Journal of Health Science 50,* 5, 556–560.

Okolo, S. (2008) 'Incidence, aetiology and epidemiology of uterine fibroids.' *Best Practice and Research Clinical Obstetrics and Gynaecology 22,* 4, 571–588.

Oqita, H., Node, K. and Kitakaze, M. (2003) 'The role of estrogen and estrogen-related drugs in cardiovascular diseases.' *Current Drug Metabolism 4,* 6, 497–504.

Park, C., Cho, K., Bae, D., Joo, N. *et al.* (2008) 'Methyl-donor nutrients inhibit breast cancer cell growth.' *In Vitro Cellular and Developmental Biology – Animal 44,* 7, 268–272.

Pino, A.M., Valladares, L.E., Palma, M.A., Mancilla, A.M., Yáñez, M. and Albala, C. (2000) 'Dietary isoflavones affect sex hormone-binding globulin levels in postmenopausal women.' *Journal of Clinical Endocrinology and Metabolism 85,* 8, 2797–2800.

Ross, R.K., Pike, M.C., Vessey, M.P., Bull, D., Yeates, D. and Casagrande, J.T. (1986) 'Risk factors for uterine fibroids: Reduced risk associated with oral contraceptives.' *British Medical Journal (Clin Res Ed) 293*, 359–362.

Rutter, M. (1999) 'Resilience concepts and findings: Implications for family therapy.' *Journal of Family Therapy 21*, 119–144.

Salih, E.Y., Zein, A.A. and Bayoumi, R.A. (1986) 'The effect of oral contraceptives on the apparent vitamin B status in some Sudanese women.' *British Journal of Nutrition 56*, 363–367.

Selva, D.M., Hogeveen, K.N., Innis, S.M. and Hammond, G.L. (2007) 'Monosaccharide-induced lipogenesis regulates the human hepatic sex hormone-binding globulin gene.' *Journal of Clinical Investigation 117*, 12, 3979.

Sharpe, R. and Irvine, D. (2004) 'How strong is the evidence of a link between environmental chemicals and adverse effects on human reproductive health?' *British Medical Journal 328*, 447–451.

Sharpe R.M. and Skakkebaek, N.E. (1993) 'Are oestrogens involved in falling sperm counts and disorders of the mail reproductive tract?' *Lancet 341*, 8857, 1392–1395.

Singh, S. and Khar, A. (2006) 'Biological effects of curcumin and its role in cancer chemoprevention and therapy.' *Anticancer Agents in Medicinal Chemistry 6*, 3, 259–270.

Smit Veninga, K. (1984) 'Effects of oral contraceptives on vitamins B6, B12, C, and folacin.' *Journal of Nurse-Midwifery 29*, 6, 386–390.

Sung K.L., Young J.W., Ji H.L., Suk H.K. *et al.* (1997) 'Altered hydroxylation of estrogen in patients with postmenopausal osteopenia.' *Journal of Clinical Endocrinology and Metabolism 82*, 4, 1001–1006.

Tan, H.L., Butler, P.C., Burke, M.D. *et al.* (2007) 'Salvestrols: A new perspective in nutritional research.' *Journal of Orthomolecular Medicine 22*, 1, 39–47.

Tham, D.M., Gardner, C.D. and Haskell, W.L. (1998) 'Potential health benefits of dietary phytoestrogens: A review of the clinical, epidemiological, and mechanistic evidence.' *Journal of Clinical Endocrinology and Metabolism 83*, 7, 2223–2235.

Toppari, J. and Skakkebaek, N.E. (1998) 'Sexual differentiation and environmental endocrine disrupters.' *Baillieres Clinical Endocrinology and Metabolism 12*, 1, 143–156.

Trock, B.J., Hilakivi-Clarke, L. and Clarke, R. (2006) 'Meta-analysis of soy intake and breast cancer risk.' *Journal of the National Cancer Institute 98*, 459–471.

Wardle, P. and Fox, R. (1989) 'Symptoms of oestrogen deficiency in women with oestradiol implants.' *British Medical Journal 299*, 1102.

Waring, R.H. (2004) 'Report on absorption of magnesium sulfate (Epsom salts) across the skin.' Available at www.epsomsaltcouncil.org/articles/Report_on_Absorption_of_magnesium_sulfate.pdf, accessed on 9 November 2009.

Weidler, C., Harle, P., Schedel, J., Schmidt, M., Scholmerich, J. and Straub, R.H. (2004) 'Patients with rheumatoid arthritis and systemic lupus erythematosus have incrased renal excretion of mitogenic estrogens in relation to endogenous antiestrogens.' *Journal of Rheumatology 31*, 3, 419–421.

Chapter *8*

DYSREGULATION OF THE IMMUNE SYSTEM: A GASTRO-CENTRIC PERSPECTIVE

Michael Ash

1. Introduction

There is no tissue or organ with a greater impact on human health than the immune system. Unlike the specialisms of gastroenterology or cardiology, the immune system is not based in one set of organised tissues, but is disparate and spread systemically throughout our bodies. The various cells of the immune system patrol every component of the body, defending against invaders and cellular damage, whilst providing continuous information to the endocrine and central nervous systems to maintain homeostasis, referred to contemporaneously as homeodynamic health (Lloyd, Aon and Cortassa 2001).

The human immune system is highly complex and possesses extensive 'plasticity'[1] in its ability to respond to pressures brought to bear on it by infectious diseases, host microbes and food availability. These external influences continuously interact with our genes, producing and defining our immunological phenotype[2] (Ferwerda *et al.* 2007). This evolutionary plasticity can be compromised, resulting in dysregulation of immune function, which may result in immunodeficiency, chronic immune activation, autoimmunity or allergy; collectively referred to as immune mediated inflammatory diseases or disorders (IMIDs) (Kuek, Hazleman and Ostör 2007).

Changes that affect human immune reactions are rarely linear processes from stimulus to response but more a complicated set of interconnected co-dependent influences. Scientific and clinical exploration of these mechanisms over the last few decades has seen an explosion of knowledge regarding how the immune system functions in health

---

1 **Plasticity**: the ability to adapt to new and immune-stimulating challenges and maintain appropriate and competent responses.

2 **Immunological phenotype**: refers to the observable physical/biochemical characteristics of an immune cell, as determined by both genetic makeup and environmental influences.

and disease, including the understanding of how pharmaceutical, lifestyle, environment and non-pharmaceutical intervention may provide opportunity for loss or restoration of immune tolerance (Haddad *et al.* 2005).

Remarkable advances in the field of innate immunity have led to a greater comprehension about the role of chronic inflammation in a wide variety of human diseases. The links between the innate immune response, inflammation and immunopathology represent a new medical paradigm explaining the role of the immune system in initiating and preventing illness.

In evolutionary terms the innate immune system is an ancient but complex and vitally important primitive system of host defence. The innate immune system remains the first line of host defence in humans, and may be of paramount importance before the acquired system has fully developed or when acquired immunity is disarmed by inherited or conditionally induced defects or disease. Innate immunity has the additional role of sorting 'self from non-self' and determining which antigen the acquired immune system responds to.

The purpose of this chapter is to explore the emerging data on the relationships between local and systemic immune responses and how natural therapies (non-pharmacological) can influence and shape the actions of these immune responses, for improved health and function. By understanding the consequences and effector changes involved in loss of immunological tolerance, practitioners can design therapy programmes targeting these immune-driven changes for their patients, with particular reference to the gastro-intestinal immune system.

1.1 What is a functional approach to innate immunity?

A functional approach to health management via the innate immune system includes the use of diet, nutrition, lifestyle changes and medicine, and recognises that exposure to environmental toxins may play a central role in illness. The innate immune system has a highly sophisticated set of receptors that are both responsive to and modifiable by the management of these exposures and the body's ability to adapt to them.

2. Immunology's developmental history

Antibodies were first discovered by Emil von Behring and Shibasaburo Kitasato in 1890, yet immunology as a clinical science only really started developing in the 1950s.

One could view the immune response as ripples in a pool of water (the water being the immune system) – the ripples will vary in size and number depending on the frequency and size of pebbles thrown into it, and the ripples will widen and converge, demonstrating the interconnectedness of the varying aspects of the immune response to multiple triggers.

The expanding 'ripples' interact to negate or amplify each other and only a comprehensive understanding of the activating triggers and responses of immune dysregulation and immune function will allow a therapeutic judgement to provide a treatment with a greater chance of success in achieving a return to tolerance, rather than inappropriate amplification or suppression (Haddad *et al.* 2005). Whilst the boosting of innate and adaptive immune responses is sometimes clinically justified, it must be undertaken in conjunction with the aim of returning the affected tissues to a state of tolerance, as loss of tolerance underlies all immunologically induced illness.

The rapidly evolving science of immunology has led to a comprehensive understanding of 'total body integration', or a 'holistic web of integration' (Jones 2005). Most, if not all, disciplines in medicine today recognise the role of the immune system in health and disease, and all healthcare practitioners aspiring to effective clinical therapy should have a detailed comprehension of its complexity.

Three principal phases exist in the evolution of clinical comprehension about the human immune system.

2.1 Phase 1

In the 1950s immunologists proposed the 'self/non-self'[3] model as the principal explanation for human immunity discrimination (Burnet and Fenner 1949). Burnet offered the classical formulation that the immune system distinguishes between 'self' and 'non-self' and responds to 'non-self' but not to 'self' (S/NS) (Burnet 1959). This S/NS discrimination model became and has remained a key component of all immunological explanation and experimentation for many years. It also generated the concept of immunological tolerance, a highly selective, essential process that disregards molecules native to the host but responds, often aggressively, to remove foreign molecules.

2.2 Phase 2

In the late 1980s Charles Janeway refined Burnet's model, suggesting that the immune system responds to 'infectious non-self' and not to 'non-infectious self' (Janeway 1992). This explanation was supported by the discovery of several highly specialised receptors embedded in the innate immune system.

Janeway hypothesised, and then proved, that, in order to identify invading pathogens[4] and the like, certain immune cells carried pattern recognition receptors (PRRs). These PRRs responded to specialised patterns embedded in bacterial cell walls, which Janeway called pathogen-associated molecular patterns (PAMPs). The PRRs are germline encoded (that is, the code has been passed down, and will continue to be passed down, through many generations). The cells that carry these PRRs are the antigen-presenting cells (APCs). Once they are triggered, the complement cascade (see 3.1 below) and the

---

3   **Non-self**: a term widely used in immunology, and covers everything which is detectably different from the host's own constituents; such as: infectious agents (bacteria, viruses and parasites); cells or organs from other sources; drugs; and foods.

4   **Pathogen**: any organism or substance, especially a microorganism, capable of causing disease, such as bacteria, viruses, protozoa or fungi.

adaptive immune response can be activated, thus allowing the shaping of an appropriate immune response and the creation of immunological memory. Without APC activation, the adaptive immune response would not be triggered.

Janeway clarified the initial S/NS concept by discovering that PRRs allowed the APCs to discriminate between 'infectious-nonself' and 'non-infectious-self' (Janeway 1992), thus triggering the immune system to respond vigorously to antigens associated with potentially pathogenic microorganisms, and effectively ignore fundamentally 'bland' antigens, self or foreign.

Janeway's work further suggested that activation of the innate immune system's APCs by a viral load or other provocative antigen reduced the rate at which the so called auto-reactive or self-harming lymphocytes are removed from the body. These are cells linked to autoimmunity and their slower deletion increases the risk for loss of tolerance.

His model also identified that cross-linked self antigens (pieces of the host) being processed by the APCs may induce some form of 'molecular mimicry' if the APC was also being co-stimulated with a nonspecific pathogen-associated molecule. Molecular mimicry is defined as the theoretical possibility that sequence similarities between foreign and self-peptides are sufficient to result in the cross-activation of autoreactive T or B cells by pathogen-derived peptides, leading to autoimmunity (Kohm, Fuller and Miller 2003). In other words the presenting cells are mixed up with host tissue and triggering cells and this combination may, in genetically susceptible people, result in their immune system attacking their own tissues.

2.3 Phase 3

Since the mid 1990s Polly Matzinger has been building upon the S/NS/PRR view. She advocates that the immune system has an additional layer of triggers: the APCs may be activated by danger/alarm signals derived from injured cells exposed to pathogens, toxins, mechanical damage, etc., which affects the 'decision-making' process, and is in part also mediated by the affected tissues (Matzinger 2007). In her model, the immune system provides increased specificity in affected tissues by distinguishing between 'dangerous and non-dangerous' entities, regardless of whether they are self or foreign, leading to her model being referred to as the 'danger model' (Matzinger 1994). Cells that die normally, using a programmed apoptosis process, are generally scavenged prior to disintegration, whereas damaged (necrotic) cells instead release their contents, any of which may act as a 'danger signal'.

This provides an important addition to the S/NS/PRR model: it means that 'selfness' is no guarantee of tolerance and the health of the affected organ is as much a mediator of immunity as the presenting trigger.

2.3.1 DANGER MODEL/ENVIRONMENT AND AUTOIMMUNE DISEASE

Matzinger's danger model provides a 'functional view' as to the cause and increase in the eighty-plus autoimmune diseases (Walsh and Rau 2000) in industrially developed countries over the last century (Bach 2002).

The danger model, by including damaged and necrotic cells as immunological triggers, suggests that environmental pathogens or toxins that cause cell stress and/ or death, or any mutations in genes governing the normal physiological death and removal process, may contribute to autoimmune diseases. These triggers are called Damage-Associated Molecular Patterns (DAMPs) (Seong and Matzinger 2004). In these cases the immune system is actually doing its job by responding to alarm signals, but inappropriately and to the detriment of the host.

As her explanation has evolved Matzinger has postulated that some evolutionary level of control is embedded within key organ tissues, which cooperatively influences and directs the immune system's responses. This feedback between immunity and organ tissues is necessary, as the complex combination of tissues are delicately balanced to perform a particular function, which may easily be compromised by the powerful effector mechanisms utilised by the immune system (Matzinger 2007).

As a consequence, organ tissues use all sorts of mechanisms to keep the cells and molecules of the immune system out until they need them and then exert some control over them when they arrive. This suggests a far greater level of complexity and variety of immune responses than has been elucidated and understood to date and this refinement to her model has already been experimentally identified to occur in lung tissue (Takabayshi *et al.* 2006).

In simple terms, Matzinger proposes that, when local tissues are 'distressed', they themselves can stimulate an immune response, and may also determine the non-local immune cells' type, duration and severity of action; thus providing an organ-specific immune response and a systemic immune balancing act. The immune response elicited, she proposes, will be determined by the health of the specific tissue in which the response is occurring, as well as by the immunological network, making no set of tissues immunologically isolated (Coutinho 1995). This establishes a paradigm in which the immune response is specific to the tissue in which the response occurs, rather than being directed by the provoking pathogen, relying instead on internal cross-talk between tissues and the immune system to determine outcome.

Matzinger's model helps us to understand why the immune system concentrates on those things that are dangerous, rather than simply foreign, and in turn allows us to:

- tolerate a lot of foreign material in the air we breathe and food we eat

- accept the occasional virus that enters a cell, makes a few copies and then leaves without committing any damage

- live with the commensal[5] bacteria in our gastro-intestinal tract

---

5   **Commensal**: a form of symbiosis in which one organism derives a benefit while the other is unaffected.
    Symbiosis: a relationship with mutual benefit between two individuals or organisms.

- grow foetuses for the future generation.

Practitioners can use this model to look at the immune system's response less as a series of apparently randomly determined sequences and more as an 'integrated web-like' driver of health and disease, where immunological health both in local tissues and systemically is a reflection of the individual's overall health. In optimal health, all relevant tissues induce tolerance, maintaining the immune system in a state of observational inactivity. Too often practitioners focus too much on the immune system responding to events, or promoting its response; they forget that for 99.99 per cent of the time, its job, when working properly, is to *not* respond to things.

For the immune system and relevant tissues to be healthy they must have adequate and optimal nutrient status. Undernourished individuals have a greater risk of adverse immune responses; and immune responses, regardless of how mild, place greater nutritional demands on the host (Scrimshaw and SanGiovanni 1997).

3. A review of key immune components

The immune system has four key aspects and many hundreds of interactive components. The principal divisions are shown in Figure 8.1.

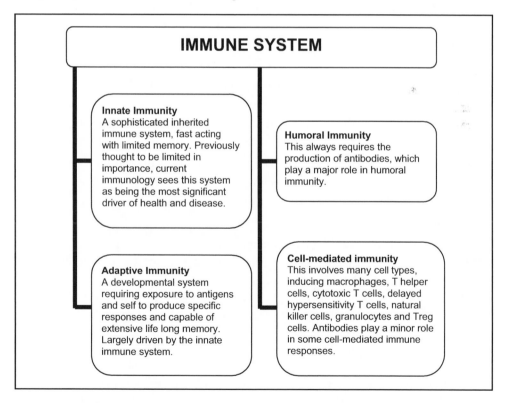

Figure 8.1 Divisions of the immune system

3.1 The innate immune system

The human innate immune system is ancient, more than 500 million years old. Elements of this system can be detected in all multicellular organisms, including vertebrates, invertebrates and plants. It is a fast-acting and surprisingly sophisticated front line defence system in which numerous strategies are employed to ensure eradication of any invader, followed by either coordination of repair and renewal, or triggering of cellular suicide (apoptosis) when the cell tissues were too damaged to salvage.

The innate immune system is dominant in the wet surfaces of the body, the principal barriers against infection. These surfaces are the mucosal immune system's territory: mucosal tissues are directly exposed to the external environment and are burdened with antigenic loads (consisting of commensal bacteria, dietary antigens, and viruses) of far greater quantities on a daily basis than the systemic immune system sees in a lifetime (Mayer 2003).

The principal components of innate immunity are: the physical barriers (skin, membranes, mucous and hair, plus characteristics such as dryness, flushing or blinking) and the chemical activities carried out by molecules, which include the secretion of salts, hydrochloric acid (HCl), lactic acid, lipids, cytokines, chemokines and enzymes. More specific cellular effects include phagocytosis – the process of engulfing and destroying particles and pathogens. This is carried out by various white blood cells, including neutrophils, monocyte/macrophages and to a lesser extent eosinophils.

In summary, the major functions of the innate immune system are:

- the recruitment of immune cells to sites of infection and inflammation, through the production of chemical factors, including specialised chemical mediators, called cytokines[6]

- the activation of the complement[7] protein cascade to identify bacteria, activate cells and to promote clearance of dead cells or antibody complexes

- the identification and removal of foreign substances present in organs, tissues, the blood and lymph, by specialised white blood cells

- the activation of the adaptive immune system through a process known as antigen presentation.

Janeway explained that the adaptive immune system, primarily dependent on T cells and B cells, has to evolve from a blank canvas; every generation has to develop its own set of adaptive immune response receptors.

One of the key elements of Dr Janeway's and later Dr Matzinger's work was to identify that innate immunity influences and directs the adaptive immune system (Agrawal, Eastman and Schatz 1998); and that this older but highly sophisticated part

---

6   **Cytokines**: non-antibody pleiotropic proteins secreted by inflammatory leukocytes and some non-leukocytic cells, which act as master immune regulators.

7   **Complement**: a series of proteins present in serum that, when activated, produce widespread inflammatory effects, as well as lysing bacteria.

of our immune system is an essential aspect of our ability to develop, activate and suppress adaptive immunity, allowing us to achieve tolerance.

To live a long and healthy life, one needs both an effective innate immune system *and* an effective adaptive immune system; defects in either one can lead to disease, difficulty living a normal, healthy life, and early death from infection.

3.1.1 THE INNATE IMMUNE SYSTEM'S PATTERN RECOGNITION RECEPTORS (PRRS)

The innate immune system has a significant role in determining antigen origination and risk, acting as a sentinel system of immunological control. By contrast with the adaptive immune system, the innate immune system distinguishes friend from foe by the use of the germline-encoded PRRs, which implies that the specificity of each receptor is genetically predetermined. Because of the complexity of identification, these key receptors recognise highly conserved (similar or identical sequences that occur within many large molecules) elements found in a large number of organisms – the PAMPs. These are highly promiscuous, providing a wide range of recognition patterns.

PRRs have four currently identified principal divisions:

1. **Toll-like receptors** (TLRs) recognise conserved molecular patterns from bacteria, viruses, protozoa and fungi; 13 have been identified so far, of which 11 are in mammals.

2. **C-type lectin receptors** (CLRs) recognise mainly fungi (Robinson *et al.* 2006); 17 have been identified so far, including the Mannose receptor (MR) (expressed primarily on macrophages and dendritic cells), which, when activated, triggers phagocytosis of the microbe.

3. **Rig-1-like receptors** (RLRs) sense viral DNA and RNA or bacterial products.

4. **Intracellular nucleotide receptors** such as the nucleotide-binding oligomerisation domain (Nod-Like) receptor (NLRs) sense endogenous products such as cytosols released by dying cells (Fritz *et al.* 2006; Inohara and Nunez 2003); 20 have been identified so far.

Because all microbes, not just pathogenic ones, possess recognisable molecular patterns, PAMPs are sometimes referred to as microbe-associated molecular patterns (MAMPs), especially when discussed in relation to health-promoting microorganisms, such as probiotics, yeasts and some nematodes (Raz 2007).

3.1.1A TLRS

TLRs are important PRRs that are designed to recognise molecules shared by groups of related microbes that are essential for the survival of those organisms and are not normally found associated with mammalian cells. In addition, unique molecules displayed on stressed, injured, infected or transformed human cells also act as PAMPs or DAMPs that are recognised by TLRs.

Table 8.1 TLR targets

Some TLR targets	Found in
Lipopolysaccharides (LPS)	Gram-negative bacterial cell walls
Peptidoglycan and lipotechoic acids	Gram-positive bacterial cell walls
Polysaccharide A (PSA-A), mannose	Microbial glycolipids and glycoproteins
Bacterial and viral unmethylated cpg DNA Bacterial flagellin amino acid N-formylmethionine	Bacterial proteins
Double-stranded and single-stranded RNA	From viruses
Glucans	Fungal cell walls

TLRs were named by Dr Christiane Nűsslein-Volhard in the 1980s, who described a drosophila (fruit fly) as looking 'weird' ('toll' is the German word for 'weird') when the toll receptor protein was missing (Anderson and Nusslein-Volhard 1984). Later research found that this protein was instrumental in immunity both in the fruit fly and human immune cells, as well as being important in the developmental stages of the fruit fly (Lemaitre *et al.* 1996). Further work has led to the understanding that humans have 11 TLRs to help drive and determine innate and adaptive immune responsiveness (Medzhitov and Janeway 1997; Raz 2007).

These small receptors, found on most structural, immune and inflammatory cells, are valid targets for immune manipulation, especially via the gastro-intestinal tract where they are found in great numbers. They are also found on neurons, allowing the immune system and nervous system to respond to microbial components in a manner called 'cross talk'.

Despite there being just 11 TLRs, these and other specialist PRRs are able to provide a comprehensive level of specificity (Aderem and Ulevitch 2000) by recruiting adaptor molecules,[8] which in turn create multi-protein collecting platforms. The TLRs capture microbes then present their pre-digested bits and pieces as 'antigen' to either naive or activated T cells. The most professional of these TLR antigen-presenting cells (APCs) are the dendritic cells (DCs) found beneath the mucous membranes in the gastro-intestinal and respiratory tracts, waiting to sample bacteria, viruses and food whilst functioning in close contact with the membranes (Maldonado-López *et al.* 1999).

3.1.2 DENDRITIC CELLS (DCS)

DCs function primarily as immune sentinels. In the periphery they actively scan surrounding interstitial spaces for pathogenic invaders and internalise (through endocytosis) foreign antigens found in the extracellular milieu. In secondary lymphoid

---

8   **TLR adaptor molecules**: specialised cell membrane proteins that are recruited in various combinations by the TLRs. Distinct combinations of TLRs and adaptor molecules allow for correct TLR signalling and lead ultimately to inflammatory gene expression.

tissues, such as lymph nodes, DCs shift their attention to presenting previously ingested antigens (as peptides) to T cells, thus alerting the immune system to an impending threat. To carry out T cell activation, DCs must migrate from peripheral non-lymphoid tissues to draining lymph nodes. During this migration, DCs degrade internalised antigen into peptide fragments that are then loaded onto special receptors called major histocompatibility complex (MHC) molecules for display at the cell surface, where they are recognised by T cells through their T-cell receptors (TCRs). This role has always suggested that DCs were promoters of defence.

New research is showing that DCs are equally responsible for a seemingly opposite role in health, that of immune tolerance, a process required to silence dangerous immune cells, preventing them from attacking innocuous materials in the body or the body's own tissues. Two mechanisms have been identified so far that allow DCs to induce tolerance.

The antigen-loaded immature DCs silence T cells by either deleting them or by inducing regulatory T cells that suppress and coordinate the reactions of other immune cells.

When the DCs subsequently mature in response to infection, the pre-existing tolerance nullifies any reaction to innocuous antigens and allows the DCs to focus the immune response on the pathogen.

These combinations lead to DC gene expressions that eventually regulate the immune response, both adaptive and innate. Modifying these innate immune system activators, and the related gene expressions, provides an exciting clinical opportunity for adaptive and systemic immune modulation (Nature Immunology 2006).

The constant sampling of the intestinal antigenic contents by the DCs provides the ability to establish tolerance to commensal bacteria, foods and self. DCs at the mucosal surface have the ability to induce the differentiation of Tregs (regulatory T cells) that produce IL-10 and Transforming growth factor-beta (TGF-β)[9] during the steady state (non-infected-non-immunised) and still retain the ability to induce effector T cells such as TH1, TH2 and TH17 in response to invasive pathogens or bacterial dysbiosis (Kelsall and Leon 2005).

3.2 The adaptive immune response

3.2.1 T CELLS

T cells are white blood cells, specifically a type of lymphocyte, and play a central role in cell-mediated immunity.[10] They are distinguished from other lymphocyte types, such as B cells and natural killer (NK) cells, by the presence of the T cell receptor (TCR) on their cell surface.

---

9   **TGF-β**: a family of signalling proteins that has over 40 members; they play major roles in the control of proliferation, cellular differentiation, and other functions in most cells.

10   **Cell-mediated immunity**: an immune response that does not involve antibodies or complement but does involve the activation of macrophages, NK cells, antigen-specific cytotoxic T-lymphocytes, and the release of various cytokines in response to an antigen.

The T in T cell stands for thymus, since it is the principal organ in the T cells' development. Not all T cells are alike: they are morphologically uniform, but their behaviour and molecular markings differ. One large set of T cells, called cytotoxic T cells (Tc) because they attack infected tissues, carries a surface protein known as cluster of differentiation 8 (CD8). A second set, the helper T cells (Th) that seem to coordinate the immunologic assault, bears the protein CD4 instead. These CD4+ or Th cells are important mediators in immune responses, acting to coordinate the other cellular components of the immune system.

3.2.1A T CELL SUBSETS

Approximately twenty years ago, two Th cell subsets were described (Mosmann and Coffman 1989), and since then numerous studies have been carried out on the TH1 and TH2 subsets (Dong and Flavell 2001). Until the mid to late 1990s these Th cells were thought to be a binary system, consisting of mutually inhibitory Th cells. Although there was suggestion of a third group of CD4+ T cell subsets, described as being derived from peripheral naive precursors, they did not fully meet the criteria to be defined as a separate lineage. However, interleukin-17 (IL-17)-expressing T cells, which are now widely known as TH17 cells, were proposed in 2006 to meet these criteria and have been recognised as a third distinct lineage of Th cells (Dong 2006; Harrington *et al.* 2005)

TH17

TH17 cells are distinct from other Th cells in their gene expression, regulation and biological function. TH17 cells, in particular, through the production of the cytokines IL-17, IL-22 and IL-17F, are considered to be pro-inflammatory (Kolls and Linden 2004). They have an important role in host defence against microbial infection especially in the mucosal tissues; by recruiting neutrophils and macrophages to infected tissues, they eliminate pathogens unaffected by TH1 and TH2 effector cells. These include pathogens such as: *Staphylococcus aureus, Bacteroides* spp., *Borrelia burgdorferi* (Lyme disease) and *Candida albicans*; all associated with widespread inflammation-associated symptoms (Chung *et al.* 2003; Huang *et al.* 2004; Infante-Duarte *et al.* 2000).

TH17 cells are now recognised as key players in autoimmune and inflammatory diseases, including rheumatoid arthritis, systemic lupus erythematosus (SLE), multiple sclerosis, asthma, psoriasis, systemic sclerosis, inflammatory bowel disease (IBD) and allograft rejection (Bettelli, Oukka and Kuchroo 2007; Steinman 2007). Because of TH17 cells' importance in disease progression and initiation, practitioners need to consider their interventions in terms of reducing IL-17 (Vojdani, Lambert and Kellermann 2008) promotion as well as increasing Treg activity and endurance.

In the gut TH17 seems to have a dual role to play as protector and possible initiator of autoimmune activation. Vitamin A as retinoic acid (Kim 2008) is used by DCs to convert naive T cells – via cytokine IL-6 suppression in conjunction with bacteria-promoted TGFβ – towards Treg cells[11] rather than TH17 cells, a development which maintains mucosal immune tolerance. Disruption of this balance via nutrient deficiency and or bacterial dysbiosis can have immune consequences far beyond the gut, including systemic autoimmune disease (Coombes *et al.* 2007).

Inflammatory events that compromise the gastro-intestinal mucosal barrier as a result of IL-17 production can also lead to increased blood brain barrier (BBB) permeability through the translocation of endotoxins, leading to activation of the nuclear inflammation enhancer, NFκB. Such endotoxins include bacterial cell walls (lipopolysaccharides) and pro-inflammatory cytokines such as IL-1. The daily consumption of environmental stressors can disrupt the gastro-intestinal barrier function, leading to a breakdown of the BBB and subsequent induction of neuroinflammation, representing a significant pathway in gut-brain axis-related pathologies (Maes, Mihaylova and Bosmans 2007). Inhibition of NFκB plays an important clinical role in the reduction of barrier permeability (Shen and Turner 2006).

3.2.2 TH1–TH2 PRINCIPAL EFFECTS

The relatively simplistic inhibitory competition view proposed by the 'hygiene theory' has merit but the inverse relationship one would expect to find between the frequency of TH1 versus TH2 diseases (see Table 8.2) has not been borne out by studies, meaning further explanations have had to be sought (Sheikh, Smeeth and Hubbard 2003; Yazdanbakhsh and Rodrigues 2001).

If the model were accurate then TH1 and TH2 diseases should not be present in the same individual, as competing cytokine production would cause inhibition of the other response. Yet patients do present with asthma (TH2), plus coeliac (TH1), rheumatoid arthritis (TH1) or psoriasis (TH1). When reviewing national data it can be seen that the increase in the incidence of allergy (TH2) in recent decades has been accompanied by similar increases in autoimmune diabetes (Stene and Nafstad 2001), Crohn's and coeliac disease (TH1) (Kero *et al.* 2001).

Table 8.2 TH1 and TH2 diseases

TH1 (cellular)-mediated autoimmune conditions	TH2 (humoral dominated)-mediated atopic diseases
Type 1 diabetes	Asthma
Rheumatoid arthritis	Eczema
IBD	Allergic rhinitis
Psoriasis	Allergies
Coeliac disease	

---

11 **Treg cells**: a special subset of T cells that regulate or suppress immune responses, preventing autoimmunity, for example.

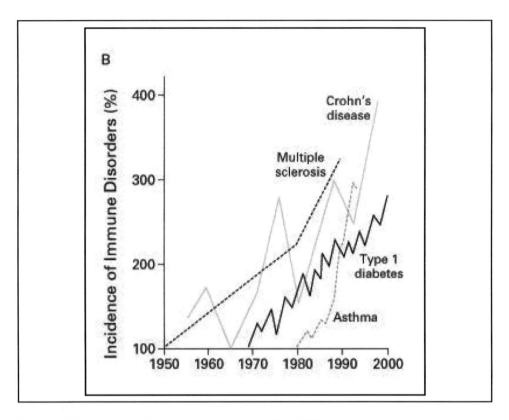

Figure 8.2 The incidence of immune disorders from 1950–2000

Because the demographics of autoimmunity are similar to those of allergy, they need to be considered together when trying to involve the potential effects of 'hygiene'. Hygiene is often misinterpreted through the populist need for simplicity; in particular, the assumption is that the critical factor is found in the home with hygiene (bathing, soaps, detergents, antibacterial kitchen accessories, etc.). Whilst these practices have a potential environmental effect on health, it is not these changes that have had the powerful immune-changing effects described here. A comprehensive study has demonstrated that domestic practices in the home have no correlation with the observed changes in the occurrence of immunoregulatory disorders (Stanwell-Smith and Bloomfield 2004).

The proposal that autoimmune and atopic diseases share risk factors that increase the propensity of the immune system to generate inappropriate TH1-, TH2- and TH17-mediated responses to well established ancient environment-sharing organisms or non-pathological antigens is gaining acceptance and represents a forward development (Sheikh *et al.* 2003). These long tolerated organisms, traceable to Paleolithic times or earlier, are required for the maturation of DCs and probably other APCs including basophils, localised inhibition of cytokine activation, development of Treg cells, adequate infection exposure control and tolerant sensory nervous system involvement (Shahabi *et al.* 2006). See 4.2.3 below for a discussion of the evolved hygiene hypothesis.[12]

3.3 Humoral immunity

Humoral immunity is named for the 'humours', or body fluids, because this is where many of its components are found. It relies on B cells, the lymphocytes that produce antibodies, which form a key part of our immune response. To remain healthy, we need to maintain an appropriate number of B cells, neither excessive nor insufficient.

B cell activation presented early immunologists, most notably Paul Ehrlich, with the effector mechanisms to be able to develop anti-toxins. They arise from a pluripotent stem cell lineage in the bone marrow, giving rise to common lymphoid progenitors which then diverge into either T or B cell lineage in the bone marrow. These cells undergo multiplication and processing in lymphoid tissue elsewhere than in the thymus gland. B cells, like T cells, have surface receptors which enable them to recognise antigens, but do not themselves neutralise or destroy antigens, apart from engulfing the pathogen/ antigen and presenting it to T cells for destruction.

B cell activation depends on one of three mechanisms:

1. **Type 1 T cell-independent activation** (also called polyclonal activation): for example, bacteria that have many repeating sequences of carbohydrate on the cell surface can cross-link the receptors on the B cell membrane.

2. **Type 2 T cell-independent activation**: macrophages present several of the same antigen in a way that causes cross-linking of antibodies on the surface of B cells.

3. **T cell-dependent activation**: an antigen presenting cell (APC) presents a processed antigen to a Th cell, priming it. When a B cell processes and presents the same antigen to the primed Th cell, the T cell releases cytokines that then activate the B cell to produce antibodies.

When B cells respond to an antigen, they take up residence in secondary lymphoid tissue called germinal centres (GC) and proliferate mitotically to form daughter B cells, identical to themselves. These B cells then develop into short-lived antibody-secreting (approx 10,000 per second) plasma cells. The GC microenvironment is the main source of memory B cells and plasma cells that produce high-affinity antibodies, necessary to protect against invading microorganisms (Maclennan 1994). GCs are found in the follicles of peripheral lymphoid tissues, including the spleen, lymph nodes, Peyer's patches and tonsils.

---

12 **Hygiene hypothesis**: the theory that exposure to microbial components, including TLR agonists, during the neonatal, infancy and early-childhood phases of development serves to polarise the immune response towards TH1, and away from TH2 responses, thereby reducing the likelihood of allergy and/ or atopy. Consistent with this hypothesis, there are inverse epidemiological relationships between the rates of infection and autoimmunity — for example, as the rates of common infections have dropped in wealthy industrialised countries, the rates of allergy and autoimmune disease have risen.

3.3.1 PRIMARY AND SECONDARY RESPONSE

In both responses, antibodies are released into the circulation at the lymph nodes. In the primary response, it takes some time (up to a few days) to produce antibodies; then some of the activated B cells become memory cells instead of plasma cells and continue to produce small amounts of the antibody long after the infection has been overcome. Their immunoglobulin production is driven in part by cytokine signalling from other immunogenic cells (Takatsu 1997). If the memory B cell comes into contact again with its specific antigen, it divides rapidly to form a clonal set of identical cells, which can produce antibodies far more quickly (secondary response).

3.3.2 ANTIBODIES

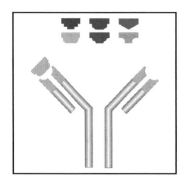

Figure 8.3 Antibody meets antigen (schematic)

Antibodies are Y-shaped molecules that circulate as part of the gamma globulin fraction of the blood plasma. At the molecular level, antibodies have a reactive site at the tip of each branch of the Y (the Fab region) which attaches to antigens on the basis of their molecular shape. This causes the infecting micro-organisms to stick together, and neutralises them until they can be dealt with by other cells. Antibodies do not destroy pathogens themselves – they merely provide markers for the effector cells (such as T cells and NK cells) to complete the elimination of the threat.

There are five classes of antibodies, known as immunoglobulins (Igs): IgG, IgA, IgM, IgD and IgE, each of which has a different function and most of which also have subclasses. Antibodies focus components of the innate immune system against the pathogen/antigen and are capable of inducing dramatic immune responses, including anaphylaxis. The roles of IgG, IgM and IgE in human health are important, but the role of secretory IgA (SIgA), the most abundant of all antibodies, has been previously underestimated and it is now receiving considerable attention as an important immunomodulator (Macpherson *et al.* 2008).

The antigen–antibody reaction forms the basis for immunisation programmes (vaccination). Here exposure to a related, weakened or dead form of a pathogenic organism, or even parts of its outer coat, provokes a primary antibody response similar to the body's normal reaction to the virulent form. This means that should the active pathogen enter the body the secondary immune response can be activated immediately, allowing much faster production of antibody and higher likelihood of rapid clearance.

3.3.3 PASSIVE IMMUNITY

Passive immunity is based on ready-made antibodies such as those provided to babies from their mother's bloodstream and first milk (colostrum). Passive immunity may also be obtained via serum – derived from blood of subjects exposed to a pathogen, who have then made antibodies to it.

3.4 Secretory IgA (SIgA)

The gut is the major lymphoid organ in the body, containing the majority of antibody-secreting plasma cells. Seventy per cent of the lymphoid tissue and most T cells are also found at mucosal surfaces. In humans IgA-producing plasma cells comprise approximately 20 per cent of total plasma cells in peripheral lymphoid tissues, whereas more than 80 per cent of plasma cells produce SIgA in mucosa-associated lymphoid tissues (MALT) (Fagarasan and Honjo 2003; Suzuki *et al.* 2004). Despite IgA being a relatively small component of serum antibodies, the abundance of IgA-secreting cells in normal mucosa means that IgA actually comprises at least 70 per cent of all immunoglobulin produced in humans. This dominance in the intestinal mucosa depends upon local colonisation with environmental microbes.

SIgA is continuously released into the lumen of the gastro-intestinal tract via the transport system of the intestinal epithelia (Mielants *et al.* 1995a); it prevents invading pathogens from binding to mucosal epithelial cells and neutralises their toxins (Lycke, Eriksen and Holmgren 1987). Natural SIgA is induced by constant antigenic stimulation, mostly of the DCs, by the intestinal commensal bacteria and other agents (Macpherson and Uhr 2004). The process of converting IgA to SIgA mainly takes place in the MALT, particularly in Peyer's patches and the lamina propria, and then IgA+ B cells recirculate through other lymphoid organs and the bloodstream (Mestecky and McGhee 1987).

SIgA acts as a triggering protein for DCs to deliver their ingested bacterial and other components to the microfold cells (MCells) found in Peyer's patches of the intestinal mucosa. These specialised cells allow for effective antigen processing and subsequent activation or suppression of immune responses, an essential component in the management of commensal bacteria. One of the MCells' primary tolerogenic (generating tolerance) roles is in the promotion of additional SIgA and Treg cells (Coombes and Powrie 2008).

Inadequate commensal populations and/or inadequate SIgA predisposes the mucosal tissues to diminished tolerance and increases the risk for loss of microbial harmony, called dysbiosis. Dysbiosis has advanced in meaning from 'altered pathogenic bacterial colonies in the gut' (Metchnikoff 1907) to more contemporary definitions, such as 'quantitative and qualitative changes in the intestinal flora, their metabolic activity and their local distribution' (Holzapfel *et al.* 1998).

From a clinical perspective the induction and maintenance of SIgA would seem a valid aim, but without suitable microbial partners SIgA levels are hard to maintain at an optimal level.

Impaired SIgA production and disturbed intestinal epithelial cell homeostasis have been observed in special lab-reared 'germ-free' mice (Rakoff-Nahoum *et al.* 2004). The DCs actually need to sample commensal bacteria at the epithelial surface and then participate in SIgA induction in the MALT through specific TLR-triggering (Niess *et al.* 2005).

This important pathway of SIgA induction is distinct from conventional T cell-dependent IgA found in serum and secretions. It demonstrates a specific mechanism that allows commensals and probiotics to attach and deliver receptor messages to our mucosal immune system, stimulating SIgA production and mediating other immune responses (Groer, Davis and Steele 2004).

Unlike the other immunoglobulins, which act only in the adaptive immune system, SIgA influences both the adaptive and innate immune systems. It can function in high-affinity modes for the neutralisation of toxins and pathogenic microbes, and as a low-affinity system to contain and manage the dense commensal microbiota within the intestinal lumen, as well as maintaining gut mucosal integrity and contributing to immune tolerance (Johansen *et al.* 1999).

4. Developing tolerance

4.1 Oral induction of tolerance

4.1.1 THE ROLE OF THE INNATE IMMUNE SYSTEM IN PEANUT ALLERGY

Over the last 20 years, the rise in childhood peanut allergy prompted the UK Food Standards Agency, between 1998 and 2000, to recommend that pregnant and breastfeeding women should avoid eating peanuts, and that weaned children should avoid eating peanuts until the age of three.

Since then it has been suggested (Lack *et al.* 2003) that this is counterproductive to inducing tolerance of peanuts, and that early oral ingestion of peanut antigens is more likely to induce tolerance via TLR activation and avoid allergy. Conversely, topical exposure to peanut antigen (such as via peanut oil in emollients used on eczema) without oral stimulation is more likely to provoke a different immune reaction that may go on to produce a hyperallergenic response. This suggests that the oral innate immune system can contribute to tolerance and small regular exposures to oral antigens early in life may avoid later allergy (Sicherer and Leung 2008).

4.1.2 THE ROLE OF THE ADAPTIVE IMMUNE SYSTEM

The oral administration of antigens (including foods, drugs and some probiotics) has long been recognised to induce peripheral tolerance of a wide range of beneficial systemic immune responses, and this has been proposed as therapy for autoimmune disease (Weiner *et al.* 1994). One of the most useful immunoregulatory mechanisms that may be induced by oral tolerance is 'bystander suppression', in which responses to a second, unrelated antigen can be inhibited when it is presented together with the antigen or food to which tolerance is already established, not only in the gut but systemically (Millington, Mowat and Garside 2004).

Vitamin A (as retinoic acid) and TGF-β have been shown to be essential partners in the production of Treg cells for the induction of mucosal tolerance (Hill *et al.* 2008). Both types of Tregs – those produced directly in the thymus and those made in the gut and elsewhere – require adequate vitamins A and D for effective local and bystander suppression and tolerance (Coombes and Maloy 2007; Izcue, Coombes and Powrie 2006).

In addition, the delivery of certain strains of probiotics stimulates DC production of IL-10 and TGF-β-promoting cells, which contribute to mucosal immunoregulation and the potential for systemic immune tolerance via the same concept of bystander suppression (Di Giacinto *et al.* 2005).

Nutrient-specific supplementation and strain-specific probiotics allow for a greater degree of DC maturation and thus the potential for controlling adverse responses to food antigens via the induction of appropriate co-stimulating anti-inflammatory cytokines. This process needs regulatory DCs and commensal organisms to work in tandem.

These potential immune-shaping effects are unlikely to be limited to the induction of tolerance to foods and have the potential for reducing autoimmune disease and others linked to adverse production of pro-inflammatory cytokines. A study looking at a mouse model of cow's milk allergy recently demonstrated that pre- and probiotics affected T cell and immunoglobulin responses to reduce the severity of skin-related symptoms (Schouten *et al.* 2009).

4.2 Environmental contributors

4.2.1 ENVIRONMENTAL TOXINS

Environmental toxins can also impact on the body's ability to maintain tolerance or develop disease, including autoimmune disease. By understanding the mechanisms involved, it may become possible to reduce the incidence of autoimmune diseases or to repair already-distressed immune systems by using natural modifiers of these mechanisms to induce immunological tolerance, as well as altering related environmental risk (Stevens and Bradfield 2008).

The cumulative effects of each subsequent generational exposure to these and other pollutants may be having as yet unknown consequences on the ability of our organ tissues and immune system to control effector cell responses to pathogens and other antigens, including damaged (dangerous) self antigens (Nakazawa 2008).

Dioxins

One such immunological trigger is the dioxin[13] group of chemicals. Human exposure to these has been increasing over the last few years and it is postulated that these chemicals

---

13 **Dioxins**: a mostly man-made family of 210 chlorinated compounds. Seventeen of the compounds are toxicologically significant and affect the aryl hydrocarbon receptor (AHR). Dioxins are a by-product of any combustion process, principally formed in the 250–400°C temperature range. The largest current sources of dioxins are industries producing chemicals, pesticides and paper products. Another suspected source is emissions from waste and toxic waste incinerators, particularly of plastic.

may be acting as part of the danger model's triggering system, which in turn may promote autoimmunity problems (Quintana *et al.* 2008).

The aryl hydrocarbon receptor (AHR)

The aryl hydrocarbon receptor (AHR) is a transcription factor that, when activated, increases the production of detoxification enzymes (Micka *et al.* 1997). It manages the detoxification of dioxins in the body and has an important role in the production of Treg cells and TH17 cells in a ligand-specific manner (Hornung *et al.* 2008). Depending on which ligand has stimulated the AHR, either Treg or T17 differentiation will be upregulated, either protecting against *or* promoting inflammatory conditions, such as EAE (experimental autoimmune encephalomyelitis, a mouse model of multiple sclerosis, MS). AHR also mutually cross regulates with another T-cell differentiation regulator, the tolerogenic cytokine TGF-β; and is known to interact with NFkB, which can influence its function (Allan 2008). The AHR also reacts with endogenous hormones and foods, affecting the immune system in a number of ways, resulting in either restraint or aggressive activation.

4.2.2 VITAMIN D

A prolific international increase in vitamin D deficiency has been identified fairly recently, contributed to by a lack of environmental sunlight exposure, and is being linked to increased risk for autoimmune disease. This micronutrient/secosteroid deficiency exemplifies how a specific deficiency can modify phenotypical risk for autoimmune disease by altering production of the immune-modulating Treg cells (Cantorna and Mahon 2004).

Vitamin D is especially important in up-regulating the expression of antimicrobial peptides (key mucous membrane defence chemicals), especially cathelicidin, which defend our mucous tissues against pathogen adhesion and survival in the gastro-intestinal tract (White 2008).

Commensal bacteria and pathogens can stimulate production of the hydroxylase enzyme that converts vitamin D into its active form 1,25(OH)2D. Once in the presence of active vitamin D, local macrophages will limit production of the pro-inflammatory cytokines TNFα, IFNγ and IL-12, and down-regulate several PAMP receptors, helping to maintain tolerance.

Thus it seems vitamin D is necessary for the local production of antibiotics and mucosal defence, and it helps to control inflammatory cytokine production in the innate immune system (Schauber *et al.* 2007).

Vitamin D deficiency therefore has many implications in the level of risk an individual may have in terms of autoimmune and CNS problems, as the principal innate immune tissues rely on it to maintain tolerance; plus it is involved in over 2000 genes, or about 10 per cent of our entire genome. Many epidemiological and retrospective analyses have demonstrated strong links between diseases and vitamin D deficiency (Holick 2007).

4.2.3 THE HYGIENE HYPOTHESIS EVOLVES

Western societal increases in the prevalence of immune-mediated diseases have been attributed to bioenvironmental factors, such as a lack of suitable ancient immuno-tolerant microbial or helminth challenges, or dietary change, or both. It was thought a result of this diminished environmental challenge included an immune deviation away from the preferred balance between the previously proposed mutually antagonistic subsets of Th cells – the 'hygiene theory' described in 3.2.2 above.

The discovery of TH17 cells and Treg cells has made this simple explanation redundant. The more evolved proposal is that environmental, nutritional, helminthic and bacterial alterations have resulted in an immune system that is more likely to produce either TH1 or TH2 responses (or both) or TH17 responses against previously benign antigens (Simpson *et al.* 2002) leading to an inappropriate expansion of inflammatory events without adequate inhibitory cytokinetic and Treg activity.

4.2.4 COUNTER-REGULATION HYPOTHESIS

The 'counter-regulation hypothesis' proposes that microbial, helminthic and some viral infections induce Treg responses. It provides an attractive explanation, although the molecular pathways induced by microbial exposure and tolerogenic responses in the host have not yet been fully identified. Newer research indicates that the relationship between the innate immune system, bacterial triggers (especially in the mucosal tissues) and an enzyme called indoleamine-2,3 dioxygenase (IDO) may provide some of the answers (Carson *et al.* 2004).

Indoleamine-2,3 dioxygenase (IDO)

IDO is released by DCs, Tregs and mucosal cells. Its role in antimicrobial resistance is well described: by catabolically depleting tryptophan (essential for the growth of microorganisms) both within the infected cell and in the surrounding milieu, IDO suppresses the growth of invasive bacteria (Gupta *et al.* 1994 Thomas *et al.* 1993). IDO also regulates maternal immune tolerance, in terms of both implantation and pregnancy; and possibly regulates more general aspects of T cell tolerance (Grohmann, Fallarino and Puccetti 2003; Mellor and Munn 2001).

As IDO inhibits T cell reactivity and induces a Treg response it is hypothesised that the induction of IDO by certain TLR triggers could provide the missing link between microbial exposure and the inhibition of allergic asthma and organ-specific autoimmunity. IDO has demonstrated unique anti-inflammatory effects within lung epithelial tissues and, in conjunction with IL-10, is both promoted by, and promotes, Treg development (Wakkach *et al.* 2003).

The clinical implication is that 'appropriate stimulation' of the key PRRs in the mucosal immune tissues, via strain-specific bacteria and helminths, will effect, amongst other immune changes, a release or suppression of IDO, and that this, along with other immunological tolerogenic effects, can mediate the risk and expansion of allergy and autoimmunity.

4.2.5 VACCINATION – GOOD OR BAD?

Vaccination strategies should perhaps be reconsidered in the context of the evolved hygiene hypothesis. The questions over vaccination are complex: they may cause immunostimulation, creating a favourable effect, or, conversely, they may actually prevent 'protective' infections, producing a negative effect. It is important to stress that there is no quantifiable evidence currently available defining either a positive or a negative role of vaccinations in the development of autoimmune or allergic diseases, but this does not exclude the possibility.

5. Contemporary understanding of microbiota and human immunity

Understanding the intricate complexity of the cells and molecules of the immune system is only the start. Scientists are now on an extended journey to understand the communication between our commensal bacteria (and other resident microbes, yeasts and helminths) and ourselves (Mullard 2008). The immune system, much like the brain, is a 'learning system' that requires regular exposure to input signals it has been designed to receive. As our way of living changes more and more, it raises this question: are our immune cells receiving the appropriate inputs to develop and maintain tolerance and health?

5.1 The microbiota and mucins – protection in the gut

Humans have innumerable micro-organisms inhabiting almost every environmentally exposed surface of the body. These organisms can be symbiotic, commensal or pathogenic; each with extensive evolutionary experience in learning how to manipulate our immune system. The human gastro-intestinal tract harbours more than 10^{14} (100,000,000,000,000) micro-organisms: at least 1800 genera and up to 40,000 species (Frank and Pace 2008); starting with small numbers in the stomach (less than 10^3/mL) and rising with the descent of the tract to the small intestine 10^6 and then 10^{11}–10^{14}/mL in the colon (Gill et al. 2006). Here the anaerobes outnumber the aerobes 100- to 1000-fold (Campieri and Gionchetti 1999).

The body's resident internal microbiota form a protective, active mulch, especially in the gut where they cohabit with an essential film of mucins, to act as our best defence against infective disease. Without them, our immune system would be on a 'hair trigger', with a nasty propensity for local and systemic mayhem. A growing scientific consensus accepts that only by understanding the way we have developed a symbiotic relationship with our long-present microbial residents can we find lasting solutions to disease, whether infectious, immune-dysfunctional or inflammatory in type.

In the intestinal mucosa this molecular 'network' functions not only to protect against pathogen intrusions but also to enable the gut flora to digest carbohydrates, especially polysaccharides, and to provide essential nutrients and vitamins to the host. It is also employed to strengthen the contiguous lining that separates the moist exterior from the host and supports effective development of the mucosa, in particular its vasculature and associated immune system.

5.1.1 INTESTINAL MUCINS AND THE GLYCOCALYX

The mucin layer is an essential part of this powerful protection. Mucin-rich glycoproteins form a gel over the epithelial tissues, protecting them against chemical, enzymatic, microbial and mechanical insult. Mucins form a relatively impervious mulch, which acts as:

- a lubricant

- a physical barrier

- a trap for microbes, thus providing a home for commensals (Linden *et al.* 2008)

- a reservoir of SIgA, providing a matrix for a rich array of endogenous antimicrobial molecules (Linden *et al.* 2008), which have broad spectrum microbicidal activity against fungi, bacteria and viruses and are highly dependent on a balanced microbiota to work effectively at eradication and mucosal tolerance.

Underneath the mucin gel is the glycocalyx;[14] the average turnover time of the human jejunal glycocalyx is 6 to 12 hours, allowing it to be constantly adjusted according to changes in the local environment due to pathogens or commensals, or population changes as seen with antibiotic usage (Madara and Trier 1987).

Commensal bacteria provide stimulation for appropriate glycoprotein production and assist with the degradation of food proteins and carbohydrates by provoking various brush border enzymes in the small intestine. The commensals also perform essential roles in: bile acid re-uptake; helping to reduce inflammation; providing better glycaemic control; reducing the risk of obesity and immunomodulation (Thomas *et al.* 2008).

---

14 **Glycocalyx**: consists of a dense forest of highly diverse glycoproteins and glycolipids that project from the apical plasma membrane of epithelial absorptive cells. It provides additional surface for absorption and includes enzymes secreted by the absorptive cells that are essential for the final steps of digestion of proteins and sugars.

5.2 Biofilms

Biofilms are aggregates of microbes with a distinct architecture, like a tiny city in which microbial cells, each only a micrometre or two long, form towers that can be hundreds of micrometres high. These dense, surface-attached bacterial communities, if the right sort of bacteria, can immunologically benefit the host, due to the increased epithelial proximity and duration of exposure, as well as through their unique communication pathways (called quorum sensing).

Biofilms can become 10–1000 times more resistant to the effects of antimicrobial agents than their non-bound counterparts (Hoyle and Costerton 1991). In substantive dysbiosis, where non-beneficial biofilms of pathogenic or pseudopathogenic bacteria may abound, adequate preparation of the microbial communities is required before the use of probiotics. Without adequate biofilm-degrading enzymes, little immunological improvement is likely, due to inhibition (by the biofilm of both DC bacterial sampling of, and TLR stimulation by, the probiotics; Bollinger *et al.* 2006).

One of the clinically essential roles of SIgA in mucosal immunology is the formation and maintenance of beneficially populated gut-associated biofilms, through the promotion of bacterial pili expression (pili help the bacteria stick together and share information).

This presents a paradox in probiotic therapy: inadequate beneficial mix of bacteria in the colon may significantly reduce SIgA production, or stimulate it so much that it washes away many of the beneficial organisms, thus preventing appropriate probiotic beneficial effects. To mediate SIgA production, the application of a different organism *Saccharomyces boulardii* (a yeast) has been shown to aid SIgA production, thus acting like a natural adjuvant to facilitate probiotic benefits via SIgA management (Rodrigues *et al.* 2000).

5.3 The microbiome

The vast numbers of microbial cells living in the human gut exceed the number of human cells in the body tenfold. Their total microbiome also contains millions of genes, compared with the 20,000 or so that makes up the human genome; we are therefore significantly outnumbered in and on our own body, both in cell numbers and in genetic code.

It has been estimated that, from a point of therapeutic drug intervention, there are only 3000 potential drug targets in humans because only a proportion of genes produce proteins that can be bound and modified by drug-like molecules. However, the microbiome has 100 times as many genes and as such represents an enormous opportunity for health intervention once the full microbiome has been translated (Hopkins and Groom 2002). It has recently been proposed that the total information encoded by the human genome is insufficient to perform all functions required to maintain health, and that products and residents of our microbiome are crucial for protection from various diseases (Zaneveld *et al.* 2008).

6. Gut and disease association

Almost every type of disease has a gastro-intestinal bacterial dysbiosis connection somewhere; from the more obvious contenders (ulcers, obesity, non-alcoholic fatty liver disease and IBD) to neurological problems (depression, autism, Tourette's syndrome and ADHD). Bacterial interaction with the mucosal immune system allows complex and fast information transfer and, because of the massive size of the bacterial genome in the human gut, there are many potential targets for intervention.

Unlike opportunistic pathogens, which mostly elicit immune responses resulting in tissue damage during infection, a range of symbiotic bacterial species have been shown to prevent inflammatory disease during colonisation. In addition, the 'normal' balanced microbiota also contains microorganisms that have been shown to induce inflammation under particular conditions. Therefore, the microbiota has the potential to exert both pro- and anti-inflammatory responses, requiring clinical judgement to take into account their separate and mutual interaction with each other and their host. It is recognised that dysbiosis can disturb the partnership between the microbiota and the human immune system, ultimately leading to altered or adverse immune responses that may underlie various human inflammatory disorders (Round and Mazmanian 2009).

There is also an increasingly well understood correlation between inflammation in the gastro-intestinal tract (with or without clinical GI symptoms) and the development and progression of interrelated rheumatological disease. These include ankylosing spondylitis (AS), infection-triggered reactive arthritis (ReA), some forms of juvenile chronic arthritis, arthritis in association with IBD, and some forms of psoriatic arthritis (PsA). Approximately two-thirds of patients suffering from spondyloarthritis have microscopic signs of gut inflammation without clinical gastro-intestinal symptoms (Mielants *et al.* 1987, 1995a, b, c). Further support for the relationship between altered mucosal tolerance and the gut-joint 'axis of conflict' is that remission of these diseases and long-term successful resolution were linked with disappearance of gastro-intestinal inflammation, whilst persistence of peripheral arthritis was also accompanied by gastro-intestinal inflammation (Mielants *et al.* 1995a, b, c).

6.1 Leaky gut

The barrier function of the gastro-intestinal tract is especially vulnerable to damage, and abruptions in its integrity or 'leaky gut' have been linked to numerous autoimmune and allergic diseases, such as IBD (Soderholm *et al.* 1999), multiple sclerosis (Yacyshyn *et al.* 1996), type 1 diabetes (Bosi *et al.* 2006) (as yet there is an unclear association with type 2 diabetes; Secondulfo *et al.* 1999) asthma (Benard *et al.* 1996) and atopic eczema (Ukabam, Mann and Cooper 1984).

The increased intestinal permeability in these patients seems to be a factor in these diseases, rather than a consequence of them, as it can precede the clinical onset of these diseases (Wyatt *et al.* 1993). It is, however, unclear as to whether it is an essential predisposing factor. One explanation is the changing communities of our resident bacteria: because the inactivation of our digestive tract's proteases depends on the presence of bacteria, a change in composition or absence of adequate bacterial nullifiers of these enzymes may lead to increased proteolytic digestion of the gut barrier (Norin, Gustafsson and Midtvedt 1986).

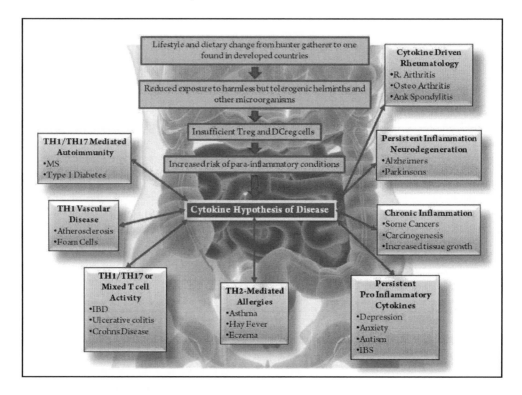

Figure 8.4 Cytokine hypothesis of disease

Protease supplements are sometimes used clinically to help patients with alterations in digestive capacity and to facilitate a change in the structure of bacterial biofilms in the gut. Proteolytic enzymes degrade microbial biofilms and increase immune penetration and the effectiveness of antimicrobial therapies. Concomitant supplementation with probiotics should resolve any inadvertent increase in barrier permeability in bacterially compromised gastro-intestinal tracts (Qin 2007).

Abruptions in the mucosal barrier may also be caused by deficiency of nutrients such as glutamine (Clark *et al.* 2003), increased TNFα production (Bruewer *et al.* 2003), pathogens (Sonoda *et al.* 1999), stress (Collins 2001), certain foods (Atisook, Carlson and Madara 1990) and medications (Rabassa *et al.* 1996).

6.2 Small intestinal bacterial overgrowth (SIBO)

The human small intestine (duodenum, jejunum and ileum) at the upper end of the digestive tract is relatively devoid of microbes under normal conditions, most likely due to a high conjugated bile acid concentration, averaging 10mMol during digestion. These acids then undergo extensive chemical modifications (deconjugation, dehydroxylation, dehydrogenation and deglucuronidation) in the colon, almost solely as a result of microbial activity (Hylemon and Glass 1983). Whilst normally low in bacterial species numbers compared to the colon, the small intestine has a major role to play in the cross-talk signalling between the host and the microbiome, and the microflora's role in this may explain some of the diverse symptoms experienced by people with small intestinal bacterial overgrowth (SIBO – defined as an abnormally high bacterial population level in the small intestine) (Grover *et al.* 2008).

The immunological clinical effects of SIBO potentially include irritable bowel syndrome (IBS) (Vanner 2008), rheumatoid arthritis (Henriksson *et al.* 1993), rosacea (Parodi *et al.* 2008a), scleroderma (Parodi *et al.* 2008b) and hypothyroidism (Lauritano *et al.* 2007). One of the explanations for this diverse set of illnesses may be found in inadequate bile acid levels, through reduced production, reduced bacterial conversion or poor flow (Masclee *et al.* 1989).

Resolving SIBO symptoms and severity can be achieved through the use of antimicrobials and probiotics. Evidence from experimental animal studies demonstrates that probiotics exert barrier-enhancing, antibacterial, immune-modulating and anti-inflammatory effects. Whilst their effect in humans has yet to be fully established, probiotics appear to represent a mucosal immune-modulating strategy of low risk in the resolution of SIBO (Quigley and Quera 2006).

7. Manipulating mucosal immunity to manage systemic health

7.1 Germ Theory vs Symbiotic Theory

It has been shown that the sophisticated families of immunological sensors and receptors do not exist simply to detect the presence of pathogens, reversing the 'all germs are bad' (Germ Theory) hypothesis that has dominated Western medicine for the last hundred years. They can also be seen to provide a useful gateway into developing ways in which mucosal immunology can affect, and be manipulated to help manage systemic immune health.

The role of the commensal organisms as systemic modifiers of human health represents a reasonable and effective point of intervention for the healthcare practitioner in the restoration of immune tolerance (Bach 2002).

To translate this model of microbial manipulation of local and systemic immune function, it can help to see humans as a superorganism: a human-microbe hybrid, with immunological and metabolic attributes of both microbial and human origin, requiring all clinical interventions to be considered as affecting the combination of these elements, rather than the human body in isolation (Sekirov and Finlay 2006). Current research is investigating 'symbiotic germ therapy', not only through the reintroduction of strain-specific probiotics, but also via the use of nematodes such as *Necator americanus* (hook worms) for the management of diseases where there has been a loss of immune tolerance (Pritchard and Brown 2001).

The Germ Theory wherein all microbes need to be destroyed is thus redundant. The 'magic bullet' concept (coined by Ehrlich) that launched the 'warfare' metaphor that has clung to drugs such as antibiotics – itself a weapons-like term – ever since, is equally outdated.

7.2 Antibiotics

The use of antibiotics for the eradication of pathogenic bacteria should be carefully considered, especially in the recent discovery that certain antibiotics can induce long-term changes to the microbiota (Antonopoulos *et al.* 2009).

In addition to the problem of antibiotic resistance, unnecessary treatment with antibiotics could reduce the quality of physiological immuno-stimulation generated by commensal bacteria, which may prove counterproductive in terms of overall health.

7.3 Probiotics

Continuing from these ideas, microbiological and immunological research is considering that the way to manage these microbial communities may be through communication changes rather than the eradication strategies employed currently (Mlot 2009). Probiotics can change the make-up of the commensal flora and improve communication by stimulating the immune response in the appropriate manner, helping to improve health.

The way that probiotics exert their effects are varied but the key clinical understanding is that probiotic bacteria are non-pathogenic, mostly Gram-positive organisms, whose very thick and sturdy cell wall (up to 50 layers) of peptidoglycans are recognised as beneficial by the PRRs; and their contents and cell patterns produce a commensally induced immunological benefit, as opposed to a potential pathogen-induced problem. Gram-negative bacteria mostly have a single peptidoglycan layer, making them easier targets for destruction by antibacterial defences, including the complement immune response. This may explain why, when using probiotic therapy, even small numbers appear to be able to induce a change in immune function.

Probiotics, along with commensal bacteria, have a definite role to play in the control of TH17 cell production as, via cytokine IL-27, they induce a key anti-inflammatory cytokine, IL-10, required for immunological tolerance through the expansion of Treg cells, which in turn inhibit or control IL-17 production (Awasthi *et al.* 2007; Stumhofer *et al.* 2007).

A recent example of this potential was demonstrated in an experimental animal model where use of the probiotics *Lactobacillus paracseii* and *L. plantarum* were found to be effective in preventing the animal version of MS, indicating that selected strains have the potential to control TH17 cell-mediated inflammation (a known agent in MS genesis; Hofstetter, Gold and Hartung 2009) via oral supplementation in sites away from the gut (Lavasani *et al.* not yet published).

7.4 Metagenomics and nutrigenomics

Although our human-derived genes are subject to a great many gene-expression control mechanisms (Pennisi 2008), our choices of foods, environment, lifestyle, stressors, medications, etc. strongly influence which genes are expressed or inhibited, in both the human and bacterial systems. This new developmental science, referred to as metagenomics[15] and nutrigenomics,[16] is being explored, along with other specialisms, in the human microbiome project (Hu and Kong 2004; Trayhurn 2003).

The human genome consists of approximately 3 billion base pairs and approximately 10 million positions in this genetic code are polymorphic in the human population at a significant frequency (Nature 2003). These sequence differences result in phenotypic differences such as height, skin colour and differential resistance to infection or disease. Some of this variation is neutral, some is advantageous and some is disadvantageous to an individual's health, dependent on context. In particular, an individual's risks of developing disease will be affected by environmental exposure. For example, sickle cell trait is not an ideal condition for any individual to have inherited, but it confers a protective advantage against *Plasmodium falciparum* malaria, and hence is allowed to persist in some African populations (Allison 2009).

Environment-induced modifiers of the immune response, as described above, can include antigenic chemicals (such as pollutants) called autogens, which are identified by the immune system as DAMPs (Halle *et al.* 2008; Hornung *et al.* 2008). These chemicals can induce immune responses that are linked to autoimmune diseases and chronic inflammatory disorders. When someone with a SNP[17] risk meets a DAMP and

---

15 **Metagenomics**: refers to all gene:food interactions between human and microbe. The food we eat impacts not only on the expression of our human genes, but also upon the expression of our bacterial genes and represents a powerful interface between our food selection and gene-expressed immunological risk. When a food choice is made and repeated the bacterial communities will adapt, and in doing so present a differing genomic concentration, which has the potential to significantly alter risk for disease.

16 **Nutrigenomics**: the study of molecular relationships between nutrition and the response of genes, with the aim of extrapolating how such subtle changes can affect human health. Nutrigenomics focuses on the effect of nutrients on the genome, proteome, and metabolome. By determining the mechanism of the effects of nutrients or of a nutritional regime, nutrigenomics tries to define the relationship between these specific nutrients and specific nutrient regimes (diets) and the effect on human health. It has been associated with the idea of personalised nutrition based on genotype.

17 **SNP – Single Nucleotide Polymorphisms**: Genetic polymorphisms are natural variations in the genomic DNA sequence present in greater than 1% of the population, with SNP representing DNA variations in a single nucleotide.

an immune challenge (such as a virus) at the same time, the cross-presentation and ensuing inflammatory cascade may initiate a chronic bout of inflammation, potentially resulting in the development of an autoimmune disease (Bevan 2006).

8. Clinical application

The clinical and functional role of nutrients, bacteria, pathogens and pollutants and their potential impact on our gene expression should now be considered in terms of both human cells and our microbiota. Healthcare practitioners will improve their clinical outcomes by expanding their concept of the human immune system away from the metaphorical model of a patrolling army, towards one of an integrated group of communicating tissues, microbes and immune-competent cells, working together to maintain human integrity and health.

To accommodate this in practice, practitioners need to intervene in a way that includes recognition of the signals from the trillions of human microflora in order to shape and maintain or destroy human immune tolerance (Gill *et al.* 2006; Pennisi 2008).

8.1 Examination thoughts

When examining a patient's health history, especially when taking a gastro-centric view, the practitioner is urged to be mindful that the health of the local tissues is as important as the overall systemic effects. In terms of the induction of tolerance, the promotion of peripherally induced Tregs and the management of unwanted IL-17 production represents a route of clinical opportunity with little risk and high reward.

When considering therapeutic interventions for a potential immune-oriented patient there are a number of investigations, as well as careful history taking, that may be of assistance.

For clarification, a working list might include the following:

- *In utero* and postnatal experiences (Wellberg and Seckl 2001) the relationships of the mother (and even grandmother) to not only immediate family but also her environment and food may have contributed risk factors to immune sensitisation. The early weeks after birth are also critical to immune maturation and retrospective and prospective investigations are continuing to explore the impact of these events on the capacity for immune balance and associated health complaints (Liu *et al.* 1997).

- Early life exposure to stressors such as medications, especially antibiotics (Garner *et al.* 2009), and stressful events in which the patient experienced loss of control over the immediate decision-making can also contribute to altered immunological status (Chrousos 2000).

- Indications or a history of gastro-intestinal infections or functional gastro-intestinal disorders. They do not need to be present or symptomatically active to exert an effect on the 'resetting' of the innate immune responsiveness to antigenic and emotive stimuli.

- Complex dietetic history in which food choice or lifestyle habits may lead to micro and macronutrient deficiency; of particular importance are foods that provide essential fatty acids, bacteria, minerals and vitamins in adequate quantities to avoid both overt and subclinical illness.

- Family history of gastro-intestinal disorders or long term medication, especially antibiotic use, by the maternal line.

- Toxin exposure – chronic and/or acute exposure to known or unknown toxins (West 2002).

- Enzymatic deficiencies, for example digestive enzymes, cholecystokinase (CCK) deficiency, HCl excess or deficiency, lack of appropriate cholinergic stimulation due to lack of CCK activity.

- Inadequate secretion of SIgA or other immunoglobulin variations; inappropriate serum levels of pro-inflammatory cytokines, raised erythrocyte sedimentation rate and C-reactive protein levels may be raised.

- Presence of a pathogen, or loss of bacterial balance known as dysbiosis; alterations in the mucosal barrier integrity and increased nitrositative and reactive oxygen species (Maes, Coucke and Leunis 2007) as well as increased translocation of bacterial cell wall lipopolysaccharides across the mucosal barrier (Groschwitz and Hogan 2009).

- Loss of immunological tolerance, characterised by increasing reactivity to food stuffs, such as disease, allergy, sensitivity and many levels of reactions in between (Verdu, Armstrong and Murray 2009). Other indications will include the development of inflammatory illnesses, including certain types of arthritis, skin complaints, chronic fatigue, neurodevelopmental conditions, certain types of depression, diabetes and/or cardiovascular disease.

- Altered organic acid excretion, including changes in nutrient-dependent and genetic-dependent enzymes and bacterially induced toxins.

Investigations may include stool analysis, immune panels, organic acid profiles, physical examination and a considered and interactive case history. An analysis of the overall trend of the evolving history, whether the patient is stable or declining, and looking for internal and external factors that press on the complexity of the immune system and the gastro-intestinal tract will allow the clinician to proceed with interventions that are of low risk to the patient's overall physiology.

The use of biological and natural modifiers of mucosal tolerance may require extensive re-evaluations and duration of therapy. Often very small changes in the cytokine balance will be adequate to impart a return to mucosal tolerance, whilst in more complex disorders it may be insufficient in strength by itself and additional pharmaceutical intervention may be required. The recommendations included in this chapter are just the starting point for this type of complementary therapy and, as further studies explore more human-related interventions, this field of healthcare will develop further.

8.2 Possible natural therapeutic agents to consider

Table 8.3 Natural therapeutic agents to consider

Natural agents	Actions	References
Retinoic acid (vitamin A)	Suppresses proinflammatory cytokine IFN-γ, increases IL-4 and reduces RORγt signalling, resulting in TH17 inhibition and Treg promotion. Improves health of peripheral sensory neurons	Batten *et al.* 2006; Mey 2001; Mucida *et al.* 2007
1α, 25-DihydroxyvitaminD	Can increase production of Regulatory DCs, inhibits NFκB expression, increases serum TGF-β and has demonstrated reduction in autoimmune conditions	Mahon *et al.* 2003; Taher *et al.* 2008; Wang *et al.* 2008
Resveratrol	Acts as an anti-inflammatory and antioxidant. Reduces NFκB expression, is neuro-protective and mucosal tissue barrier-protective	Gonzales and Orlando 2008
Probiotics	*Bifidobacterium breve* and *Streoptococcus thermophilus* release metabolites exerting an anti-TNF-α effect capable of crossing the intestinal barrier Reduce gut permeability *Lactobacillus GG* and VSL#3 increase IL-10 expression and Treg numbers Early experimentation, using probiotics in mice that were genetically susceptible for diabetes, saw the prevention of the disease development, most probably due to the increased production of IL-10	Calcinaro *et al.* 2005; Galdeano *et al.* 2007; Hermelijn *et al.* 2005; Menard 2004
	Probiotics have many effects on the gastro-intestinal immune system, some are summarised here: (strain-specific application remains vital to outcome) Production of antioxidants Increased production of SIgA Production of antimicrobial substances (bacteriocins and others) Transcription of NF-κB Induction of pro- and/or anti-inflammatory cytokines Bacterial DNA-induced TLR9 signalling → anti-inflammatory effect in colitis Elevation of serum IL-10 levels Induction of dendritic cell (DC) maturation	Ljungh and Wadström 2006; Wallace 2009

Natural agents	Actions	References
	Enhancement of serum antibody response to orally and systemically administered antigens Enhanced immunoreactivity of spleen cells and phagocytes Activation of the gene for human beta defensin 2 in intestinal mucosa Induction of oral tolerance to β-lactoglobulin Production of β-galactosidase→ improvement of lactose intolerance Induction of PPARγ to reduce local inflammation in GIT	
Saccharomyces boulardii	Assists improved growth and proliferation of mucosal cells Increases SIgA production Reduces gut permeability Increase brush border enzyme activity Neutralises pathogenic toxins Suppresses the pro-inflammatory IL-8 Chemokine PPARγ inducer Increases spermines to maintain mucosal integrity Inhibits excess zonulin – reducing gut permeability	Lee *et al.* 2005; McFarland *et al.* 1994
Garlic (allicin), beta carotene, curcumin, quercetin, green tea, boswellia	Suppression of NFκB, IL-1, TH17 and IL-17 production, making them potential support products for the reduction of cytokine induced and abrogated loss of tolerance. May also manage IL-6 and so support increased production of TGF- β to aid IL17 suppression and generation of Tregs	Guruvayoorappan and Kuttan 2007; Husan *et al.* 2007; Kasinski *et al.* 2008; Ruiz *et al.* 2007; Siddiqui *et al.* 2008; Syrovets *et al.* 2005
Butyric acid	Anti-inflammatory short chain fatty acid, also important for epithelial cell health. Increases production of PPARγ	Wachtershauser, Loitsch and Stein 2000
Colostrum	Reduces gut permeability, supports immunoglobulin defence, maintains immunglobulin function	Pironi *et al.* 1990
Glutamine, slippery elm, epithelial growth factor	Reduces inflammation, repairs the epithelial barrier in the gastro-instestinal tract. Glutamine is an important amino acid for cellular health	Langmead *et al.* 2002; Murnin *et al.* 2000
Omega-3 FAs	PPARγ induction. It also acts as a gastro-intestinal anti-inflammatory, reduces NFκB promotion and expression and aids Treg promotion	Bassaganya-Riera *et al.* 2004

References

Aderem, A. and Ulevitch, R.J. (2000) 'Toll-like receptors in the induction of the innate immune response.' *Nature 406*, 6797, 782–7.

Agrawal, A., Eastman, Q.M. and Schatz, D.G. (1998) 'Transposition mediated by RAG1 and RAG2 and its implications for the evolution of the immune system.' *Nature 394*, 744–751.

Allan, S. (2008) 'T cells: Tuning T cells through the aryl hydrocarbon receptor.' *Nature Reviews Immunology 8*, 326.

Allison, A.C. (2009) 'Genetic control of resistance to human malaria.' *Current Opinion in Immunology 21*, 5, 499–505.

Anderson, K.V. and Nüsslein-Volhard, C. (1984) 'Information for the dorsal–ventral pattern of the Drosophila embryo is stored as maternal MRNA.' *Nature 311*, 5983, 223–227.

Antonopoulos, D.A., Huse, S.M., Morrison, H.G., Schmidt, T.M., Sogin, M.L. and Young, V.B. (2009) 'Reproducible community dynamics of the gastrointestinal microbiota following antibiotic perturbation.' *Infection and Immunity 77*, 6, 2367–2375.

Atisook, K., Carlson, S. and Madara, J.L. (1990) 'Effects of phlorizin and sodium on glucose-elicited alterations of cell junctions in intestinal epithelia.' *American Journal of Physiology 258*, C77–85.

Awasthi, A., Carrier, Y., Peron, J.P., Bettelli, E. *et al.* (2007) 'A dominant function for interleukin 27 in generating interleukin 10-producing anti-inflammatory T cells.' *Nature Immunology 8*, 1380–1389.

Bach, J.F. (2002) 'The effect of infections on susceptibility to autoimmune and allergic diseases.' *New England Journal of Medicine 347*, 12, 911–920.

Bassaganya-Riera, J., Reynolds, K., Martino-Catt, S., Cui, Y. *et al.* (2004) 'Activation of PPAR gamma and delta by conjugated linoleic acid mediates protection from experimental inflammatory bowel disease.' *Gastroenterology 127*, 777–791.

Batten, M., Li, J., Yi, S., Kljavin, N.M *et al.* (2006) 'Interleukin 27 limits autoimmune encephalomyelitis by suppressing the development of interleukin 17-producing T cells.' *Nature Immunology 7*, 9, 929–936.

Benard, A., Desreumeaux, P., Huglo, D., Hoorelbeke, A., Tonnel, A.B. and Wallaert, B. (1996) 'Increased intestinal permeability in bronchial asthma.' *Journal of Allergy and Clinical Immunology 97*, 1173–1178.

Bettelli, E., Oukka, M. and Kuchroo, V.K. (2007) 'TH-17 cells in the circle of immunity and autoimmunity.' *Nature Immunology 8*, 345–350.

Bevan, M.J. (2006) 'Cross priming.' *Nature Immunology 7*, 363–365.

Bollinger, R.R., Everett, M.L., Wahl, S.D., Lee, Y.H., Orndorff, P.E. and Parker, W. (2006) 'Secretory iga and mucin-mediated biofilm formation by environmental strains of Escherichia coli: Role of type 1 pili.' *Molecular Immunology 43*, 378–387.

Bosi, E., Molteni, L., Radaelli, M.G., Folini, L. *et al.* (2006) 'Increased intestinal permeability precedes clinical onset of type 1 diabetes.' *Diabetologia 49*, 2824–2827.

Bruewer, M., Luegering. A., Kucharzik, T., Parkos, C.A. *et al.* (2003) 'Proinflammatory cytokines disrupt epithelial barrier function by apoptosis-independent mechanisms.' *Journal of Immunology 171*, 6164–6172.

Burnet, F.M. (1959) *The Clonal Selection Theory of Acquired Immunity.* London: Cambridge University Press.

Burnet, F.M. and Fenner, F. (1949) *The Production of Antibodies*, 2nd edn. Monograph of the Walter and Eliza Hall Institute, Melbourne. Melbourne: Macmillan.

Calcinaro, F.D.S., Marinaro, M., Candeloro, P., Bonato, V. *et al.* (2005) 'Oral probiotic administration induces interleukin-10 production and prevents spontaneous autoimmune diabetes in the non-obese diabetic mouse.' *Diabetologia 48*, 1565–1575.

Campieri, M. and Gionchetti, P. (1999) 'Probiotics in inflammatory bowel disease: New insights to pathogenesis or a possible therapeutic alternative.' *Gastroenterology 116*, 1246–1249.

Cantorna, M.T. and Mahon, B.D. (2004) 'Mounting evidence for vitamin D as an environmental factor affecting autoimmune disease prevalence.' *Experimental Biology and Medicine 229*, 11, 1136–1142.

Carson D.A., Raz, E., Hayashi, T., Beck, L. *et.al.* (2004) 'Inhibition of experimental asthma by indoleamine 2,3-dioxygenase.' *Journal of Clinical Investigation 114*, 2, 270–279.

Chrousos, G.P. (2000) 'The stress response and immune function: Clinical implications.' The 1999 Novera H. Spector Lecture. *Annals of the New York Academy of Sciences 917*, 38–67.

Chung, D.R., Kasper, D.L., Panzo, R.J., Chitnis, T. *et al.* (2003) 'CD4+ T cells mediate abscess formation in intra-abdominal sepsis by an IL-17-dependent mechanism.' *Journal of Immunology 170*, 1958–1963.

Clark, E.C., Patel, S.D., Warhurst, G., Curry, A., Carlson, G.L and Chadwick, P.R. (2003) 'Glutamine deprivation facilitates tumour necrosis factor induced bacterial translocation in Caco-2 cells by depletion of enterocyte fuel substrate.' *Gut 52*, 224–230.

Collins, S.M. (2001) 'Stress and the gastrointestinal tract IV. Modulation of intestinal inflammation by stress: Basic mechanisms and clinical relevance.' *American Journal of Physiology Gastrointestinal and Liver Physiology 280*, G315–318.

Coombes, J.L. and Maloy, K.J. (2007) 'Control of intestinal homeostasis by regulatory T cells and dendritic cells.' *Seminars in Immunology 19*, 116–126.

Coombes J.L. and Powrie, F. (2008) 'Dendritic cells in intestinal immune regulation.' *Nature Reviews Immunology 8*, 6, 435–446.

Coombes, J.L., Siddiqui, K.R., Arancibia-Cárcamo, C.V., Hall, J. *et al.* (2007) 'A functionally specialized population of mucosal CD103+ DCs induces Foxp3+ regulatory T cells via a TGF- and retinoic acid-dependent mechanism.' *Journal of Experimental Medicine 204*, 1757–1764.

Coutinho, A. (1995) 'The network theory: 21 years later.' *Scandinavian Journal of Immunology 42*, 1, 3–8.

Di Giacinto, C., Marinaro, M., Sanchez, M., Strober, W. and Boirivant, M. (2005) 'Probiotics ameliorate recurrent Th1-mediated murine colitis by inducing IL-10 and IL-10-dependent TGF-β-bearing regulatory cells.' *Journal of Immunology 174*, 3237–3246.

Dong, C. (2006) 'Diversification of T-helper-cell lineages: Finding the family root of IL-17-producing cells.' *Nature Review of Immunology 6*, 329–334.

Dong, C. and Flavell, R.A. (2001) 'TH1 and TH2 cells.' *Current Opinion in Hematology 8*, 47–51.

Fagarasan, S. and Honjo, T. (2003) 'Intestinal iga synthesis: Regulation of front-line body defences.' *Nature Review of Immunology 3*, 63–72.

Ferwerda, B., McCall, M.B., Alonso, S., Giamarellos-Bourboulis, E.J. *et al.* (2007) 'TLR4 polymorphisms, infectious diseases, and evolutionary pressure during migration of modern humans.' *The Proceedings of the National Academy of Science (US) 104*, 42, 16645–16650.

Frank, D.N. and Pace, N.R. (2008) 'Gastrointestinal microbiology enters the metagenomics era.' *Current Opinion in Gastroenterology 24*, 1, 4–10.

Fritz, J.H., Ferrero, R.L., Philpott, D.J. and Girardin, S.E. (2006) 'Nod-like receptors in innate immunity and inflammation.' *Nature Immunology 7*, 1250–1257.

Galdeano, C.M., de Moreno de Le Blanc, A., Vinderola, G., Bonet, M.E.B. and Perdigon, G. (2007) 'Proposed model: Mechanisms of immunomodulation induced by probiotic bacteria.' *Clinical and Vaccine Immunology 14*, 485–492.

Garner, C.D., Antonopoulos, D.A., Wagner, B., Duhamel, G.E. *et al.* (2009) 'Perturbation of the small intestine microbial ecology by streptomycin alters pathology in a Salmonella enterica serovar typhimurium murine model of infection.' *Infection and Immunity 77*, 7, 2691–2702.

Gill, S.R., Pop, M., Deboy, R.T., Eckburg, P.B. *et al.* (2006) 'Metagenomic analysis of the human distal gut microbiome.' *Science 312*, 5778, 1355–1359.

Gonzales, A.M. and Orlando, R.A. (2008) 'Curcumin and resveratrol inhibit nuclear factor-kappaB-mediated cytokine expression in adipocytes.' *Nutrition and Metabolism 5*, 17–30.

Groer, M., Davis, M. and Steele, K. (2004) 'Associations between human milk siga and maternal immune, infectious, endocrine, and stress variables.' *Journal of Human Lactation 20*, 2, 153–158; quiz 159–163.

Grohmann, U., Fallarino, F. and Puccetti, P. (2003) 'Tolerance, DCs and tryptophan: Much ado about IDO.' *Trends in Immunology 24*, 242–248.

Groschwitz, K.R. and Hogan, S.P. (2009) 'Intestinal barrier function: Molecular regulation and disease pathogenesis.' *Journal of Allergy and Clinical Immunology 124*, 1, 3–20; quiz 21–22.

Grover, M., Kanazawa, M., Palsson, O.S., Chitkara, D.K. *et al.* (2008) 'Small intestinal bacterial overgrowth in irritable bowel syndrome: Association with colon motility, bowel symptoms, and psychological distress.' *Neurogastroenterology and Motility 20*, 9, 998–1008.

Gupta, S.L., Carlin, J.M., Pyati, P., Dai, W., Pfefferkorn, E.R. and Murphy, M.J. (1994) 'Antiparasitic and antiproliferative effects of indoleamine 2,3-dioxygenase enzyme expression in human fibroblasts.' *Infection and Immunity 62*, 2277–2284.

Guruvayoorappan, C. and Kuttan, G. (2007) 'Beta-carotene inhibits tumor-specific angiogenesis by altering the cytokine profile and inhibits the nuclear translocation of transcription factors in B16F-10 melanoma cells.' *Integrated Cancer Therapy 6*, 258–270.

Haddad, P.S., Azar, G.A., Groom, S. and Boivin, M. (2005) 'Natural health products, modulation of immune function and prevention of chronic diseases.' *Evidence Based Complementary and Alternative Medicine 2*, 513–520.

Halle, A., Hornung, V., Petzold, G.C., Stewart, C.R. *et al.* (2008) 'The NALP3 inflammasome is involved in the innate immune response to amyloid-β.' *Nature Immunology 9*, 857–865.

Harrington, L.E., Hatton, R.D., Mangan, P.R., Turner, H. *et al.* (2005) 'Interleukin-17-producing CD4+ effector T cells develop via a lineage distinct from the T helper type 1 and 2 lineages.' *Nature Immunology 6*, 1123–1132.

Henriksson, A.E., Blomquist, L., Nord, C.E., Midtvedt, T. and Uribe, A. (1993) 'Small intestinal bacterial overgrowth in patients with rheumatoid arthritis.' *Annals of the Rheumatic Diseases 52*, 7, 503–510.

Hermelijn, H.S., Engering, A., van der Kleij, D., de Jong, E.C. *et al.* (2005) 'Selective probiotic bacteria induce IL-10-producing regulatory T cells in vitro by modulating dendritic cell function through dendritic cell-specific intercellular adhesion molecule 3-grabbing nonintegrin.' *Journal of Allergy and Clinical Immunology 115*, 1260–1267.

Hill J.A., Hall, J.A., Sun, C.M., Cai, Q. *et al.* (2008) 'Retinoic acid enhances Foxp3 induction indirectly by relieving inhibition from CD4+CD44hi cells.' *Immunity 29*, 5, 758–770.

Hofstetter, H., Gold, R. and Hartung, H.P. (2009) 'Th17 cells in MS and experimental autoimmune encephalomyelitis.' *International MS Journal 16*, 1, 12–18.

Holick, M.F. (2007) 'Vitamin D deficiency.' *New England Journal of Medicine 19*, 357, 3, 266–281.

Holzapfel, W.H., Haberer, P., Snel, J., Schillinger, U., Huis in't, Veld, J.H. *et al.* (1998) 'Overview of gut flora and probiotics.' *International Journal of Food Microbiology 41*, 85–101.

Hopkins, L. and Groom, C. (2002) 'The druggable genome.' *Nature Reviews Drug Discovery 1*, 727–730.

Hornung, V., Bauernfeind, F., Halle, A., Samstad, E.O. *et al.* (2008) 'Silica crystals and aluminum salts activate the NALP3 inflammasome through phagosomal destabilization.' *Nature Immunology 9*, 847–856.

Hoyle, B.D. and Costerton, W.J. (1991) 'Bacterial resistance to antibiotics: The role of biofilms.' *Progress in Drug Research 37*, 91–105.

Hu, R. and Kong, A.N. (2004) 'Activation of MAP kinases, apoptosis and nutrigenomics of gene expression elicited by dietary cancer prevention compounds.' *Nutrition 20*, 1, 83–88.

Huang, W., Na, L., Fidel, P.L. and Schwarzenberger, P. (2004) 'Requirement of interleukin-17A for systemic anti-Candida albicans host defense in mice.' *Journal of Infectious Diseases 190*, 624–631.

Husan, N., Mashiat, U.S., Toossi, Z., Khan, S., Iobal, J. and Islam, N. (2007) 'Allicin-induced suppression of Mycobacterium tuberculosis 85B mRNA in human monocytes.' *Biochemical and Biophysical Research Communications 335*, 471–476.

Hylemon, P.B. and Glass, T.L. (1983) 'Biotransformation of Bile Acids and Cholesterol by the Intestinal Microflora.' In D.J. Hentges (ed.) *Human Intestinal Microflora in Health and Disease.* New York: Academic Press.

Infante-Duarte, C., Horton, H. F., Byrne, M. C. and Kamradt, T. (2000) 'Microbial lipopeptides induce the production of IL-17 in Th cells.' *Journal of Immunology 165*, 6107–6115.

Inohara, N. and Nunez, G. (2003) 'Nods: intracellular proteins involved in inflammation and apoptosis.' *National Review of Immunology 3*, 371–382.

Izcue, A., Coombes, J.L. and Powrie, F. (2006) 'Regulatory T cells suppress systemic and mucosal immune activation to control intestinal inflammation.' *Immunology Review 212*, 256–271.

Janeway, C.A. Jr (1992) 'The immune system evolved to discriminate infectious non-self from non-infectious self.' *Immunology Today 13*, 1, 11–16.

Johansen, F.E., Pekna, M., Norderhaug, I.N., Haneberg, B. *et al.* (1999) 'Absence of epithelial immunoglobulin A transport, with increased mucosal leakiness, in polymeric immunoglobulin receptor/secretory component-deficient mice.' *Journal of Experimental Medicine 190*, 915–922.

Jones, D. (ed.) (2005) *Textbook of Functional Medicine.* Gig Harbor, WA: Institute for Functional Medicine.

Kasinski, A.L., Du, Y., Thomas, S.L., Zhao, J. *et al.* (2008) 'Inhibition of IkappaB kinase-nuclear factor-kappaB signaling pathway by 3,5-bis (2-flurobenzylidene)piperidin-4-one (EF24), a novel monoketone analog of curcumin.' *Molecular Pharmacology 74*, 654–661.

Kelsall, B.L. and Leon, F. (2005) 'Involvement of intestinal dendritic cells in oral tolerance, immunity to pathogens, and inflammatory bowel disease.' *Immunology Review 206*, 132–148.

Kero, J., Gissler, M., Hemminki, E. and Isolauri, E. (2001) 'Could T_H1 and T_H2 diseases coexist? Evaluation of asthma incidence in children with coeliac disease, type 1 diabetes, or rheumatoid arthritis: A register study.' *Journal of Allergy and Clinical Immunology 108*, 781–783.

Kim, C.H. (2008) 'Regulation of FoxP3+ regulatory T cells and Th17 cells by retinoids.' *Clinical and Developmental Immunology.* Article ID 416910. Available at www.ncbi.nlm.nih.gov/pubmed/18389070, accessed 13 March 2010.

Kohm, A., Fuller, K. and Miller, S. (2003) 'Mimicking the way to autoimmunity: An evolving theory of sequence and structural homology.' *Trends in Microbiology 11*, 3, 101–105.

Kolls, J.K. and Linden, A. (2004) 'Interleukin-17 family members and inflammation.' *Immunity 21*, 467–476.

Kuek, A., Hazleman, B.L. and Ostör, A.J. (2007) 'Immune-mediated inflammatory diseases (imids) and biologic therapy: A medical revolution.' *Postgraduate Medical Journal 83*, 978, 251–260.

Lack, G., Fox, D., Northstone, K., Golding, J. and Avon Longitudinal Study of Parents and Children Study Team (2003) 'Factors associated with the development of peanut allergy in childhood.' *New England Journal of Medicine 348*, 11, 977–985.

Langmead, L., Dawson, C., Hawkins, C., Banna, N., Loo, S. and Rampton, D.S. (2002) 'Antioxidant effects of herbal therapies used by patients with inflammatory bowel disease: An in vitro study.' *Alimentary Pharmacology and Therapeutics 16*, 2, 197–205.

Lauritano, E.C., Bilotta, A.L., Gabrielli, M., Scarpellini, E. *et al.* (2007) 'Association between hypothyroidism and small intestinal bacterial overgrowth.' *Clinical Endocrinology and Metabolism 92*, 11, 4180–4184.

Lavasani, S., Buske S., Fåk F., Dzhambazov B., Molin G., Alenfall J., and Weström B. (unpublished) 'Oral administration of unique probiotic strains successfully ameliorates experimental autoimmune encephalomyelitis.' Submitted to *Nature Medicine.*

Lee, S.K., Kim, H.J., Chi, S.G., Jang, J.Y. *et al.* (2005) 'Saccharomyces boulardii activates expression of peroxisome proliferator-activated receptor-gamma in HT-29 cells.' *Korean Journal of Gastroenterology 45*, 328–334.

Lemaitre, B., Nicolas, E., Michaut, L., Reichhart, J. and Hoffmann, J. (1996) 'The dorsoventral regulatory gene cassette spaetzle/toll/cactus controls the potent antifungal response in Drosophila adults.' *Cell 86*, 973–983.

Linden, S.K., Sutton, P., Karlsson, N.G., Korolik, V. and McGuckin, M.A. (2008) 'Mucins in the mucosal barrier to infection.' *Mucosal Immunology 1*, 3, 183–197.

Liu, D., Diorio, J., Tannenbaum, B., Caldji, C. *et al.* (1997) 'Maternal care, hippocampal glucocorticoid receptors, and hypothalamic-pituitary-adrenal responses to stress.' *Science 277*, 1659–1662.

Ljungh, A. and Wadström, T. (2006) 'Lactic acid bacteria as probiotics.' *Current Issues in Intestinal Microbiology 7*, 73–90.

Lloyd, D., Aon, M.A. and Cortassa, S. (2001) 'Why homeodynamics, not homeostasis?' *Scientific World Journal 4*, 1, 133–145.

Lycke, N., Eriksen, L. and Holmgren, J. (1987) 'Protection against cholera toxin after oral immunization is thymus-dependent and associated with intestinal production of neutralizing iga antitoxin.' *Scandinavian Journal of Immunology 25*, 4, 413–419.

Maclennan, I.C. (1994) 'Germinal centers.' *Annual Review of Immunology 12*, 117–139.

Macpherson, A.J. and Uhr, T. (2004) 'Induction of protective IgA by intestinal dendritic cells carrying commensal bacteria.' *Science 303*, 1662–1665.

Macpherson, A.J., McCoy, K.D., Johansen, F.E. and Brandtzaeg, P. (2008) 'The immune geography of IgA induction and function.' *Mucosal Immunology 1*, 1, 11–22.

Madara, J. and Trier, J. (1987) 'Functional morphology of the mucosa of the small intestine.' In L.R. Johnson (ed.) *Physiology of the Gastrointestinal Tract.* New York: Raven Press.

Maes, M., Coucke, F. and Leunis, J.C. (2007) 'Normalization of the increased translocation of endotoxin from gram negative enterobacteria (leaky gut) is accompanied by a remission of chronic fatigue syndrome.' *Neuroendocrinology Letters 28*, 6, 739–744.

Maes, M., Mihaylova, I. and Bosmans, E. (2007) 'Not in the mind of neurasthenic lazybones but in the cell nucleus: Patients with chronic fatigue syndrome have increased production of nuclear factor kappa beta.' *Neuroendocrinology Letters 28*, 4, 456–462.

Mahon, B.D., Gordon, S.A., Cruz, J., Cosman, F. and Cantorna, M.T. (2003) 'Cytokine profile in patients with multiple sclerosis following vitamin D supplementation.' *Journal of Neuroimmunology 134*, 128–132.

Maldonado-López, R., De Smedt, T., Michel, P., Godfroid, J. *et al.* (1999) 'CD8alpha+ and CD8alpha-subclasses of dendritic cells direct the development of distinct T helper cells in vivo.' *Journal of Experimental Medicine 189*, 3, 587–592.

Masclee, A., Tangerman, A., van Schaik, A., van der Hoek, E.W. and van Tongeren, J.H. (1989) 'Unconjugated serum bile acids as a marker of small intestinal bacterial overgrowth.' *European Journal of Clinical Investigation 19*, 4, 384–389.

Matzinger, P. (1994) 'Tolerance, danger, and the extended family.' *Annual Review of Immunology 12*, 991–1045.

Matzinger P. (2007) 'Friendly and dangerous signals: Is the tissue in control?' *Nature Immunology 8*, 1, 11–13.

Mayer, L. (2003) 'Mucosal immunity.' *Pediatrics 111*, 6, 3, 1595–1600.

McFarland, L.V., Surawicz, C.M., Greenberg, R.N., Fekety, R. *et al.* (1994) 'A randomized placebo-controlled trial of *Saccharomyces boulardii* in combination with standard antibiotics for *Clostidium difficile* disease.' *Journal of the American Medical Association 271*, 1913–1918.

Medzhitov R. and Janeway, C.A. (1997) 'Innate immunity: Impact on the adaptive immune response.' *Current Opinion in Immunology 9*, 1, 4–9.

Mellor, A.L. and Munn, D.H. (2001) 'Tryptophan catabolism prevents maternal T cells from activating lethal antifetal immune responses.' *Journal of Reproductive Immunology 52*, 5–13.

Menard, S. (2004) 'Lactic acid bacteria secrete metabolites retaining anti-inflammatory properties after intestinal transport.' *Gut 53*, 821–828.

Mestecky, J. and McGhee, J.R. (1987) 'Immunoglobulin A (iga, molecular and cellular interactions involved in IgA biosynthesis and immune response.' *Advances in Immunology 40*, 153–245.

Metchnikoff, E. (1907) *The Prolongation of Life: Optimistic Studies.* London: William Heinemann.

Mey, J. (2001) 'Retinoic acid as a regulator of cytokine signaling after nerve injury.' *Zeitschrift fur Naturforschung 56*, 3–4, 163–176.

Micka, J., Milatovich, A., Menon, A., Grabowski, G.A., Puga, A. and Nebert, D.W. (1997) 'Human Ah receptor (AHR) gene: Localization to 7p15 and suggestive correlation of polymorphism with CYP1A1 inducibility.' *Pharmacogenetics 7*, 2, 95–101.

Mielants, H., Veys, E.M., Joos, R., Cuvelier, C. and De Vos, M. (1987) 'Repeat ileocolonoscopy in reactive arthritis.' *Journal of Rheumatology 14*, 456–458.

Mielants, H., Veys, E.M., De Vos, M., Cuvelier, C. *et al.* (1995a) 'The evolution of spondyloarthropathies in relation to gut histology. I. Clinical aspects.' *Journal of Rheumatology 22*, 12, 2266–2272.

Mielants, H., Veys, E.M., Cuvelier, C., De Vos, M. *et al.* (1995b) 'The evolution of spondyloarthropathies in relation to gut histology. II. Histological aspects.' *Journal of Rheumatology 22*, 12, 2273–2278.

Mielants, H., Veys, E.M., Cuvelier, C., De Vos, M. *et al.* (1995c) 'The evolution of spondyloarthropathies in relation to gut histology. III. Relation between gut and joint.' *Journal of Rheumatology 22*, 12, 2279–2284.

Millington, O.R., Mowat, A.M. and Garside, P. (2004) 'Induction of bystander suppression by feeding antigen occurs despite normal clonal expansion of the bystander T cell population.' *Journal of Immunology 173*, 10, 6059–6064.

Mlot, C. (2009) 'Antibiotics in nature: Beyond biological warfare.' *Science 324*, 5935, 1637–1639.

Mosmann, T.R. and Coffman, R.L. (1989) 'TH1 and TH2 cells: Different patterns of lymphokine secretion lead to different functional properties.' *Annual Review of Immunology 7*, 145–173.

Mucida, D., Park, Y., Kim, G., Turovskaya, O. (2007) 'Reciprocal TH17 and regulatory T cell differentiation mediated by retinoic acid.' *Science 317*, 5835, 256–260.

Mullard, A. (2008) 'Microbiology: The inside story.' *Nature 453*, 578–580.

Murnin, M., Kumar, A., Li, G.D., Brown, M., Sumpio, B.E. and Basson, M.D. (2000) 'Effects of glutamine isomers on human (Caco-2) intestinal epithelial proliferation, strain-responsiveness, and differentiation.' *Journal of Gastrointestinal Surgery 4*, 4, 435–442.

Nakazawa, D.J. (2008) *The Auto Immune Epidemic: Bodies Gone Haywire in a World out of Balance.* New York: Touchstone.

Nature (2003) 'The international hapmap project.' *Nature 426*, 789–796.

Nature Immunology (2006) 'Editorial. The innate immune system "puzzle".' *Nature Immunology 7*, 1235.

Niess, J.H., Brand, S., Gu, X., Landsman, L. *et al.* (2005) 'CX3CR1-mediated dendritic cell access to the intestinal lumen and bacterial clearance.' *Science 307*, 254–258.

Norin, K.E., Gustafsson, B.E. and Midtvedt, T. (1986) 'Strain differences in faecal tryptic activity of germ-free and conventional rats.' *Laboratory Animals 20*, 67–69.

Parodi, A., Paolino, S., Greco, A., Drago, F. *et al.* (2008a) 'Small intestinal bacterial overgrowth in rosacea: Clinical effectiveness of its eradication. *Clinical Gastroenterology and Hepatology 6*, 7, 759–64.

Parodi, A., Sessarego, M., Greco, A., Bazzica, M. *et al.* (2008b) 'Small intestinal bacterial overgrowth in patients suffering from scleroderma: Clinical effectiveness of its eradication.' *Journal of Gastroenterology 103*, 5, 1257–1262.

Pennisi, E. (2008) 'Microbiology. Bacteria are picky about their homes on human skin.' *Science 320*, 5879, 1001.

Pironi, L., Miglioli, M., Ruggeri, E., Levorato, M. *et al.* (1990) 'Relationship between intestinal permeability to EDTA and inflammatory activity in asymptomatic patients with Crohn's disease.' *Digestive Diseases and Sciences 35*, 5, 582–588.

Pritchard, D.I. and Brown, A. (2001) 'Is Necator Americanus approaching a mutualistic symbiotic relationship with humans?' *Trends in Parasitology 17*, 4, 169–172.

Qin, X. (2007) 'Inactivation of digestive proteases: Another mechanism that probiotics may have conferred a protection.' *American Journal of Gastroenterology 102*, 9, 2109.

Quigley, E.M. and Quera, R. (2006) 'Small intestinal bacterial overgrowth: Roles of antibiotics, prebiotics, and probiotics.' *Gastroenterology 130*, 2 suppl. 1, S78–S90.

Quintana, F.J., Basso, A.S., Iglesias, A.H., Korn, T. *et al.* (2008) 'Control of T(reg) and T(H)17 cell differentiation by the aryl hydrocarbon receptor.' *Nature 453*, 7191, 65–71.

Rabassa, A.A., Goodgame, R., Sutton, F.M., Ou, C.N., Rognerud, C. and Graham, D.Y. (1996) 'Effects of aspirin and Helicobacter pylori on the gastroduodenal mucosal permeability to sucrose.' *Gut 39*, 2, 159–163.

Rakoff-Nahoum, S., Paglino, J., Eslami-Varzaneh, F., Edberg, S. and Medzhitov, R. (2004) 'Recognition of commensal microflora by toll-like receptors is required for intestinal homeostasis.' *Cell 118*, 229–241.

Raz, E. (2007) 'Organ-specific regulation of innate immunity.' *Nature Immunology 8*, 1, 3–4.

Robinson, M.J., Sancho, D., Slack, E.C., LeibundGut-Landmann, S., Reis, E. and Sousa, C. (2006) 'Myeloid C-type lectins in innate immunity.' *Nature Immunology 7*, 12, 1258–1265.

Rodrigues, A.C., Cara, D.C., Fretez, S.H., Cunha, F.Q. *et al.* (2000) 'Saccharomyces boulardii stimulates siga production and the phagocytic system of gnotobiotic mice.' *Journal of Applied Microbiology 89*, 3, 404–414.

Round, J.L. and Mazmanian, S.K. (2009) 'The gut microbiota shapes intestinal immune responses during health and disease.' *Nature Reviews Immunology 9*, 5, 313–323.

Ruiz, P.A., Braune, A., Hölzlwimmer, G., Quintanilla-Fend, L. and Haller, D. (2007) 'Quercetin inhibits TNF-induced NF-kappaB transcription factor recruitment to proinflammatory gene promoters in murine intestinal epithelial cells.' Journal of Nutrition *137*, 1208–1215.

Schauber, J., Dorschner, R.A., Coda, A.B., Büchau, A.S. *et al.* (2007) 'Injury enhances TLR2 function and antimicrobial peptide expression through a vitamin D-dependent mechanism.' *Journal of Clinical Investigation 117*, 3, 803–811.

Schouten, B., van Esch, B.C., Hofman, G.A., van Doorn, S.A. *et al.* (2009) 'Cow milk allergy symptoms are reduced in mice fed dietary synbiotics during oral sensitization with whey.' *Journal of Nutrition 139*, 7, 1398–1403.

Scrimshaw, N.S. and SanGiovanni, J.P. (1997) 'Synergism of nutrition, infection and immunity: An overview.' *American Journal of Clinical Nutrition 66*, 2, 464s–477s.

Secondulfo, M., de Magistris, L., Sapone, A., Di Monda, G., Esposito, P. and Carratu, R. (1999) 'Intestinal permeability and diabetes mellitus type 2.' *Minerva Gastroenterology Dietology 45*, 187–192.

Sekirov, I. and Finlay, B.B. (2006) 'Human and microbe: United we stand.' *Nature Medicine 12*, 736–737.

Seong, S.Y. and Matzinger, P. (2004) 'Hydrophobicity: An ancient damage-associated molecular pattern that initiates innate immune responses.' *National Review of Immunology 4*, 6, 469–478.

Shahabi, S., Hassan, Z.M., Jazani, N.H. and Ebtekar, M. (2006) 'Sympathetic nervous system plays an important role in the relationship between Immune mediated diseases.' *Medical Hypotheses 67*, 4, 900–903.

Sheikh, A., Smeeth, L. and Hubbard, R.J. (2003) 'There is no evidence of an inverse relationship between TH2-mediated atopy and TH1-mediated autoimmune disorders: Lack of support for the hygiene hypothesis.' *Journal of Allergy and Clinical Immunology 111*, 1, 131–135.

Shen, L. and Turner, J.R. (2006) 'Role of epithelial cells in initiation and propagation of intestinal inflammation. Eliminating the static: Tight junction dynamics exposed.' *American Journal of Physiology – Gastrointestinal and Liver Physiology 290*, 4, G577–G582.

Sicherer, S.H. and Leung, D.Y. (2009) 'Advances in allergic skin disease, anaphylaxis, and hypersensitivity reactions to foods, drugs, and insects in 2008.' *Journal of Allergy and Clinical Immunology 123*, 2, 319–327.

Siddiqui, I.A., Shukla, Y., Adhami, V.M., Sarfaraz, S. *et al.* (2008) 'Suppression of NFkappaB and its regulated gene products by oral administration of green tea polyphenols in an autochthonous mouse prostate cancer model.' *Pharmacology Research 25*, 9, 2135–2142.

Simpson, C.R., Anderson, W.J., Helms, P.J., Taylor, M.W. *et al.* (2002) 'Coincidence of immune-mediated diseases driven by TH1 and TH2 subsets suggests a common aetiology. A population megabased study using computerized general practice data.' *Clinical and Experimental Allergy 32*, 1, 37–42.

Soderholm, J.D., Olaison, G., Lindberg, E., Hannestad, U. *et al.* (1999) 'Different intestinal permeability patterns in relatives and spouses of patients with Crohn's disease: An inherited defect in mucosal defence?' *Gut 44*, 96–100.

Sonoda, N., Furuse, M., Sasaki, H., Yonemura, S. *et al.* (1999) 'Clostridium perfringens enterotoxin fragment removes specific claudins from tight junction strands: Evidence for direct involvement of claudins in tight junction barrier.' *Journal of Cell Biology 147*, 195–204.

Stanwell-Smith R. and Bloomfield, S. (2004) *The Hygiene Hypothesis and its Implications for Home Hygiene.* Milan: NextHealth.

Steinman, L. (2007) 'A brief history of TH17, the first major revision in the TH1/TH2 hypothesis of T cell–mediated tissue damage.' *Nature Medicine 13*, 139–145.

Stene, L.C. and Nafstad, P. (2001) 'Relation between occurrence of type 1 diabetes and asthma.' *Lancet 357*, 607–608.

Stevens, E.A. and Bradfield, C.A. (2008) 'Immunology: T cells hang in the balance.' *Nature 453*, 46–47.

Stumhofer, J.S., Silver, J.S., Laurence, A., Porrett, P.M. *et al.* (2007) 'Interleukins 27 and 6 induce STAT3-mediated T cell production of interleukin 10.' *Nature Immunology 8*, 1363–1371.

Suzuki, K., Meek, B., Doi, Y., Muramatsu, M. *et al.* (2004) 'Aberrant expansion of segmented filamentous bacteria in IgA-deficient gut.' *Proceedings of the National Academy of Sciences USA 101*, 1981–1986.

Syrovets, T., Buchele, B., Krauss, C., Laumonnier, Y. and Simmet, T. (2005) 'Acetyl-boswellic acids inhibit LPS-mediated TNF-{alpha} induction in monocytes by direct interaction with I{kappa}B kinases.' *Journal of Immunology 174*, 1, 498–506.

Taher, Y.A., van Esch, B.C.A.M., Hofman, G.A., Henricks, P.A.J. and van Oosterhout, A.J.M. (2008) '1{alpha},25-Dihydroxyvitamin D3 potentiates the beneficial effects of allergen immunotherapy in a mouse model of allergic asthma: Role for IL-10 and TGF-β1.' *Journal of Immunology 180*, 5211–5221.

Takabayshi, K., Corr, M., Hayashi, T., Redecke, V. (2006) 'Induction of a homeostatic circuit in lung tissue by microbial compounds.' Immunity 24, 4, 475–487.

Takatsu, K. (1997) 'Cytokines involved in B-cell differentiation and their sites of action.' *Proceedings of the Society for Experimental Biology and Medicine 215*, 2, 121–133.

Thomas, C., Pellicciari, R., Pruzanski, M., Auwerx, J. and Schoonjans, K. (2008) 'Targeting bile-acid signalling for metabolic diseases.' *Nature Reviews Drug Discovery 7*, 678–693.

Thomas, S.M., Garrity, L.F., Brandt, C.R., Schobert, C.S. *et al.* (1993) 'IFOMEGA-mediated antimicrobial response: indoleamine 2,3-dioxygenase-deficient mutant host cells no longer inhibit intracellular Chlamydia spp. or Toxoplama growth.' *Journal of Immunology 150*, 5529–5534.

Trayhurn, P. (2003) 'Nutritional genomics – "Nutrigenomics".' *British Journal of Nutrition 89*, 1–2.

Ukabam, S.O., Mann, R.J. and Cooper, B.T. (1984) 'Small intestinal permeability to sugars in patients with atopic eczema.' *British Journal of Dermatology 110*, 649–652.

Vanner, S. (2008) 'The small intestinal bacterial overgrowth. Irritable bowel syndrome hypothesis: Implications for treatment.' *Gut 57*, 9, 1315–1321.

Verdu, E.F., Armstrong, D. and Murray, J.A. (2009) 'Between celiac disease and irritable bowel syndrome: The 'no man's land' of gluten sensitivity.' *American Journal of Gastroenterology 104*, 6, 1587–1594.

Vojdani, A., Lambert, J. and Kellermann, G. (2008) 'The role of Th17 in neuroimmune disorders: A target for CAM therapy. Part I, II, III.' *Evidence Based Complementary and Alternative Medicine* [Epub ahead of print]

Wachtershauser, A., Loitsch, S.M. and Stein, J. (2000) 'PPAR-gamma is selectively upregulated in Caco-2 cells by butyrate.' *Biochemical and Biophysical Research Communications 272*, 380–385.

Wakkach, A., Fournier, N., Brun, V., Breittmayer, J.P., Cottrez, F. and Groux, H. *et al.* (2003) 'Characterization of dendritic cells that induce tolerance and T regulatory 1 cell differentiation in vivo.' *Immunity 18*, 605–617.

Wallace, B. (2009) 'Clinical use of probiotics in the pediatric population.' *Nutrition in Clinical Practice 24*, 1, 50–59.

Walsh, S.J. and Rau, L.M. (2000) 'Autoimmune diseases: A leading cause of death among young and middle-aged women in the United States.' *American Journal of Public Health 90*, 1463–1466.

Wang, J.T., Pencina, M.J., Booth, S.L., Jacques, P.F. *et al.* (2008) 'Vitamin D deficiency and risk of cardiovascular disease.' *Circulation 117*, 503–511.

Weiner, H., Friedman, A., Miller, A., Khoury, S.J. *et al.* (1994) 'Oral tolerance: Immunologic mechanisms and treatment of animal and human organ-specific autoimmune diseases by oral administration of autoantigens.' *Annual Review of Immunology 12*, 809.

Wellberg, L.A.M. and Seckl, J.R. (2001) 'Prenatal stress, glucocorticoids and the programming of the brain.' *Journal of Neuroendocrinology 13*, 113–128

West, L.J. (2002) 'Defining critical windows in the development of the human immune system.' *Human and Experimental Toxicology 21*, 9–10, 499–505.

White J.H. (2008) 'Vitamin D signaling, infectious diseases, and regulation of innate immunity.' *Infection and Immunity 76*, 9, 3837–3843.

Wyatt, J., Vogelsang, H., Hubl, W., Waldhoer, T. and Lochs, H. (1993) 'Intestinal permeability and the prediction of relapse in Crohn's disease.' *Lancet 341*, 1437–1439.

Yacyshyn, B., Meddings, J., Sadowski, D. and Bowen-Yacyshyn, M.B. (1996) 'Multiple sclerosis patients have peripheral blood CD45RO+ B cells and increased intestinal permeability.' *Digestive Disease Science 41*, 2493–2498.

Yazdanbakhsh, M. and Rodrigues, L.C. (2001) 'Allergy and the hygiene hypothesis: The TH1/TH2 counter regulation cannot provide an explanation.' *Wien Klin. Wochenschrift 113*, 23–24, 899–902.

Zaneveld, J., Turnbaugh, P.J., Lozupone, C., Ley, R.E. *et al.* (2008) 'Host–bacterial coevolution and the search for new drug targets.' *Current Opinion in Chemical Biology 12*, 109–114.

Chapter 9

POOR ENERGY PRODUCTION AND INCREASED OXIDATIVE STRESS

Surinder Phull

Introduction

Oxidative stress is now considered to play a major role in the pathogenesis of many diseases including chronic, degenerative conditions (Bandyopadhyay *et al.* 2004; Beal 1995; Thompson 2004). Emerging research in this field is forging a new era of healthcare that will offer practitioners novel approaches to both treatment and prevention of major illness.

This chapter will assess the role of oxidative stress in disease and outline how it is intricately linked to energy production. It will review mitochondrial energy metabolism, oxidation and the underlying mechanisms that connect these processes. Most importantly, the text will highlight the role of nutrition in minimising the impact of oxidative injury and identify interventions that address this issue on a cellular level.

The first part of the chapter examines the major causes of oxidative stress and how mitochondrial energy production can play a significant role in increasing oxidative load. Oxygen may be vital for life, but it is also potentially hazardous. It routinely disrupts the stability of other chemicals within the body through **oxidation**, the removal of electrons from cells. These reactions can create highly reactive oxygen species (ROS), which propagate a chain of tissue injury. Given that 85 per cent of cellular oxygen is consumed by the mitochondria (Fukagawa 1999), these organelles are considered to be the most important cellular source of free radical oxidants, hence playing a significant role in oxidative stress (Turrens 2003).

The second part examines the body's antioxidant protection system and the integral role of nutrition in its function. It explores nutritional protocols that support both antioxidant mechanisms and mitochondrial function, with the dual aim of reducing oxidative stress. Central to this theme is the evaluation of methods for clinically assessing antioxidant status and the controversy surrounding antioxidant supplementation. This section will integrate biochemical, epidemiological and clinical evidence to create clear nutritional strategies for clinicians and practitioners.

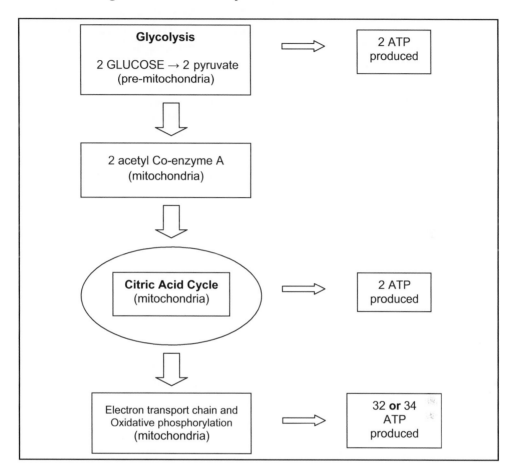

Figure 9.1 From glucose to ATP: Summary of cellular respiration

Part 1 Oxidation and oxidative stress

1. Mitochondrial energy production

Aptly termed the 'power house of the cell', the mitochondrion is the principal site of cellular respiration, the metabolic process by which energy is derived from food. Each mitochondrion is comprised of two membranes in a complex structure that facilitates the process of energy production. A number of biochemical functions take place within the cells' mitochondria, including calcium metabolism, amino acid synthesis, the citric acid cycle and apoptosis. The mitochondrial process of key interest in regard to oxidative stress is oxidative phosphorylation. This is an end-stage enzymatic procedure of cellular respiration that leads to the production of adenosine triphosphate (ATP), the predominant cellular fuel (see Figure 9.1). Although other mitochondrial processes are oxygen-dependent, it is only during this process that oxygen is routinely employed as a direct oxidising agent. Oxidative phosphorylation is accomplished via the electron transport chain, a complex network of carrier systems and enzymatic complexes embedded in the inner mitochondrial membrane.

This transport system involves the systematic exchange of electrons through oxidation and reduction. These electrons are ultimately delivered to oxygen, the terminal electron acceptor. The electron transport process channels free energy obtained from these reactions into the synthesis of ATP.

1.1 Micronutrients in mitochondrial metabolism

Micronutrients play a key role in every stage of mitochondrial metabolism. They act as co-factors for the catalytic activity of enzymes, structural components and autonomous substances that facilitate metabolic procedures.

The mitochondrial-hosted citric acid cycle, which precedes electron transport, is dependent on a range of B vitamins, lipoic acid, iron and magnesium as enzymatic co-factors.

Additionally, the principal transport structures and enzyme systems that form the electron transport chain are dependent on another range of nutrients, including vitamins B2, B3, C and K, and magnesium, zinc, copper and iron. Coenzyme Q10 also plays an independent role as a carrier system that facilitates electron transport and is needed in high concentrations in mitochondria-rich cells (Liska *et al.* 2004). These nutrient-dependent mechanisms highlight the importance of adequate micronutrient supply in maintaining an efficient energy-producing system. The following sections will explore how failure to maintain this supply might play a critical role in the development of chronic disease.

2. The drawbacks of aerobic energy production

Aerobic energy production is the body's most effective means of energy production but it also has its drawbacks. ROS are potentially dangerous by-products of aerobic metabolism (Fosslien 2001). The process is analogous to burning fuel for fire: the heat produced is a valuable energy source but the fumes are potentially dangerous.

The oxidation/reduction reactions that take place as part of electron transport involve stripping electrons from the outer orbit of cells, sometimes resulting in free electrons escaping from the chain (Figure 9.2). Electrons are at their most stable in pairs and free electrons may scavenge electrons from other pairs to regain stability. The newly broken pair will seek to destroy another electron partnership and, if the body is unable to halt this self-perpetuating process, a chain of destruction ensues. Electrons that escape from the chain to join oxygen form ROS. It is estimated that somewhere between 1 and 5 per cent of the oxygen consumed by the mitochondria is converted to ROS, such as super oxide, hydrogen peroxide and the hydroxyl radical (Hsin-Chen and Yau-Huei 2007). These highly aggressive chemicals can incite a cascade of tissue injury and degeneration. Biological antioxidant defence mechanisms keep levels of ROS relatively low under healthy physiological conditions; however, inherited or acquired defects to the mitochondria can increase levels of oxidative stress (Yau-Huei and Hsin-Chen 2002). So, by virtue of its function, the mitochondrion is not simply the power house vital for the processes of life but, paradoxically, the principal source of potentially life-threatening oxidants.

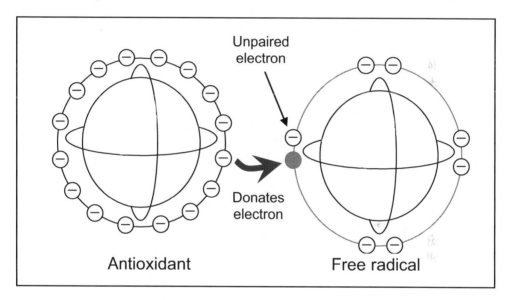

Figure 9.2 Antioxidant behaviour

2.1 Other sources of endogenous oxidants

Mitochondrial metabolism is certainly one of the most important internal sources of oxidative stress but by no means the only source. From a clinical perspective, it is important to identify other endogenous and exogenous sources of ROS. Several biological processes increase radical production, including prostaglandin synthesis, P450-dependent enzymatic reactions, inflammation, infection, and physiologic stress. The principal sources of endogenous oxidants can be categorised as follows.

2.1.1 IMMUNE RESPONSES

Blood-borne immune cells such as neutrophils and macrophages play a critical role in preventing bacterial and viral infection. However they routinely release ROS as a necessary part of phagocytosis. This can cause secondary damage to cells (Ji 1999). Oxidative stress can therefore be both cause and effect of many disease processes.

2.1.2 FATTY ACID OXIDATION

Fatty acid oxidation can occur within the mitochondria but also takes place in peroxisomes. The metabolism of fatty acids by these cellular organelles results in the formation of extra-mitochondrial oxidative by-products. These may be elevated in situations where the body increases its use of this form of energy production, such as in periods of starvation (Godin and Wohaieb 1988).

2.1.3 INSUFFICIENT OXYGEN SUPPLY

Paradoxically, under conditions of insufficient oxygen supply – such as ischaemia, hypoxia or anaemia – oxidative stress increases (Bertuglia and Giusti 2003). Several mechanisms have been proposed for this shift, including inhibition of certain stages of electron transport and enzymatic reactions that occur in response to the hypoxic environment.

2.1.4 INCREASED ENERGY DEMANDS

Although moderate exercise has been shown to be beneficial in terms of oxidative stress, research indicates that high intensity activity can incite endogenous production of ROS in the skeletal muscle and myocardium. Reasons for this include: increased demands on mitochondrial metabolism; activation of oxidative processes through tissue injury and inflammation; and increased fatty acid metabolism (Ji 1999).

2.2 Environmental sources of reactive oxygen species

There is a great deal of information in the popular press regarding 'free radicals' in the environment. From a clinical perspective, our understanding needs to go beyond the sources of these chemicals to examine where specific chemicals take effect and the duration and nature of their action. The major sources of oxidative stress are examined below.

2.2.1 ENVIRONMENTAL POLLUTANTS AND SMOKING

Chemicals inhaled from industrial pollution, exhaust fumes and cigarette smoke can cause a chain reaction of oxidative stress. In some individuals, even natural particles such as pollen can act as oxidants. ROS can be generated as a direct effect of these substances or by inciting physiological reactions, such as an inflammatory response. Primary generation of ROS can continue even when the pollutant is removed. This is clinically significant, as exposure to these pollutants can initiate a cycle of oxidative stress that significantly outlasts exposure (see Chapter 3 on detoxification for a fuller discussion). Previous exposure to such pollutants is therefore an important aspect of taking the case history for clinicians and practitioners. The mechanism by which particulate matter enters the cell has been shown to react favourably to high concentrations of cellular antioxidants (Schroder and Krutmann 2005).

2.2.2 UV RADIATION

The main source of UV radiation is sunlight, although tanning booths and therapeutic UV treatment are additional sources. During exposure to UV radiation, ROS are generated but afterwards primary production of ROS stops (Schroder and Krutmann 2005). In other words, if the body's antioxidant defence is able to curtail damage during short term exposure, UV radiation may cause little long-term damage. However, prolonged exposure has been shown to cause mitochondrial DNA damage, leading to poor energy metabolism and oxidative stress.

2.2.3 DIET

In the second section of this chapter we will explore the potential of diet as a protective factor in oxidative stress; however diet may also play a part in oxidative damage. Ingestion of oxidised lipids has been linked to increased oxidative stress. It has been proposed that foods that are susceptible to oxidation, such as chemically heated polyunsaturated fats, may contribute to this process (Turek *et al.* 2003). This implicates heated or chemically treated unsaturated fats. Research on animal models has implicated hydrogenated (*trans* fats) in increased oxidative stress (Sanchez Moreno *et al.* 2004, p.665). Burnt food and certain cured meats also contain nitrosamines, chemicals linked to increased oxidative load (Bartsch, Hietanen and Malaveille 1989).

2.2.4 MEDICATION

Certain medications may interact with the electron transport chain and increase the production of the super oxide anion through two distinct mechanisms. Some compounds interfere with the mechanisms of electron transport, whereas others accept electrons from the chain and donate them to oxygen. The anti-tumour drug Adriamycin and other anthracyclines constitute good examples of this second mechanism (Turrens 2003). The antiretroviral drug zidovudine depletes muscle mitochondrial DNA, which might also initiate a cycle of oxidative stress (Dalakas *et al.* 1990).

2.3 Oxidative stress and disease

ROS indiscriminately target components of the cells, particularly lipid membranes, DNA and enzymes. Membrane-associated unsaturated fatty acids are particularly vulnerable, due to the high quantity of unstable bonds. The site of oxidative injury in the body, or even within the cell, influences the pathological consequences. For example, damage to circulating triglycerides has been implicated in cardiovascular disease. Oxidation of low density lipoprotein (LDL) cholesterol has been shown to incite inflammatory mechanisms that are detrimental to vascular cells (Tribble 1999). This has established the belief that free radical-mediated oxidative stress plays a key role in atherogenesis and cardiovascular disease.

ROS can also damage cellular DNA, initiating changes that have been implicated in cancer (Toyokuni *et al.* 1994). However, it cannot be presumed that persistent oxidative stress is a causal factor in all individuals with chronic disease. Tissue injury and inflammation have been shown to increase free radical production and therefore the presence of these chemicals may be secondary to a pathological process (see Figure 9.3).

2.4 Mitochondria as targets of oxidative injury

There are a number of factors that make the mitochondria especially susceptible to oxidative damage. They are packed with membranes made up of unsaturated fatty acids that are vulnerable from electron transport leakage. Yet the key area of concern is the unique genetic material within this organelle. Mitochondria are unique from other components of the cell in that they have their own DNA. One scientific theory for this is that mitochondria were once foreign organisms that penetrated the cell (Baker *et al.* 2005). Their genetic material is indeed structured very much like that of bacterial DNA. Mitochondrial DNA is highly vulnerable, due to both its structure and function. First, it lacks histones, protective structural components that hold together nuclear DNA, and has relatively poor repair mechanisms when damage does occur. Second, the DNA is at close proximity to oxidative reactions in the inner mitochondrial membrane (Hsin-Chen and Yau-Huei 2007). Studies have shown that damage to mitochondrial DNA accumulates more oxidative damage than nuclear DNA, with injury occurring at a frequency around 20 times greater in mitochondrial genetic material (Richter, Park and Ames 1988, p.6465).

Genes in the mitochondria govern the processes of energy production. Consequently mutations as a result of oxidative stress may lead to impaired oxidative phosphorylation, inciting further production of ROS. Mitochondria are highly concentrated in aerobic cells such as cardiocytes, hepatocytes and musculoskeletal cells. These tissues, therefore, are particularly sensitive to defects in oxidative phosphorylation.

Mitochondrial DNA also plays a role in signalling appropriate cell apoptosis (cell suicide) by releasing their oxidative potential. This is a vital protective mechanism that halts the replication of damaged cells. However, if mitochondrial function is altered by oxidative stress, healthy cells may be indiscriminately subjected to apoptosis (Orrenuis, Gogvadze and Zhivotovsky 2007); or, conversely, unhealthy cells may escape apoptosis. In summation, mitochondrial vulnerability to oxidative stress may cause vital cellular functions to be impaired, leading to tissue degeneration and disease.

3. Cycle of oxidative stress

The inter-relationship between oxidative stress, mitochondrial metabolism and energy production is extremely complex (Figure 9.3). We have established that free radical-induced defects in electron transport can perpetuate oxidative stress. However, trying to pinpoint the catalyst in this process can be problematic. In certain cases genetic mitochondrial DNA may act as the initiator of a disease process, which is exacerbated by the cycle of oxidative injury. This may be the case in documented mitochondrial encephalomyopathies (Johns 1995). However, new research indicates that mitochondrial dysfunction as a result of oxidative stress may be an initiating factor in disease processes (Fukagawa 1999). Overall it appears that ROS are *both* an indicator and a causal factor of cumulative mitochondrial damage and a range of degenerative diseases.

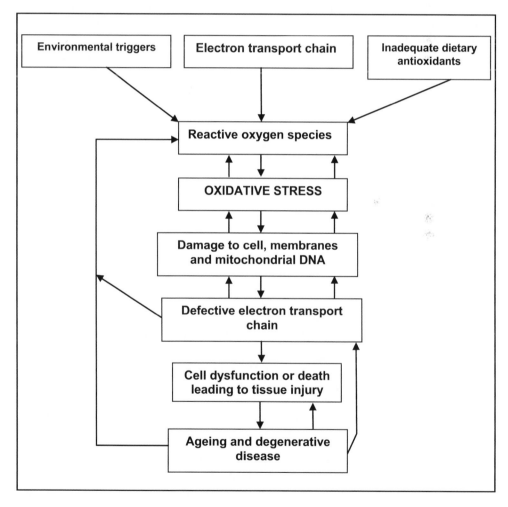

Figure 9.3 Cycle of oxidative stress: The complex interplay between energy production, oxidative stress and disease

In many respects the most important factor for clinicians to note is that ROS can have deleterious effects on health. Therefore therapeutic strategies that reduce their formation, minimise their impact and support mitochondrial function offer the potential to reduce morbidity as well as increase the healthy lifespan of individuals.

Part 2 Antioxidant defences

4. Antioxidant defence – an overview

Until now we have regarded oxidative stress as an accumulation of cell injury incited by endogenous and exogenous sources of reactive oxidants. Yet, although production of ROS might be inevitable, cell injury and tissue degeneration are not. The body possesses a complex antioxidant defence system designed to neutralise the effects of routine oxidative onslaught. Damage occurs only when there is a shift in equilibrium between the pro- and antioxidants, in favour of the former. Antioxidants act by preventing oxidant formation, interacting with formed oxidants and repairing oxidative injury. The antioxidant system can be categorised into two broad lines of defence:

- endogenous antioxidants, including protective enzymes and antioxidant compounds
- micronutrient antioxidants.

Each of these systems is outlined below.

4.1 Endogenous antioxidants

4.1.1 ANTIOXIDANT ENZYMES

Antioxidant enzymes are a diverse group of compounds that facilitate the decrease of cellular oxidants. The three main enzymes are super oxide dismutase (SOD), glutathione peroxidase and catalase. SOD plays a central role in the neutralisation of the super oxide radical. In the cytoplasm, this enzyme is zinc- and copper-dependent, whereas mitochondrial SOD is manganese-associated. Studies on rodents suggest that depletion of manganese-dependent SOD plays a more critical role in endogenous oxidative stress and mitochondrial function (Van Remmen *et al.* 2003, p.29). Glutathione peroxidase is a selenium-containing enzyme that removes hydrogen peroxide as well as lipid/non-lipid peroxides and aids in the regeneration of vitamin C. Its catalytic activity requires the polypeptide glutathione, which is discussed below. Catalase is an iron-dependent enzyme located predominantly in the peroxisomes and inner mitochondrial membrane. It also plays a prominent role in the elimination of hydrogen peroxide.

4.1.2 ANTIOXIDANT COMPOUNDS

Antioxidant compounds are substances that are synthesised in the body from substances present in the diet. The thiol compounds (glutathione, cysteine, methionine) are perhaps the most significant group in this category. They can react directly with hydroxyl radicals in both aqueous and lipid environments. Thiols located in cell membrane proteins (such as glutathione) aid the function of micronutrient antioxidants such as vitamin E. Glutathione can also be absorbed in small amounts from the small intestine, so it is both an endogenous and exogenous antioxidant. Levels of this polypeptide compound are known to decrease as a result of age-related mitochondrial decline (Clayton 2001). Low glutathione might lead to an increase in ROS, causing levels of the antioxidant to be further depleted. (Further discussion of glutathione can be found in Chapter 3 on detoxification.)

Another remarkable thiol compound with potent antioxidant activity is alpha lipoic acid (A-LA). As well as scavenging hydroxyl radicals, hydrogen peroxide and other reactive species, A-LA plays a critical role in the recycling of other antioxidants. Likewise, co-enzyme Q10 (ubiquinol) is an antioxidant compound that plays a significant role in antioxidant regeneration. In addition to its function in electron transport, this vitamin-like compound carries out important antioxidant activity in lipid membranes.

4.2 Micronutrient antioxidants

The major micronutrient antioxidants act directly as antioxidants within the cytoplasm, the cell membrane and extra-cellular space. The established nutrients in this category are vitamins C and E, and beta carotene.

4.2.1 VITAMIN E AND CAROTENOIDS

Due to its lipid solubility, vitamin E is particularly useful in membrane protection. Likewise, beta carotene is an important carotenoid antioxidant in membranes. It has the ability to react with peroxyl radicals involved in lipid peroxidation, although it is believed to be less potent than vitamin E. Other carotenoids, such as lycopene and alpha carotene, may quench singlet molecular oxygen in solution and membrane systems.

4.2.2 VITAMIN C (ASCORBIC ACID)

This is an efficient antioxidant that scavenges free radicals within the aqueous compartments of the cell and in extra-cellular fluids. The role of vitamin C in protecting membrane damage is twofold. First, it can interact directly with radicals in the cytoplasm before they reach the membrane and, second, it enhances the antioxidant activity of vitamin E by regenerating its reduced form.

4.2.3 FLAVONOIDS

In addition to the established micronutrients, flavonoids are a more recently recognised group of polyphenolic compounds found in fruits, vegetables and certain beverages that also demonstrate antioxidant activity. Flavonoids fall into sub-categories according to chemical structure, including: flavanols, flavanones, isoflavones, catechins, anthocyanidins and chalcones. Within these categories over 4000 types of compounds have been identified. Flavonoids have been shown to reduce oxidative stress through a number of mechanisms. They are able to directly neutralise cellular free radicals, prevent the cascade of lipid peroxidation in cell membranes and stabilise free oxygen species (Buhler and Miranda 2000).

Flavonoids may also act as pro-oxidants, signalling appropriate apoptosis and preventing tumour growth, as well as acting synergistically with other antioxidant compounds (Scalbert, Johnson and Saltmarsh 2005). Investigation into the precise antioxidant effects of flavonoids is problematic, partly due to their diverse and ubiquitous nature. Furthermore, many of the beneficial effects of flavonoids are believed to be a result of metabolites that they conjugate in the body. This suggests that *in vitro* studies may not reflect the full potential of these compounds. In spite of these issues, the role of flavonoids as antioxidants and disease-protective agents appears to be very promising.

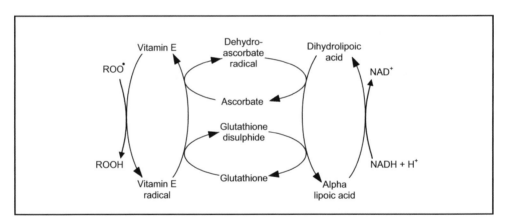

Figure 9.4 Antioxidant regeneration
Vitamin E neutralises a free radical, thereby becoming one itself. Vitamin C (ascorbate) and glutathione restore Vitamin E, and are in turn recycled by dihydrolipoic acid, which is oxidised to alpha-lipoic acid; this is then reduced back to dihydrolipoic acid (the more powerful of the two in antioxidant terms) by NADH.

4.3 Antioxidant regeneration

The antioxidant system involves complex strategies to neutralise radical species but the components of this system do not work in isolation, they work in a complex synergistic arrangement (Figure 9.4). In order to stabilise a free radical, an antioxidant will often donate an electron, leading to the antioxidant itself becoming a reactive species. Therefore, a process of recycling needs to occur to neutralise any harmful effects. The end result may be a molecule with an unpaired electron but one that is more energetically stable than a free radical. Dihydrolipoic acid and its redox partner, alpha lipoic acid, are possibly the most potent substances in this regard. They are involved in the recycling of the major micronutrient antioxidants vitamins C and E, as well as Co Q10 and glutathione. Vitamin C, Co Q10 and glutathione also play important roles in recycling. The synergistic interaction of these nutrients will vary according to the reaction involved but one example is highlighted below.

5. Therapeutic intervention – antioxidants in the diet

We have observed that micronutrients may act as autonomous antioxidants as well as being components of endogenous antioxidant mechanisms. Given the complex interactions between these molecules, therapeutic interventions are by no means straightforward. Any strategy to increase antioxidant potential must take into account the synergy of compounds. In many respects, antioxidant-rich plant foods are ideal for this purpose. Plants contain their own integrated antioxidant systems to protect their cellular components from oxidative damage. It has been suggested that synergistic co-operation of plant antioxidants can be replicated in humans through the ingestion of antioxidant-rich foods (Halvorsen *et al.* 2006). Research indicates that dietary antioxidants can reduce oxidative damage in humans. Epidemiological studies support the hypothesis that consuming a diet high in antioxidant-rich foods is inversely associated with chronic disease (Stanner, Hughes and Kelly 2004, p.422). Of course it is impossible to extrapolate exactly which components of these plant foods confer favourable effects and it is most likely that benefits are multi-factorial. Nevertheless, the diversity of the micronutrient antioxidants, co-factors and synergistic compounds in plant foods is immense. Plant foods are rich sources of carotenoids, tocopherols, tocotrienols and ascorbic acid, as well as containing thousands of phenolic compounds, all of which help protect cell components against oxidation (Benzie 2003). For all these reasons, targeting antioxidant-rich foods must be a priority in nutritional intervention to improve antioxidant status.

5.1 Rating antioxidant potential of food

Several methodologies have been developed to measure the antioxidant capacity of foods, none of them offering complete precision.

5.1.1 ORAC

The oxygen radical absorbance capacity (ORAC) is the best known of these methods but has not proved to be entirely consistent across different laboratories. Shortcomings of the methodology include relatively high selectivity of molecules and a tendency to detect protein thiols that are poorly absorbed intestinally.

5.1.2 FRAP

Another technology, the ferric reducing ability of plasma (FRAP) assay, measures the reduction of ferric iron to ferrous iron. This method shows less selectivity and therefore may be more appropriate for measuring general antioxidant activity (Blomhoff 2005, p.51).

Table 9.1 shows the highest ranking foods in different food groups from a recent large scale study using FRAP methodology (Halvorsen *et al.* 2006, p.95). Most analytical methods have found the same food groups to be highest in antioxidants: herbs, seeds, nuts, berries, fruits. Spices rank highest overall per weight but as these are consumed in minute quantities, this score is not an accurate reflection of their dietary potential. Table 9.2 ranks the top 15 foods according to serving size to demonstrate realistic consumption.

Table 9.1 Sources of antioxidant-rich foods by food category

Herbs and spices	Berries	Other fruits	Nuts and seed	Vegetables	Other
Cloves	Blackberries	Sour cherries	Walnuts	Kale	Dark
Oregano	Cranberries	Pomegranate	Pecans	Red cabbage	chocolate
Ginger	Raspberries	Red grapes	Flaxseed	Spinach	Red wine
Cinnamon	Strawberries	Plums	Sunflower	Artichokes	Green tea
Turmeric	Blueberries	Kiwi fruit	seeds	Broccoli	Black coffee
Basil		Prunes	Pistachios		

Source: Adapted from Halvorsen *et al.* 2006, p.99

Table 9.2 Sources of antioxidant-rich foods by serving size

Top 15 foods per serving size
Blackberries
Walnuts
Strawberries
Artichokes
Cranberries
Coffee
Raspberries
Pecans
Blueberries
Ground cloves
Grape juice
Baking chocolate
Cranberry juice
Sour cherries
Red wine

Source: Adapted from Halvorsen *et al.* 2006, p.99

5.2 Guidelines for improving baseline antioxidant status using foods

The data from Tables 9.1 and 9.2 give us general indications as to the type of foods that have highest antioxidant potential and therefore can inform guidelines for improving baseline antioxidant status as listed below.

5.2.1 INCREASE THE PROPORTION OF PLANT BASED FOODS IN THE DIET

Plant foods in the diet generally have significantly higher antioxidant content than most animal-based foods. Individuals should be encouraged to increase their consumption of a variety of brightly coloured fruits and vegetables, including those listed in Tables 9.1 and 9.2. In addition, green leafy vegetables, red peppers, carrots, squash and sweet potato are excellent sources of beta carotene, an antioxidant which is better absorbed in the presence of dietary fat. Cooked tomatoes are an excellent source of the carotenoid lycopene, which again is better absorbed with fat. Citrus fruits, peppers, berries and tomatoes are good sources of vitamin C.

5.2.2 SELECT PLANT SOURCES WITH HIGH FLAVONOID CONTENT

Highlighting flavonoid-rich foods in the diet is recommended to increase the therapeutic effect. Flavonoid consumption varies considerably across the general population, compared to other dietary antioxidants, with intakes ranging from 50–800mg a day, thus offering significant scope for dietary intervention (Buhler and Miranda 2000). Flavonoids are found in a variety of fruits, vegetables, nuts, beverages and herbs. Concentrations are greatest in the skin and seeds of a plant and therefore these elements of foods should not be discarded. Many of the foods listed in Tables 9.1 and 9.2 are high in flavonoids. Good sources of these compounds are dark purple and red berries, grapes and red wine, apples, cocoa (dark chocolate), onions, tea (black, green and white), broccoli, kale, soya and pulses. Research into the properties of individual flavonoids is ongoing and individual compounds may be also used for specific therapeutic aims. A number of these are discussed below. However, for the purpose of improving general antioxidant status, consumption of a variety of these synergistic compounds is recommended.

5.2.3 INCREASE USE OF CULINARY SPICES

A number of culinary spices have been shown to possess potent antioxidant activity at levels comparable to established micronutrient antioxidants. Clove extract has demonstrated significant reduction potential and free radical scavenging activity at levels similar to alpha tocopherol. Additionally, clove extract has the ability to chelate pro-oxidant trace metals (Gülçin et al. 2004). Components of oregano (thymol and rosmarinic acid) have also been shown to function as potent antioxidants. Studies have identified sage, peppermint, garden thyme, lemon balm, clove, allspice, cinnamon and turmeric as having significant antioxidant action (Dragland et al. 2003, p.1286).

Obviously, doses used in clinical trials may not always reflect quantities used in everyday cooking. However in conjunction with other dietary support, these herbs and spices can act as additional protective agents in maintaining a strong antioxidant base. For specific therapeutic actions, concentrated supplement forms may be considered.

5.2.4 INCLUDE POLYUNSATURATED FATTY ACIDS AND SOURCES OF VITAMIN E

Traditionally unsaturated fatty acids are perceived as targets of oxidative stress rather than protective agents against free radical damage. However, studies *in vivo* have indicated reduced excretion of lipid peroxidation products following omega-3 intake. *In vitro* research confirms the idea that long-chain fatty acids, especially of the omega-3 series, might act as indirect antioxidants, although the precise mechanism of action is not understood (Richard *et al.* 2008, p.451). Interestingly, in food analysis, omega-3-rich walnuts have been shown to confer high antioxidant activity, whereas omega-3-rich fish have not (Halvorsen *et al.* 2006, p.99) This may be due to the synergistic activity of other components such as ellagic acid and mixed tocopherols. When increasing unsaturated fatty acids in the diet it is advisable to increase intake of mixed tocopherols, which act as important antioxidants in lipids. Food sources include nuts, seeds and wheat germ. Additionally, adequate intake of supporting antioxidants such as selenium, carotenoids and vitamin C should be ensured to allow sufficient vitamin E regeneration. A favourable balance of unsaturated fatty acids and tocopherols in the diet may also serve the dual purpose of improving membrane fluidity and therefore aiding mitochondrial function.

5.2.5 INCREASE FOODS THAT INDUCE ANTIOXIDANT ENZYMES

Sulphur-containing compounds and metabolites from vegetables in the brassica family can induce antioxidant enzymes and enzymes necessary for phase II liver detoxification. Phase II enzymes demonstrate indirect antioxidant activity through the conversion of toxic metabolites to compounds that can be easily excreted from the body. Foods to increase include broccoli, Brussels sprouts, cabbage, kale, cauliflower, onions and garlic (Fahey, Zhang and Talalay 1997; Talalay 2000)

5.3 Antioxidants – foods in focus

5.3.1 TEA

Tea is a rich source of polyphenols, including theaflavins, thearubigins and catechins, the latter having the most potent antioxidant activity. The fermentation process of black tea lowers its catechin content, whereas green tea contains relatively high concentrations of this flavonoid group. Tea catechins are effective scavengers of ROS (Nakagawa and Yokozawa 2002). Individual catechins and theaflavins have also been shown to inhibit pro-oxidant enzymes such as nitric oxide synthase. In addition to its direct antioxidant effects, green tea polyphenol extract has been shown to induce the enzymes of phase II liver detoxification and thus promote the excretion of potentially toxic chemicals (Balz and Higdon 2003). Furthermore, studies on animal models have identified the ability of green tea catechins to spare endogenous alpha tocopherol and prevent decreases in tissue glutathione concentrations, thus working as an effective synergistic agent (Skrzydlewska *et al.* 2002, p.232). Green tea appears to have greater antioxidant potential than black varieties and *in vitro* studies suggest that the addition of milk to tea may diminish its total antioxidant capacity. However it is unclear whether this effect is replicated *in vivo* (Arts *et al.* 2002, p.1184).

5.3.2 TURMERIC (CURCUMIN)

Turmeric is a widely used spice that ranks highly in terms of antioxidant content. In addition to its potent antioxidant activity, turmeric has been shown to possess anti-inflammatory properties (Surh 2002). Preliminary research also indicates that it has antithrombotic and immunostimulatory actions (Shah, Nawaz and Pertanin 1999). Current scientific understanding replicates many of the traditional therapeutic values attributed to this spice in traditional Ayurvedic medicine. A recent study investigating the antioxidant activity of turmeric showed that intake of 200mg per day led to a marked decrease in lipid peroxide levels, as well as high density lipoprotein (HDL) and LDL cholesterol peroxidation. This effect was accompanied by antioxidant-induced regulation of fibrinogen levels, which may also be protective in cardiovascular disease. Turmeric was shown to potentiate the atherogenic activity of alpha tocopherol (Miquel *et al.* 2002, p.46). Although intervention studies are limited, there is indication that turmeric may also play a useful role in colorectal cancer stabilisation (Sharma *et al.* 2001, p.1894) as well as in the symptomatic treatment of rheumatoid arthritis (Deodahr, Sethi and Srimal 1980). There appear to be no safety concerns with turmeric used in foods and in fact studies have revealed that cooking with the spice may increase its antioxidant potential (Tiwari *et al.* 2006, p.1313). There is no consensus for dosage in supplemental form but doses of 500–4000mg have been used in various therapeutic interventions. It would be advisable to use this herb in dietary form or at the low end of the dosage range for general antioxidant support.

5.3.3 RED WINE

Epidemiological data suggests that moderate red wine consumption reduces the risks of cardiovascular disease. Although there is some indication that alcohol itself may be moderately cardio-protective, red wine's antioxidant capacity appears to play a much more significant role. It is rich in polyphenolic flavonoids, the most abundant of which are procyanidins. Procyanidins act directly to quench ROS, as well as acting as protective agents in blood vessels, inhibiting cell-mediated LDL oxidation and atherogenic plaque formation. Procyanidins equally act as anti-hypertensive agents in vascular endothelium by increasing nitric oxide synthesis and promoting vasodilation. The literature supports consumption of red wine in preference to other alcohol to promote cardiovascular health (Rifici *et al.* 1999, p.143).

6. Antioxidant supplements – the controversy

There appears to be scientific consensus that consuming a range of antioxidant-dense plant-based foods plays a preventive role in chronic disease. Research into antioxidant supplements, on the other hand, is rather more ambiguous. The main body of research in this domain has focused on vitamins A (beta carotene), C and E. Research in this area has shown very mixed results. A recent high-profile Cochrane review concluded that supplementation of vitamin A, beta-carotene, and vitamin E might increase mortality (Bjelakovic *et al.* 2008). Such studies highlight the potential safety issues of antioxidant supplementation and should be taken very seriously by practitioners who prescribe such supplements.

However that is not to say that such reviews should not be closely scrutinised. Indeed, this review attracted a great deal of methodological criticism (Albanes 2007; Hemila 2007; Huang, Teutsch and Bass 2007, p.400). Clinically, our interest is not so much in critiquing the methodology of the review as it is in reviewing the nutritional methodology used universally in antioxidant intervention trials.

First, the studies reviewed only examined a small section of the antioxidants needed for antioxidant activity: vitamins A, C and E and beta carotene. It did not include any of the trace minerals, nutrient-dependent compounds or other substances previously highlighted in this chapter. This may have impaired the synergistic activity of nutrients. Indeed, many studies used nutrients in isolation, which may have led to the production of pro-oxidant substances.

Second, the paper does not differentiate between different molecular forms of vitamin E and therefore fails to acknowledge the potentially adverse effects of synthetic forms of alpha tocopherol used in most studies. Likewise, it made no reference to the various forms of carotenoids that act as vitamin A precursors. There has been previous suggestion that synthetic forms of beta carotene have negative effects (Ben Amotz and Levy 1996, p.734). Again, in the majority of studies reviewed, synthetic beta carotene was used.

These criticisms do not dismiss the potential dangers of antioxidant supplementation but simply highlight that overall benefits are perhaps currently being overlooked. Although randomised controlled trials are hailed as the 'gold standard' in scientific research, by their very nature they tend to favour the use of a limited number of compounds. However, as this chapter has highlighted, a broad range of dietary antioxidants are required to achieve synergistic efficacy. At present, clinicians must take prudent decisions informed by the current evidence base, as well as an understanding of antioxidant biochemistry. The following generic guidelines have been formed on that basis.

6.1 General guidelines for antioxidant supplementation

DIETARY INTERVENTION SHOULD BE THE BASIS OF ANTIOXIDANT THERAPY

Supplementation should be an adjunct, not a substitute, to dietary support in order to ensure an intake of a wide range of synergistic micronutrient and phytochemical compounds. Supplementation should only be considered in cases of excessive oxidative load and protocols should be based on supporting evidence for the specific combination of compounds used.

ANTIOXIDANT SUPPLEMENTATION SHOULD TAKE INTO ACCOUNT THE NUTRIENTS REQUIRED FOR SYNERGISTIC REGENERATION (SEE TABLE 9.3)

In general practitioners should avoid using nutrients in isolation and identify overall requirements for antioxidant and mitochondrial function.

THE ANTIOXIDANTS BETA CAROTENE AND VITAMIN E SHOULD ONLY BE SUPPLEMENTED IN NATURAL FORM

Vitamin C does not present an issue as it is identical in both synthetic and natural forms (Mangels *et al.* 1993).

ANTIOXIDANTS SHOULD ONLY BE USED AT THERAPEUTIC LEVELS WHERE THERE ARE HUMAN TRIALS TO SUPPORT THIS PRACTICE

6.2 Special nutrients for antioxidant support

While the traditional focus in antioxidant trials has been on micronutrient antioxidants, the following section highlights a number of antioxidant compounds that support antioxidant function and mitochondrial energy production. Table 9.3 highlights how nutrients may form part of a larger therapeutic framework.

6.2.1 CO-ENZYME Q10 (UBIQUINOL)

The minute amounts of Co-enzyme Q10 in dietary sources are not considered to have therapeutic effects. However, supplementation appears to have significant value. As an antioxidant, Co Q10 acts primarily in lipid protection and has been proved to reduce LDL oxidation and maintain cell membrane integrity. Research also indicates that it is able to reduce oxidative damage in congestive heart failure (Morisco, Trimarco and Condorelli 1995, p.136) and exert antihypertensive effects (Langsjoen, Willis and Folkers 1994, p.265). Therefore it offers great potential in cardiovascular disease prevention. Where Co Q10 stands outs from other antioxidants is in its capacity to promote efficient mitochondrial function, thereby offering bi-directional intervention against oxidative stress. Indeed, Co Q10 has proven effective in the treatment of genetic

Table 9.3 Benefits of antioxidant micronutrients: The role of major antioxidants in mitochondrial metabolism

Antioxidant supplement	Works with synergistic antioxidants	Antioxidant activity	Role in mitochondrial metabolism	Recommended doses	Safety and interactions
Alpha lipoic acid	Regenerates: Vitamin C Vitamin E glutathione Co Q10	Acts in lipid and aqueous environments Key in regenerating other antioxidants	ATP production, carbohydrate metabolism	No RNI 600–800mg therapeutically for diabetic neuropathy (Reljanovic et al. 1999, p.171)	May decrease blood glucose levels
Beta carotene as part of mixed carotenoids (use natural form)	Acts with carotenoids: including alpha carotene lycopene, lutein and vitamins C and E	Reduces lipid peroxidation Reduces oxidative damage to DNA	No direct role but important synergistic function (see left)	No RNI for carotenoids 5–10mg where fruit and vegetable intake is low or requirements are increased	Synthetic beta carotene may increase mortality in smokers
Co Q10	Regenerates vitamins C and E Recycled by alpha lipoic acid	Reduces lipid peroxidation and LDL oxidation	Carrier in electron transport chain	No RNI 50–100mg in cardiac conditions 60mg x2/d in hypertension 150mg in diabetes 300–1200mg in Parkinson's (Jellin 2004, p.364)	No clear side-effects reported to date

Antioxidant supplement	Works with synergistic antioxidants	Antioxidant activity	Role in mitochondrial metabolism	Recommended doses	Safety and interactions
Manganese	Antagonistic to copper and zinc so broad mineral range should be ensured	Co-factor in mitochondrial SOD	Co-factor in carbohydrate metabolism	No RNI 1.4mg safe intake Avoid higher doses	High doses may be related to mitochondrial degeneration
Selenium	Vitamin E	Component of antioxidant enzyme glutathione peroxidase	Component of membrane protein in electron transport chain	RNI 70mcg for men 60mcg for women	Excess can be toxic
Vitamin C (ascorbic acid)	Vitamin E Carotenoids Bioflavonoids Co Q10	Regenerates vitamin E Acts in plasma	Co-factor in electron transport chain	RNI 40mg Larger doses may be used for specific therapeutic purposes	Excess can cause gastric symptoms, loose stools
Vitamin E (tocopherols and tocotrienols)	Recycled by vitamin C, alpha lipoic acid, Co Q10 Works with selenium	Potent antioxidant in cell membranes	No direct role but vital synergistic actions	No RNI 10mg considered safe but doses of up to 900mg have been used in diabetic neuropathy (Jellin 2004, p.1321)	May cause nausea, gastric upset, rash, and may increase bleeding in excess
Zinc	Excess zinc may inhibit copper absorption	Antagonises redox-active metals iron and copper. Co-factor in SOD	Co-factor in electron transport chain	RNI 9.5mg men 7mg women	Copper deficiency Nausea, vomiting in excess

or acquired disorders of mitochondrial function, the latter possibly being related to increased oxidative stress. The function of Co Q10 in the electron transport chain may explain its efficacy in Parkinson's (Shults *et al.* 1998), which has been linked to defects in this system. It also increases plasma levels of vitamin E (Kagan, Fabisiak and Quinn 2006).

In patients with cardiac-related conditions, doses of approximately 50–100mg a day have been used, and in Parkinson's, doses of between 300 and 1200mg per day. It is recommended that practitioners generally use the lower levels of supplementation to minimise adverse effects and that if doses of higher than 100mg a day are administered, this should be in divided doses (Jellin *et al.* 2004, p.364).

6.2.2 ALPHA LIPOIC ACID

Endogenous alpha lipoic acid (A-LA) plays a vital role in cellular respiration and also acts as an important antioxidant. Although A-LA is found naturally in the diet within organ meats, red meat and yeast, research indicates that it offers increased functional capacity in supplemental form (Wollin and Jones 2003, p.3327). A-LA and its derivative, dihydrolipoic acid, have been shown to counteract a variety of ROS, both in lipids and aqueous cellular space. This versatility enables A-LA to regenerate other antioxidants, such as vitamins E and C and glutathione, acting as a valuable safety net when prescribing antioxidants in supplement form. It has been suggested that its ability to recycle other antioxidants may explain the reason that A-LA offers protection against oxidation of LDL cholesterol (Kagan *et al.* 1992). This antioxidant action might also explain the protective role it appears to play in diabetes and related conditions. Supplementation has a proven role in the reduction of symptoms of peripheral neuropathy and in improving insulin sensitivity (Konrad *et al.* 1999, p.280; Reljanovic *et al.* 1999, p.171).

There is also preliminary data to suggest that its antioxidant mechanisms exert protection in numerous conditions associated with mitochondrial dysfunction. The ability of this compound to support mitochondrial function offers dual protection against oxidative damage.

In the treatment of diabetic neuropathy doses of 600–800mg have been used with no clear consensus as to optimum levels (Jellin *et al.* 2004). Theoretically this compound may have hypoglycaemic potential and therefore may interact with anti-diabetic drugs. Appropriate medical consultation should precede supplementation in diabetics or patients taking any other prescribed medication. However, for baseline antioxidant support, doses of around 100mg are commonly used.

7. Guidelines for chronic disease

Having examined the role of a number of specific antioxidant compounds, below are examples of how antioxidant therapy may be applicable to two specific conditions.

7.1 Case study 1

Janice, aged 52, has a family history of type 2 diabetes. A test conducted by her GP two months ago indicated that her fasting blood glucose levels were high. Her blood pressure was also slightly elevated. She was referred to a dietitian to help her lose weight and help manage her blood sugar. She made significant changes to her diet but decided to visit a nutritionist again to check her progress. Her typical diet following her visit to the dietitian was as follows:

Breakfast: *Bran Flakes or sugar-free muesli or porridge with semi-skimmed milk*

Mid-morning: *Apple, small piece of cheese*

Lunch: *4 Ryvita with cottage cheese, lettuce, cucumber, tomato*

Mid-afternoon: *Yoghurt and cereal bar (or biscuit and tea)*

Dinner: *Boiled potatoes, fish and vegetables (combination of frozen sweetcorn, peas, carrots) or brown rice with chilli con carne and salad*

Drinks: *Occasional water, 3 cups of tea per day (alcohol rarely)*

Dietary advice given: She was advised to make the following simple changes to improve her antioxidant status:

- *Add a variety of mixed berries and walnuts to breakfast cereal.*
- *Vary cheese at snack time to mixed nuts/seeds.*
- *Replace lettuce and cucumber at lunch with any of the following: spinach leaves, artichokes, rocket, watercress, grated red cabbage.*
- *Try to introduce spices into food: add fresh basil to salads, turmeric to chilli sauces, oregano to tomato-based dishes, and use cinnamon to sweeten porridge.*
- *Try to cook fresh green leafy vegetables such as broccoli, cabbage and spinach.*
- *Try green tea as an alternative to tea occasionally.*

Supplements:

Alpha lipoic acid: 150mg per day. This is much lower than the therapeutic doses for diabetes but as she does not yet have frank diabetes, this is used at a lower dose to improve insulin sensitivity.

Co Q10: 50mg twice a day. This is based on the lower end of therapeutic doses for diabetes and hypertension (see Table 9.3).

7.2 Case study 2

Michael, aged 65, had been diagnosed with early stage Parkinson's disease. He was unable to provide a food diary but admitted his meal patterns were erratic and he rarely consumed any fruit or vegetables. His diet was high in convenience foods (pizza, fish and chips, and ready-meals), bread, chocolate, cakes and processed meat.

Dietary advice given: Michael and his wife were advised of simple ways to improve his baseline antioxidant status:

- *Increase vegetable and fruit intake through soups, smoothies, vegetables on pizzas and frozen vegetables.*

- *Replace sweet snacks with dried berries and nuts and dark chocolate, for their higher nutritional and antioxidant value.*

- *Drink tea on a regular basis and include green tea wherever possible.*

Supplements:

Co Q10: 300mg per day in 3 separate doses (see Table 9.3 for dosage range).

Mixed low dose antioxidant supplement with beta carotene, vitamins C and E due to poor diet. Natural vitamin E has been shown to be of benefit in Parkinson's (Jellin 2004 et al., p.1316).

8. Assessing oxidative stress

Practitioners can assess oxidative stress through clinical case history and functional tests. The endogenous and exogenous factors that may increase oxidative load are summarised in Figure 9.5 below.

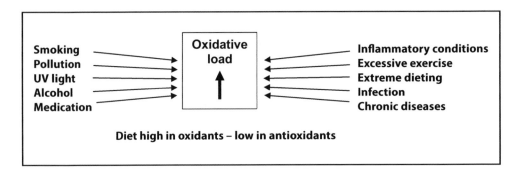

Figure 9.5 Oxidative load

For a more accurate picture of oxidative load and antioxidant status, functional testing can be used. Functional tests can measure antioxidant reserves, lipid peroxidation (as an indication of oxidative damage) and mitochondrial function via levels of organic acids in the urine. However, research has shown that different technologies that are used to measure antioxidant status do not produce the same results. Overall, the ORAC assay appears to have high specificity and respond to a wide range of antioxidants, as well as being able to differentiate between lipid soluble and aqueous components (Cao and Prior 1998, p.1309). When ordering tests, practitioners should therefore investigate which technology is used and request suitable evidence to support the use of this methodology.

9. Conclusion

There is compelling evidence to suggest that oxidative stress is implicated in chronic disease and that impaired mitochondrial function may be both a cause and result of this process. Clinical studies suggest that dietary antioxidants act directly as protective agents in oxidative injury and indirectly through supporting energy production structures. Observational research has associated consumption of antioxidant-rich foods with a reduction in disease risk. However, intervention trials using antioxidant supplementation have shown mixed results, possibly due to the failure to examine the broad spectrum of antioxidants found in food. It is recommended that future trials review the synergistic activity of a wider range of micronutrient and phytochemical compounds. Trials should also look at assessing baseline levels of oxidative stress to identify individuals most likely to benefit from preventative therapy, rather than focusing exclusively on secondary intervention. In the absence of such trials, there is sufficient evidence to support increases in specific antioxidant-rich foods in aiding disease prevention. Potential issues with antioxidant supplementation can be minimised by judicious use of synergistic nutrients by practitioners who have a clear biochemical appreciation of oxidative stress.

References

Albanes, D. (2007) 'Antioxidant supplements and mortality.' Letter. *Journal of the American Medical Association 298*, 4, 400.

Arts, M.J., Haenen, G.R., Wilms, L.C., Beestra, S.A. *et al.* (2002) 'Interactions between flavonoids and proteins: Effect on total antioxidant capacity.' *Journal of Agriculture and Food Chemistry 50*, 1184–1187.

Baker, S.M., Bennett, P., Bland, J., Galland, L. *et al.* (2005) *Textbook of Functional Medicine.* Washington: Institute for Functional Medicine.

Balz, F. and Higdon, J.V. (2003) 'Antioxidant effect of tea polyphenols in vivo: Evidence from animal studies.' *Journal of Nutrition 133*, 3275S–3284S.

Bandyopadhyay, D., Chattopadhay, A., Ghosh, G. and Datta, A.G. (2004) 'Oxidative stress induced ischemic heart disease: Protection by antioxidants.' *Current Medicinal Chemistry 11*, 369–387.

Bartsch, H., Hietanen, E. and Malaveille, C. (1989) 'Carcinogenic nitrosamines: Free radical aspects of their action.' *Free Radical Biology and Medicine 7*, 6, 637–644.

Beal, F. (1995) 'Aging, energy and oxidative stress in neurodegenerative diseases.' *Annals of Neurology 38*, 357.

Ben Amotz, A. and Levy, Y. (1996) 'Bioavailability of natural isomer mixture compared with synthetic all trans beta carotene in human serum.' *American Journal of Clinical Nutrition 63*, 729–734.

Benzie, I.F. (2003) 'Evolution of dietary antioxidants.' *Comparative Biochemistry and Physiology 136*, 113–126.

Bertuglia, S. and Giusti A (2003) 'Microvascular oxygenation, oxidative stress, NO suppression, and superoxide dismutase during post ischemic reperfusion.' *American Journal of Physiology: Heart and Circulation Physiology 285*, 1064–1071.

Bjelakovic, G., Nikolova, D., Gluud, L.L., Simonetti, R.G. and Gluud, C. (2008) 'Antioxidant supplements for prevention of mortality in healthy participants and patients with various diseases.' *Cochrane Database of Systematic Reviews 16*, 2, CD007176.

Blomhoff, R. (2005) 'Dietary antioxidants and cardiovascular disease.' *Current Opinion in Lipidology 16*, 47–54.

Buhler, D.R. and Miranda, C, (2000) 'Antioxidant activities of flavonoids.' *Linus Pauling Institute Newsletter* (fall/winter).

Cao, G. and Prior, R.L. (1998) 'Comparison of different analytical methods for assessing total antioxidant capacity of human serum.' *Clinical Chemistry 44*, 6, 1309–1315.

Clayton, P. (2001) *Health Defence*. London: Accelerated Learning Systems.

Dalakas, M.C., Illa, I., Pezeshkpourn, G.H., Laukaitis, J.P., Cohen, B. and Griffin, J.L. (1990) 'Mitochondrial myopathy caused by long term Zidovudine therapy.' *New England Journal of Medicine 322*, 1098–1105.

Deodahr, S.D., Sethi, R. and Srimal, R.C. (1980) 'Preliminary study on antirheumatic activity of curcumin.' *Indian Journal of Medical Research 71*, 632–634.

Dragland, S., Senoo, H., Wake, K., Holte, K. and Blomhoff, R. (2003) 'Several culinary and medicinal herbs are important sources of antioxidants.' *Journal of Nutrition 133*, 1286–1290.

Fahey, J.W., Zhang, Y. and Talalay, P. (1997) 'Broccoli sprouts: An exceptionally rich source of inducers of enzymes that protect against chemical carcinogens.' *Proceedings of the National Academy of Sciences USA 94*, 10367–10372.

Fosslien, E. (2001) 'Mitochondrial medicine – molecular pathology of oxidative phosphorylation.' *Annals of Clinical and Laboratory Science 31*, 25–67.

Fukagawa, N.K. (1999) 'Aging: Is oxidative stress a marker or causal?' *Experimental Biology and Medicine 222*, 293–298.

Godin, D.V. and Wohaieb, S.A. (1988) 'Nutritional deficiency, starvation and tissue antioxidant status.' *Free Radical Biology and Medicine 5*, 165–176.

Gülçin, I., Ukrü, A., Beydemir, U., Elmasta, M. and Küfreviolu, R. (2004) 'Comparison of antioxidant activity of clove (*Eugenia caryophylata* Thunb) buds and lavender (*Lavandula stoechas* L.).' *Food Chemistry 87*, 3, 393–400.

Halvorsen, B.L., Carlsen, M.H., Phillips, K.M., Bohn, S.K. *et al.* (2006) 'Content of redox-active compounds (i.e. antioxidants) in foods consumed in the United States.' *American Journal of Clinical Nutrition 84*, 95–135.

Hemila, H. (2007) 'Antioxidant supplements and mortality.' Letter. *Journal of the American Medical Association 298*, 4, 401.

Hsin-Chen, L. and Yau-Huei, W. (2007) 'Oxidative stress, mitochondrial DNA and apoptosis in aging.' *Experimental Biology and Medicine 232*, 592–606.

Huang, H.Y., Teutsch, S. and Bass, E. (2007) 'Antioxidant supplements and mortality.' Letter. *Journal of the American Medical Association 298*, 4, 400.

Jellin, J.M., Gregory, P.J., Batz, F., Hitchens, K. *et al.* (2004) *Pharmacist's Letter/Prescriber's Letter: Natural Medicines Comprehensive Database*, 6th edn. Stockton, CA: Therapeutic Research Faculty.

Ji, L.L. (1999) 'Antioxidants and oxidative stress in exercise.' *Experimental Biology and Medicine 222*, 283–292.

Johns, D.R. (1995) 'Mitochondrial DNA and disease.' *New England Journal of Medicine 333*, 638–644.

Kagan, V.E., Fabisiak, J.P. and Quinn, P.J. (2006) 'Coenzyme Q and vitamin E need each other as antioxidants.' *Protoplasma 214*, 11–18.

Kagan, W., Kulinski, B., Ruhlmann, C. and Plotz, C. (1992) 'Recycling of vitamin E in human low density lipoproteins.' *Journal of Lipid Research 33*, 385–397.

Konrad, T., Vicini, P., Kusterer, K., Höflich, A. *et al.* (1999) 'A-lipoic acid treatment decreases serum lactate and pyruvate concentrate ions and improves glucose effectiveness in lean and obese patients with type 2 diabetes.' *Diabetes Care 22*, 280–287.

Langsjoen, P., Willis, R. and Folkers, K. (1994) 'Treatment of essential hypertension with coenzyme Q10.' *Molecular Aspects of Medicine 15*, 1, S265–272.

Liska, D., Quinn, S., Lukaczer, D., Jones, D.S. and Lerman, R.H. (2004) *Clinical Nutrition. A Functional Approach*, 2nd edn. Washington: Institute for Functional Medicine.

Mangels, A.R., Block, G., Frey, C.M., Patterson, B.H. *et al.* (1993) 'The bioavailability to humans of ascorbic acid from oranges, orange juice and cooked broccoli is similar to that of synthetic ascorbic acid.' *Journal of Nutrition 123*, 6, 1054.

Miquel, J., Bernd, A., Sempere, J.M., Díaz-Alperi, J. and Ramírez, A. (2002) 'The curcuma antioxidants: Pharmacological effects and prospects for future clinical use. A review.' *Archives of Gerontology and Geriatrics 34*, 1, 37–46.

Morisco, C., Trimarco, B. and Condorelli, M. (1995) 'Effect of coenzyme Q10 therapy in patients with congestive heart failure: A long term, multicenter, randomized study.' *Clinical Investigation 71*, S134–136.

Nakagawa, T. and Yokozawa, T. (2002) 'Direct scavenging of nitric oxide and superoxide by green tea.' *Food Chemistry and Toxicology 40*, 1745–1750.

Orrenuis, S., Gogvadze, V. and Zhivotovsky, B. (2007) 'Mitochondrial oxidative stress: Implications for cell death.' *Annual Review of Pharmacology and Toxicology 47*, 143–183.

Reljanovic, M., Reichel, G., Rett, K., Lobisch, M. *et al.* (1999) 'Treatment of diabetic polyneuropathy with the antioxidant thiotic acid (alpha lipoic acid). A 2 year multicenter, randomized, double-blind, placebo-controlled trial.' *Free Radical Research 31*, 171–177.

Richard, D., Kefi, K., Barbe, U., Bausero, P. and Visioli, F. (2008) 'Polyunsaturated fatty acids as antioxidants.' *Pharmacological Research 57*, 6, 451–455.

Richter, C., Park, J.W. and Ames, B.N. (1988) 'Normal oxidative damage to mitochondrial and nuclear DNA is extensive.' *Proceedings of the National Academy of Sciences 85*, 6465–6467.

Rifici, V.A., Stephan, E.M., Schneider, S.H. and Khachadurian, A.K. (1999) 'Red wine inhibits the cell mediated oxidation of LDL and HDL.' *Journal of the American College of Nutrition 18*, 2, 137–143.

Sanchez-Moreno, C., Dorfman, S.E., Lichenstein, A.H. and Martin, A. (2004) 'Dietary fat type affects vitamin C and E and biomarkers of oxidative status in peripheral and brain tissues of Golden Syrian Hamsters.' *Journal of Nutrition 134*, 665–660.

Scalbert, A., Johnson, I.T. and Saltmarsh, M, (2005) 'Polyphenols: Antioxidants and beyond.' *American Journal of Clinical Nutrition 81*, 215S–217S.

Schroder, P. and Krutmann, J. (2005) 'Environmental oxidative stress – environmental sources of reactive oxygen species.' *Handbook of Environmental Chemistry 2*, 19–31.

Shah, B.H., Nawaz, Z. and Pertanin, S.A. (1999) 'Inhibitory effect of curcumin, a food spice from turmeric, on platelet activating factor and arachidonic acid-mediated platelet aggregation through inhibition of thromboxane formation and Ca2+ signalling.' *Biochemical Pharmacology 58*, 1167–1172.

Sharma, R.A., McLelland, H.R., Hill, K.A., Ireson, C.R. *et al.* (2001) 'Pharmacodynamic and pharmacokinetic study of oral Curcuma extract in patients with colorectal cancer.' *Clinical Cancer Research 7,* 7, 1894–1900.

Shults, C.W., Oakes, D., Kieburtz, K., Beal M.F. *et al.* (1998) 'Absorption, tolerability and effects on mitochondrial activity of oral coenzyme Q10 in early Parkinson's disease: Evidence of slowing of functional decline.' *Archives of Neurology 59,* 1541–1550.

Skrzydlewska, E., Ostrowska, J., Farbiszewwski, R. and Michalak, K. (2002) 'Protective effect of green tea against lipid peroxidation in the rat liver, blood serum and the brain.' *Phytomedicine 9,* 232–238.

Stanner, S.A., Hughes, J. and Kelly, C.N. (2004) 'A review of the epidemiological evidence for the "antioxidant hypothesis".' *Public Health Nutrition 7,* 407–422.

Surh, Y.J. (2002) 'Anti-tumor promoting potential of selected spice ingredients with antioxidative and anti-inflammatory activities: A short review.' *Food Chemistry and Toxicology 40,* 1091–1097.

Talalay, P. (2000) 'Chemoprotection against cancer by induction of phase 2 enzymes.' *Biofactors 12,* 5–11.

Thompson, H.J. (2004) 'DNA oxidation products, antioxidant status and cancer prevention.' *Journal of Nutrition 134,* 3186.

Tiwari, V., Shanker, R., Srivastava, J. and Vankar, S. (2006) 'Change in antioxidant activity of spices – turmeric and ginger on heat treatment.' *Electronic Journal of Environmental, Agricultural and Food Chemistry 5,* 2, 1313–1317.

Toyokuni, S., Okamoto, K., Yodoi, J. and Hiai, H. (1994) 'Persistent oxidative stress in cancer.' *Federation of European Biochemical Societies 358,* 1–3.

Tribble, D.L. (1999) 'Antioxidant consumption and cardiovascular disease. Emphasis on vitamin C, vitamin E, and beta carotene: A statement for healthcare professionals from the American Heart Association.' *Circulation 99,* 591–595.

Turek, J.J., Watkins, B.A., Schoenlein, I.A., Allen, K.G., Hayek, M.G. and Aldrich, C.G. (2003) 'Oxidized lipid depresses canine growth, immune function, and bone formation.' *Journal of Nutritional Biochemistry 14,* 1, 24–31.

Turrens, J.F. (2003) 'Mitochondrial formation of reactive oxygen species.' *Journal of Physiology 552,* 2, 335–344.

Van Remmen, H., Ikeno, Y., Hamilton, M., Pahlavani, M. *et al.* (2003) 'A life-long reduction in MnSOD activity results in increased DNA damage and higher incidence of cancer but does not accelerate ageing.' *Physiological Genomics 16,* 29–37.

Wollin, S.D. and Jones, P.J.H. (2003) 'Alpha lipoic acid and cardiovascular disease.' *Journal of Nutrition 133,* 3327–3320.

Yau-Huei, W. and Hsin-Chen, L. (2002) 'Oxidative stress, mitochondrial DNA mutation and impairment of antioxidant enzymes.' *Experimental Biology and Medicine 227,* 671–682.

Chapter **10**

DYSREGULATED NEUROTRANSMITTER FUNCTION

Basant K. Puri and Helen Lynam

Introduction

This chapter begins by explaining key aspects of normal neurotransmission, including the oft-ignored but highly important role of membrane phospholipids in this function. Changes in neurotransmission function in a variety of neurological and psychiatric diseases, including depression, schizophrenia and Alzheimer's disease, are then described. Investigations are discussed. Finally, practical interventions to help treat compromised neurotransmitter function are considered, in respect of both conventional pharmacological approaches and nutritional and lifestyle changes.

Note that adrenaline and noradrenaline are also known as epinephrine and norepinephrine – the former will be used throughout the chapter.

1. Neurotransmission

1.1 Neurotransmitters

Neurotransmitters are important mediators of the process of neurotransmission. A strict definition of what constitutes a neurotransmitter has been summarised by Deutch and Roth (2008, p.134).

1. A neurotransmitter must be synthesised by and released from neurons. This means that the presynaptic neuron should contain a transmitter and the appropriate enzymes need[ed] to synthesise that transmitter. Synthesis in the *axon terminal* is not an absolute requirement. For example, peptide transmitters are synthesised in the *cell body* and transported to distant sites, where they are released.

2. The substance should be released from nerve terminals in a chemically or pharmacologically identifiable form. Thus, one should be able to isolate the transmitter and characterise its structure using biochemical or other techniques.

3. A neurotransmitter should reproduce at the postsynaptic cell the specific events (such as changes in membrane properties) that are seen after stimulation of the presynaptic neuron.

4. The effects of a putative neurotransmitter should be blocked by competitive antagonists of the receptor for the transmitter in a dose-dependent manner. In addition, treatments that inhibit synthesis of the transmitter candidate should block the effects of presynaptic stimulation.

5. There should be active mechanisms to terminate the action of the putative neurotransmitter. Such mechanisms include uptake of the transmitter by the presynaptic neuron or glial cells through specific transporter molecules, or alternatively enzymatic inactivation of the chemical messenger.

Recognised forms of neurotransmitters are shown in Table 10.1.

Table 10.1 Different types of neurotransmitters

Class of neurotransmitter	Examples
Acetylcholine	
Proteinogenic amino acids	• Glutamate (central nervous system (CNS) excitatory neurotransmitter) • Glycine (CNS inhibitory neurotransmitter)
Biogenic amines	• Catecholamines (ultimately derived from the amino acid tyrosine); GABA (gamma-aminobutyric acid or 4-aminobutyrate, from the amino acid glutamate) • Serotonin or 5-hydroxytryptamine (5-HT, from the amino acid tryptophan) • Histamine (from the amino acid histidine)
Peptides	Beta-endorphin, met-encephalin, leu-encephalin, substance P, somatostatin, thyroliberin, gonadoliberin, angiotensin II, cholecystokinin (CCK)
Derivatives of purines	Adenosine triphosphate (ATP), adenosine diphosphate (ADP), adenosine monophosphate (AMP) and adenosine
Soluble gases	Nitrogen monoxide (NO)

1.2 Receptor chemistry

There are two main types of neurotransmitter receptors:

1.2.1 IONOTROPIC RECEPTORS

These include nicotinic receptors for acetylcholine, GABA-A receptors, glycine receptors, 5-HT$_3$ receptors, and AMPA, NMDA and kainite glutamate receptors. They are ligand-gated ion channels. (Ion channels are potential openings through lipid membranes which allow the selective passage of ions.) In the case of excitatory neurotransmitters, such as glutamate, binding of the neurotransmitter to the ionotropic receptor allows cationic inflow of predominantly sodium cations (Na$^+$) from the extracellular space into the cytosol, which in turn leads to postsynaptic membrane depolarisation and therefore an increased probability of the occurrence of an action potential in the postsynaptic neurone. Conversely, in the case of inhibitory neurotransmitters, such as glycine, binding of the neurotransmitter to the ionotropic receptor allows inflow of predominantly chloride anions (Cl$^-$) from the extracellular space into the cytosol, which in turn leads to postsynaptic membrane hyperpolarisation and therefore a decreased probability of the occurrence of an action potential in the postsynaptic neurone.

1.2.2 METABOTROPIC RECEPTORS

These include: M1, M2, M3, M4 and M5 muscarinic receptors for acetylcholine; alpha-1, alpha-2, beta-1, beta-2 and beta-3 receptors for noradrenaline; 5-HT$_1$, 5-HT$_2$ and 5-HT$_4$ receptors for serotonin; D$_1$, D$_2$, D$_3$, D$_4$ and D$_5$ receptors for dopamine; and delta, kappa and mu opioid receptors. They are G-protein coupled receptors. (These are membrane receptors which are able to recognise and combine with neurotransmitters.) Neurotransmitter binding that activates G proteins leads to increased intracellular levels of the second messenger cAMP; activation of G$_i$ proteins leads to decreased intracellular cAMP levels; activation of G$_q$ proteins leads to increased intracellular levels of calcium cations (Ca^{2+}), which also act as second messengers. (cAMP is 3,5'-cyclo-adenosine monophosphate, which can be formed from ATP via the action of the enzyme adenylate cyclase.)

1.3 Compromised neurotransmission

From the viewpoint of biochemical imbalances, there are several ways in which neurotransmission can become compromised.

1.3.1 DEFICIENCY OF NEUROTRANSMITTERS AND ASSOCIATED RECEPTOR CHANGES

In theory, a deficiency of the substrates needed for forming neurotransmitters could lead to impaired neurotransmission function. These would include choline in the case of acetylcholine; the amino acids mentioned above for proteinogenic amino acids that have neurotransmitter actions and for biogenic amines and peptides. In practice, however, this is unlikely to occur except under conditions of extreme dietary deprivation, or in the case of phenylketonuria, where a lack/shortage of phenylalanine hydroxylase can lead to a shortage of tyrosine. Nevertheless, an increased dietary intake of a neurotransmitter dietary precursor may help increase levels of the respective neurotransmitter. In conventional pharmacotherapy, for example, L-tryptophan has been successfully used for helping treat depression (but see below).

A dietary deficiency of sodium ions and chloride ions is also unlikely to occur under normal circumstances, and therefore would not cause ionotropic receptor function to be compromised. In respect of metabotropic receptor function, while a deficiency of calcium intake certainly may occur, even in the Western world, in practice the bone mineral of the body can act as a reservoir of calcium, from which this mineral can be removed for use in other functions, including its second messenger actions, at the expense of the structural integrity of the skeletal system.

The biosynthetic pathways of several neurotransmitters involve co-enzymes and co-factors. Deficiency of one of these may compromise biosynthesis of the relevant neurotransmitter, while any suspicion of a particular neurotransmitter deficiency may suggest the possibility, clinically, of ensuring that a patient has a sufficient intake of the relevant factors. Examples of the involvement of co-enzymes are provided by the biosynthetic pathway of the catecholamines. Beginning with the aromatic amino acid tyrosine, hydroxylation by the enzyme tyrosine hydroxylase (tyrosine-3-monooxygenase) yields dopa (3,4-dihydroxyphenylalanine). The co-enzyme tetrahydrobiopterin is needed for this hydroxylation reaction alongside iron. Following decarboxylation of dopa by L-aromatic amino acid decarboxylase to the neurotransmitter dopamine, the dopamine in turn is hydroxylated, in (nor)adrenergic neurones and in the suprarenal (adrenal) glands into noradrenaline by dopamine-beta-monooxygenase. Ascorbic acid (vitamin C) and copper are needed for this hydroxylation reaction. The subsequent N-methylation of noradrenaline to adrenaline by phenylethanolamine N-methyltransferase requires the co-enzyme S-adenosylmethionine (SAM).

1.3.2 RECEPTOR INADEQUACY

There is yet another way in which neurotransmission may be compromised: by a deficiency of appropriate long-chain polyunsaturated fatty acids (PUFAs) in the phospholipid molecules that make up the cell membrane phospholipid bilayer in which the neurotransmitter receptors are actually located. The importance of this was emphasised many times by the late Professor David F. Horrobin. For example, just before his untimely death in 2003, he and his colleague Crispin Bennett published the following (Horrobin and Bennett 2003, pp.14–15):

> Phospholipids are molecules which usually contain a 3-carbon backbone, two fatty acids, a phosphorus atom and a water-soluble head group... Given the ubiquity of phospholipids, one is entitled to ask why more attention has not been paid to them?

Part of the reason is a simple matter of inadvertent propaganda. Because of their chemistry, phospholipids in an aqueous environment naturally form bilayers. All their hydrophobic fatty acid tails face to the inner part of the membrane, and all their hydrophilic head groups face towards the water – either of the extracellular fluid (ECF) or of the various aqueous compartments of the intracellular fluid. Textbook after textbook, and research paper after research paper, almost invariably show pictures of these bilayers in diagrams of misleading oversimplicity. Proteocentric or genocentric biologists portray these simplistic bilayers as mere carriers for what is really important, i.e. gene or protein [including neurotransmitter receptor] function. Nothing could be further from the truth. Membranes are enormously complex, with thousands of functional components which can be arranged in millions of different ways. Far from being mere scaffolding, phospholipids and their derivatives are central to cellular function.

...

The quaternary structures of proteins [including neurotransmitter receptors], the final modelling and folding, often depend on the precise nature of the lipid environment of that protein. As an example, the addition of two carbon atoms on a single double bond to fatty acids in the vicinity of a benzodiazepine receptor can so modulate the final structure of that receptor that its ligand-binding capacity can be substantially changed.

Horrobin and Bennett pointed out that, for example, Witt and Nielsen had demonstrated the profound influence of unsaturated fatty acids on the brain GABA-benzodiazepine receptor chloride channel complex *in vitro* (Witt and Nielsen 1994). Certainly, as predicted by Horrobin, changes in long-chain PUFAs in cell membranes have been implicated in cerebral disorders as diverse as depression, attention-deficit hyperactivity disorder (ADHD) and myalgic encephalomyelitis (ME) (Puri, Tsaluchidu and Treasaden 2009; Richardson and Puri 2000). The key fatty acids which have been found to be important are the omega-3 long-chain PUFA eicosapentaenoic acid (EPA) and the omega-6 long-chain PUFA gamma-linolenic acid (GLA). Thus, ultra-pure EPA has been found to be effective in treating depression, while a combination of EPA-rich omega-3 fatty acids plus evening primrose oil (supplying GLA) has been found to help ADHD-symptomatology in children. (Interestingly, the higher the ratio of EPA to docosahexaenoic acid (DHA) in the formulation tested, the better the response of ADHD symptomatology.)

1.3.3 ERRORS IN INACTIVATION OF NEUROTRANSMITTERS

Once neurotransmitters have completed their function, they are inactivated to prevent accumulation; this is done variously via diffusion, degradation, reuptake, astrocytic removal and enzymatic degradation. Monoamine oxidase (MAO) and catechol-O-methyl transferase (COMT) are both enzymes used to break down catecholamines, MAO through oxidative deamination and COMT by the transfer of a methyl group from SAM to oxygen. MAO needs the co-factors vitamin B6, zinc, manganese and copper, whilst COMT needs vitamins B3 and C, folic acid and magnesium. MAO also breaks down serotonin and histamine and excess MAO has been linked to depression, whilst deficient MAO has been associated with psychiatric problems, paranoid schizophrenia and increased risk of suicide (Edelman 2001). Conjugated oestrogen inhibits MAO activity, thereby elevating mood (Krieger and Hughes 1990), and these pathways are used by conventional medications to increase low levels of neurotransmitters, as described later.

2. Cerebral disorders

When treating individuals with cerebral disorders, it is important to first take a detailed life history. This will include looking at the predisposing, precipitating and mediating factors.

2.1 Depression

The criteria of the *Diagnostic and Statistical Manual of Mental Disorders, Fourth Edition, Text Revision* (DSM-IV-TR) of the American Psychiatric Association for a major depressive episode include (American Psychiatric Association 2000, p.356):

- At least five of the following symptoms have been present during the same two-week period and represent a change from previous functioning; at least one of the symptoms is either (1) depressed mood or (2) loss of interest or pleasure.

1. Depressed mood most of the day, nearly every day; this can be irritable mood in the case of children and adolescents.

2. Markedly diminished interest or pleasure in all, or almost all, activities most of the day, nearly every day.

3. Significant weight loss when not dieting or weight gain (e.g. a change of more than five per cent of body weight in a month), or decrease or increase in appetite nearly every day.

4. Insomnia or hypersomnia nearly every day.

5. Psychomotor agitation or retardation nearly every day.

6. Fatigue or loss of energy nearly every day.

7. Feelings of worthlessness or excessive or inappropriate guilt nearly every day (not merely self-reproach or guilt about being sick).

8. Diminished ability to think or concentrate, or indecisiveness, nearly every day.

9. Recurrent thoughts of death (not just fear of dying), recurrent suicidal ideation without a specific plan, or a suicide attempt or a specific plan for committing suicide.

- The symptoms cause clinically significant distress or impairment in social, occupational or other important areas of functioning.

- The symptoms are not caused by the direct physiological effects of a substance (e.g. a drug of abuse, or a medication) or a general medical condition (e.g. hypothyroidism).

- The symptoms are not better accounted for by bereavement.

Changes in CNS functional noradrenaline or serotonin are two of the important perpetuating and mediating factors implicated in the aetiology of major depression. A more detailed summary of the aetiology of depressive episodes and bipolar disorders has been given by one of the authors of this chapter (Puri 2008) below.

2.1.1 PREDISPOSING FACTORS

These include genetic factors (family, twin and adoption studies) and personality (cyclothymic or cycloid personality disorder may predispose to bipolar disorder). (Cyclothymic personality disorder is characterised by persistent mood instability with numerous periods of mild depression and mild elation.)

2.1.2 PRECIPITATING FACTORS

These include psychosocial stresses (life events) and physical illnesses (e.g. viral infections are associated with depression).

2.1.3 PERPETUATING AND MEDIATING FACTORS

These include social factors, psychological factors (e.g. cognitive dysfunction), the patient's family (high expressed emotion at home is associated with an increased risk of relapse of depression), neurotransmitters (changes in central functional noradrenaline and serotonin), psychoneuroendocrinological factors, water and electrolyte changes and photic changes.

2.2 Schizophrenia

The criteria of the DSM-IV-TR of the American Psychiatric Association for schizophrenia include (American Psychiatric Association 2000, p.312):

A. *Characteristic symptoms*: At least two of the following, each present for a significant portion of time during a one-month period (or less, if successfully treated):

   o   Delusions

   o   Hallucinations

   o   Disorganised speech

   o   Grossly disorganised or catatonic behaviour

○ Negative symptoms (i.e. affective flattening, alogia, or avolition).

If the delusions are bizarre or the hallucinations consist of either a voice keeping up a running commentary on the patient's behaviour or thoughts, or two or more voices conversing with each other, then Criterion A is sufficient to make a DSM-IV-TR diagnosis of schizophrenia. Otherwise, the following criteria are also required.

B. *Social/occupational dysfunction:*

In the case of adult onset, for a significant portion of the time since onset at least one major area of social/occupational functioning is markedly below the level achieved before onset of the illness. These areas include:

○ Work

○ Interpersonal relations

○ Self-care.

In the case of onset during childhood or adolescence, there is a failure to achieve the expected level of achievement in the following areas:

○ Interpersonal

○ Academic

○ Occupational.

C. *Duration:* Continuous signs of the disturbance persist for at least six months, including at least one month of symptoms (or less if successfully treated) that meet Criterion A and may include periods of prodromal or residual symptoms.

D. *Exclude schizoaffective disorder and mood disorder.*

E. *Exclude substance-related disorder and general medical conditions.*

F. *Relationship to a pervasive developmental disorder.* If there is a history of autistic disorder or another pervasive developmental disorder, the additional diagnosis of schizophrenia is made only if prominent delusions or hallucinations are also present for at least a month (or less, if successfully treated).

Several neurotransmitters have been implicated in the aetiology of schizophrenia, particularly dopamine and serotonin. A more detailed summary of the aetiology of schizophrenia is given below (Puri 2008).

2.2.1 PREDISPOSING FACTORS

These include genetic factors (family, twin and adoption studies), prenatal factors (higher incidence in late winter and early spring births, particularly in cases of maternal viral infection), perinatal factors (obstetric complications commoner) and personality (schizotypal personality disorder is commoner in first-degree relatives).

2.2.2 PRECIPITATING FACTORS

Psychosocial stresses (life events) have been suggested.

2.2.3 PERPETUATING FACTORS

These include social factors (e.g. poverty of social milieu is associated with increased negative symptoms in chronic schizophrenia) and the patient's family if there is high expressed emotion (relatives make critical comments and become over-involved emotionally).

2.2.4 MEDIATING FACTORS

These may include neurotransmitters (the dopamine hypothesis, which suggests central dopaminergic hyperactivity in the mesolimbic-mesocortical system; or central serotonergic dysfunction), neurodegeneration, psychoneuroimmunological and psychoneuroendocrinological factors. (The mesolimbic-mesocortical system is a dopaminergic pathway originating in dopaminergic neurones of the ventral tegmental area of the midbrain. The axons of this system pass, via the medial forebrain bundle, to various parts of the limbic system and cerebral cortex.)

2.3 Alzheimer's disease

Alzheimer's disease (AD) is the commonest cause of dementia in those over the age of 65 years and is also particularly common amongst younger people who have Down syndrome. The clinical presentation is usually with memory impairment and then gradual deterioration. In early-onset AD, that is, onset before the age of 65 years, symptoms usually progress rapidly and disorders of higher cortical function are likely to occur; these may include aphasia, agraphia, alexia and apraxia. Alzheimer's disease is known to be associated with accumulation in the brain parenchyma of Abeta (beta-amyloid protein), leading to the formation of neurofibrillary tangles and neuritic plaques. Impairment of functional cholinergic activity in the central nervous system appears to occur in AD.

2.4 Indirect illnesses

2.4.1 GUT-BRAIN DISORDERS

The gut-brain connection is a large research area under the heading of psychoneuroimmunology. Many neurotransmitters actually act as secretagogues in the gut, in other words, they regulate the secretion of digestive enzymes and electrolytes. Examples include histamine, which is a potent stimulator of hydrochloric acid (HCl) secretion; acetylcholine, which elicits salivary, gastric and pancreatic enzymes; and serotonin. There are estimated to be 100 million neurons in the gut, and the organ with the greatest amount of serotonin is believed to be in the gut rather than the brain (Arehart-Treichel 2001).

Researchers have theorised that opioids such as casomorphins and gliadomorphins can be derived from the incomplete digestion of the proteins casein (from milk) and gliadin (from wheat), respectively, and when abnormally porous intestinal membranes increase the passage of these peptides into the CNS, this has been linked to autism (Whiteley *et al.* 1999). The action seems to be that these opioids bind to opioid receptors, and affect the stress response, peripheral autonomic and central nervous system. It is also theorised that autistic children may be lacking dipeptidyl peptidase IV (DPP IV), an enzyme needed to break down casomorphin and gliadomorphin. This enzyme is also lacking in people suffering from alcoholism, schizophrenia and depression, where the patients' enterocytes have been damaged (Campbell-McBride 2006). If a client appears to be addicted to wheat or dairy, or if testing (see later) confirms that casomorphins and gliadomorphins are present, then eliminating wheat and dairy from the diet is recommended. This would need to be done slowly, remembering that the client is effectively withdrawing from addictive drugs. The client's diet should also be reviewed to ensure that they are not left with a nutrient-deficient diet.

Researchers at Reading University have concluded that yeast and the *Clostridia* bacteria seem to be relevant in autism, and that abnormal bacterial metabolites of tyrosine seem to contribute to the overgrowth of *Clostridia* species. They found that when yeast and *Clostridia* are under control, clinical improvement and even complete remission of autistic symptoms can be experienced (Bingham 2008).

Some food additives, such as tartrazine, sunset yellow and monosodium glutamate (MSG) have been found to exert some effects on the brain. While reviews by bodies such as Joint FAO/WHO Expert Committee on Food Additives (JECFA), the Scientific Committee for Food (SCF), the Europe Commission (EC) and the Federal Drug Administration (FDA) have not found any specific toxic effect due to MSG, they have not discounted the existence of a sensitive subpopulation (Walker and Lupein 2000). A study of healthy 3-year-olds and 8/9-year-olds using mixes containing sunset yellow, carmoisine, tartrazine, ponceau 4R and sodium benzoate, quinoline yellow and allura red found an adverse effect of food additives on the hyperactive behaviour of the children (McCann *et al.* 2007).

2.4.2 TOXICITY

Mineral toxicity from mercury, cadmium, lead and aluminium has been implicated in some aspects of mental health, particularly in its ability to interfere with neurotransmitter functioning. Lead competes with calcium, inhibiting the release of neurotransmitters, and interferes with the regulation of cell metabolism by binding to second-messenger calcium receptors (Goyer 1995). Animal studies have demonstrated that mercury affects dopamine and MAO. The removal of dental amalgam from schizophrenic patients has shown significant improvement in their symptoms and behaviour, implying that mercury from the amalgam had entered the brain and affected neurotransmitters (Siblerud, Motl and Kienholz 1999). Links between aluminium toxicity and AD continue to be investigated, with research in America finding that past consumption of foods containing large amount of aluminium additives differed between people with AD and controls, indicating that dietary intake of aluminium, may affect the risk of developing AD (Rogers and Simon 1999). It is interesting to note that aluminium is used in the production of vaccinations including influenza vaccines, as it can enable lower doses of antigen to be used during production (Hehme *et al.* 2004).

2.4.3 HISTADELIA

Histadelia has many characteristics, which can include suicidal depression, obsessiveness, compulsiveness, mental fogginess and hyperactivity. It is also indicated by increased salivation, elevated metabolic rate, seasonal and respiratory allergies, frequent headaches, diminished pain threshold, heightened sexual responsiveness and strong cravings for sugar. Elevated blood histamine levels (greater than 70ng/mL) confirm the diagnosis of histadelia (Prousky and Lescheid 2002), and 20 per cent of patients with schizophrenia are found to be histadelic, along with many depressed patients. Histamine in the blood has the ability to chelate copper and zinc (Pfeiffer 1975) which may account for some of its detrimental actions. Inactivation of histamine occurs through either diamine oxidase (DAO), also known as histaminase, which uses copper and pyridoxal phosphate as cofactors, or histamine methyltransferase (HMT) which catalyses the transfer of a methyl group from S-adenosyl-L-methionine (SAMe) to form N-methylhistamine.

2.4.4 HISTAPENIA/PYRROLURIA

Excess copper decreases blood histamine and can create histapenia through the up-regulation of the copper-dependent enzymes histaminase and ceruloplasmin. Histapenics tend to have paranoia and hallucinations accompanied by racing thoughts. Their typical appearance includes stubby fingers and plentiful hair; it is also indicated by slow metabolism and associated tendency to obesity, food and environmental allergies, low salivary flow and dental caries. Forty to fifty per cent of schizophrenics were found to be histapenic (Edelman 2001).

Pyrroluria is associated with psychiatric symptoms such as schizophrenia; it occurs in 30–40 per cent of patients with schizophrenia and 5–10 per cent of 'normals' (Pfeiffer *et al.* 1974). Pyrroluria occurs when a specific pyrrole, 2, 4, dimethyl-3-ethylpyrrole (kryptopyrrole) is produced and excreted in the urine. Kryptopyrroles combine with pyridoxal, which then complexes with zinc – this depletes the body stores of B6 and zinc and they are thought to promote the loss of essential fatty acids in the urine.

Pyrroluria appears to be familial and so possibly has a genetic predisposition, with the usual age of onset being 15–20 years. Symptoms and signs of pyrroluria are in line with those of B6 and zinc deficiency: general loss of appetite, morning nausea, impaired collagen synthesis, cold hands and feet, tendency to stretch marks and macrocytic anaemia. Neurological symptoms include low stress tolerance and depression.

Both histapenia and pyrroluria are rarely discussed as there has been little published research since Carl Pfeiffer's work in the 1970s.

2.4.5 FUNGAL DYSBIOSIS

Candida albicans is a natural inhabitant of the intestinal tract, and under certain circumstances can proliferate into overgrowth. *Candida* can become systemic and invade organs beyond the intestinal tract, and mycotoxins are secreted that can enter the blood stream and cross the blood–brain barrier (BBB). Brain symptoms include poor memory, inability to concentrate, anxiety, insomnia, depression and mood swings. One theory on how *Candida* can have such effects is that in anaerobic conditions it can convert sugar into acetaldehyde, which, in the brain, can impair the synthesis and release of acetylcholine and change nerve cell membrane permeability (Truss 1984).

3. Investigations

3.1 Electronic scanning

Direct investigation of the functional levels of some CNS neurotransmitters, including dopamine and serotonin, can be carried out using positron emission tomography (PET) and, to a lesser extent, single-photon emission (computerised) tomography (SPECT or SPET). However, both of these investigations are expensive and expose the subject to ionizing radiation. Furthermore, the radio-labelled ligands used usually have to be created relatively close to the PET or SPECT scanner, before the level of radioactivity diminishes too much to make the radioligand of use. Certainly, at the time of writing PET and SPECT are not routinely used in diagnosing or investigating depression, schizophrenia or Alzheimer's disease; their use in such disorders is currently confined to the research domain.

3.1.1 NEUROSPECTROSCOPY

An alternative functional neuroimaging method that may be used is neurospectroscopy. This has the advantage of not using ionizing radiation. However, this is a very specialised technique that is not readily available in most hospitals at the current time. Furthermore, being a magnetic resonance-based technique, there are safety issues related to the need to ensure that subjects are free of ferromagnetic substances that might pose a danger when in the vicinity of the powerful magnetic fields of scanners. For example, the safety checklist that the first author of this chapter employs before carrying out neurospectroscopy investigations on anyone is to check for the presence of the following:

- cardiac pacemaker
- mechanical heart valve
- history of foreign body in eye
- occupation as a metal worker, grinder, welder
- metallic implant, metal prosthesis, orthopaedic plates, screws

- shrapnel

- aneurysm clip/haemostatic clip

- ear implant

- artificial eye

- coloured contact lens

- interventional radiological device

- pregnancy

- IUCD

- implantable pumps or neurostimulators

- allergies – if the subject is to receive a contrast agent

- a watch

- any jewellery

- anything in their pockets (such as keys, etc.).

Proton neurospectroscopy

Proton neurospectroscopy allows levels of free choline to be measured. Its measurement can give us a valuable understanding of the cause of, and therefore potentially useful treatment intervention in, brain diseases. For example, three independent proton neurospectroscopy studies of ME, also known as chronic fatigue syndrome (CFS), have shown that the levels of free choline in the brain are significantly raised in this devastating neurological disorder. Since choline is often the polar head group of membrane phospholipid molecules, this rise in free (unbound) choline is consistent with a functional deficiency of omega-3 and omega-6 long-chain PUFAs (also part of phospholipid molecules). This is consistent with evidence suggesting that a chronic viral infection may occur in many patients with ME. Such viral infections might inhibit the ability of cells to biosynthesise long-chain PUFAs (via inhibition of the enzyme delta-6-desaturase). A clear therapeutic implication is that supplementation with long-chain PUFAs (particularly GLA and EPA) may prove helpful.

Radioactive phosphorus neurospectroscopy

Similarly, 31-phosphorus neurospectroscopy allows nucleotide triphosphate levels to be measured; this allows energy metabolism to be studied, again potentially helping us understand aetiological factors and potentially leading to appropriate therapeutic interventions. However, given the current lack of facilities and the shortage of suitably trained personnel, neurospectroscopy is, like PET and SPECT, mainly confined to the research domain.

3.2 Other tests

3.2.1 VOLUMETRIC NIACIN RESPONSE

While the volumetric niacin response (VNR) – a measure of the amount of skin flushing when given continuous niacin – gives an index of arachidonic acid (AA)-related signal transduction (Puri *et al.* 2002), this only gives an indirect measure of neurotransmitter activity and is therefore not an investigation of choice when trying to determine whether neurotransmitter function has been compromised.

3.2.2 URINE TESTS

Urine tests are a useful non-invasive method of testing bodily functionality.

- *Amino acid urine tests*: These can be used to check levels of the base amino acids such as tyrosine and tryptophan needed to make neurotransmitters, whilst an organic acid urine test can check the functional pathways of tyrosine and tryptophan metabolism for co-factor deficiency and neurotransmitter function (Bralley and Lord 2002). For example vanilmandelic acid, homovanillic acid, and 3-methyl-4-hydroxyphenylglycol are end products of catecholamine metabolism and 5-hydroxyindoleacetic acid is an end product of serotonin metabolism. These compounds are expected to be in urine at certain levels, if they are too high, or too low, then co-factor deficiencies can be derived.

- *Kryptopyrroles*: Urine can also be used to test for the presence of kryptopyrroles; normally there should be none present in the urine (Biolab 2009).

- *Toxic metals*: Urine is tested using a chelating agent as a challenge, where a urine sample is taken before and after the challenge agent. Agents used include Biomer, ethylenediaminetetraacetic acid (EDTA), 2,3 dimercapto succinic acid (DMSA), 2,3-dimercapto-1-propane sulphonate (DMPS) and D-Penicillamine. This type of test can help to measure the level of toxicity and also the type of metal present.

3.2.3 HAIR MINERAL ANALYSIS

Another test for toxic metals is hair mineral analysis. This can be used as a convenient, non-invasive and painless test, but the accuracy of this type of testing is often questioned, and a review of laboratories in America revealed significant inconsistencies in the results (Seidel *et al.* 2001). However, it has since been argued that good quality laboratory practices will generate precise, accurate and reliable results (Quig and Urek 2001).

4. Treatment

4.1 Conventional

4.1.1 DEPRESSION

There is good evidence that there is a functional reduction in levels of serotonin in certain parts of the brain in major depression. One way that has been employed to improve the levels of central serotonin is to increase the level of tryptophan, from which serotonin is biosynthesised *in vivo*. As mentioned above, L-tryptophan is therefore available as an antidepressant medication. Unfortunately, a few years ago there was a problem with a batch of synthetic L-tryptophan: a contaminated batch had a propensity to cause the dangerous condition of eosinophilia-myalgia syndrome. Ever since, caution has been exercised by the medical profession before prescribing L-tryptophan; such treatment is withheld if the patient develops an increased eosinophil count, myalgia, arthralgia, pyrexia, dyspnoea, neuropathy, oedema or dermatological lesions, until the possibility that they are developing this syndrome is satisfactorily excluded.

Another way of improving the levels of central serotonin at the synaptic cleft is to inhibit the neuronal re-uptake of serotonin. This approach gave rise to several selective serotonin re-uptake inhibitors (SSRIs), including citalopram, escitalopram, fluoxetine, fluvoxamine, paroxetine and sertraline. They are prone to cause gastrointestinal side-effects, such as nausea, vomiting, dyspepsia, abdominal pain, diarrhoea or constipation, and a variety of other side-effects, including sexual dysfunction, galactorrhoea, movement disorders and visual disturbance. Worryingly, there is evidence that they may be associated with suicidal and even homicidal thoughts in a minority; the March 2009 *British National Formulary* comments:

> The use of antidepressants has been linked with suicidal thoughts and behaviour; children, young adults, and patients with a history of suicidal behaviour are particularly at risk. Where necessary, patients should be monitored for suicidal behaviour, self-harm, or hostility, particularly at the beginning of treatment, or if the dose is changed. (p.206)

It is now recommended that SSRIs should not, in general, be prescribed to children and adolescents.

4.1.2 SCHIZOPHRENIA

Conventional (also known as 'typical') antipsychotic drugs have been used for many decades in the treatment of schizophrenia and work primarily by blocking dopamine receptors in certain pathways in the brain (particularly the mesolimbic–mesocortical system mentioned above). These drugs include chlorpromazine, haloperidol, benperidol, flupentixol, pimozide and trifluoperazine. Unfortunately, dopamine receptors elsewhere in the brain are also blocked by drugs such as chlorpromazine and haloperidol. Blockage of dopamine receptors in the nigrostriatal pathway gives rise to symptoms and signs similar to those seen in Parkinson's disease, including tremor. Other extrapyramidal side-effects include dystonia, akathisia and tardive dyskinesia (a distressing chronic movement disorder). Blockage of dopamine receptors in the tuberoinfundibular system (which projects from the hypothalamus to the pituitary gland) leads to an increase in prolactin levels, and therefore to other unpleasant side-effects such as galactorrhoea (inappropriate lactation), menstrual disturbances and gynaecomastia (enlargement of mammary gland tissue leading, for example, to the appearance of more female-looking breasts in men). Some of these drugs also act on other neurotransmitters, so that a host of other unwanted side-effects may also occur, such as drowsiness, convulsions, hypotension, impaired temperature regulation, and anti-muscarinic side-effects (that is, side-effects associated with blockage of muscarinic cholinergic receptors) including dry mouth, constipation, difficulties with passing urine and blurring of the vision. (These anti-muscarinic actions are also side-effects that occur with the tricyclic antidepressants.)

A range of newer, so-called 'atypical', antipsychotic drugs have become available which do not primarily act on dopamine neurotransmission; therefore they are less likely than the typical antipsychotic drugs to cause extrapyramidal side-effects when prescribed for patients with schizophrenia. These atypical antipsychotic drugs include amisulpride, aripiprazole, clozapine, olanzapine, paliperidone, quetiapine, risperidone and zotepine. Unfortunately, some of the atypical antipsychotics can cause the QT interval (which is a particular cardiac function parameter that can be readily measured using electrocardiography) to be unduly prolonged, and therefore should be used with caution in patients with a history of cardiovascular disease or epilepsy. (We feel it is good practice to carry out regular electrocardiographic investigations in patients being treated with certain atypical antipsychotic drugs.) The drug clozapine, although particularly effective at treating 'treatment-resistant' schizophrenia, may unfortunately cause the potentially fatal side-effect of a particular depletion of white blood cells known as agranulocytosis. It should therefore only be prescribed under strict conditions in which patients are registered with an appropriate clozapine patient monitoring service so that leucocyte and differential blood counts are regularly monitored. Certain atypical antipsychotic drugs may cause metabolic syndrome (see Chapter 5) and the development of type 2 diabetes mellitus.

It is important to note that antipsychotics of both the typical and atypical classes may, rarely, cause neuroleptic malignant syndrome. The features of this condition can include hyperthermia, fluctuating consciousness level, muscle rigidity, pallor, lability of blood pressure, tachycardia, urinary incontinence and sweating. The development of this syndrome constitutes a medical emergency. Without prompt treatment, a patient may die.

4.1.3 ALZHEIMER'S DISEASE

Three of the major drugs currently licensed for AD work by inhibiting acetylcholinesterases (enzymes which break down acetylcholine), thereby increasing the central levels of acetylcholine. These drugs are donepezil, galantamine and rivastigmine. Common side-effects include nausea, vomiting and diarrhoea.

- Donepezil may also cause anorexia, fatigue, insomnia, headache, dizziness, syncope, hallucinations, agitation, aggression, muscle cramps, urinary incontinence, rashes and pruritus and, less commonly, seizures and gastro-intestinal haemorrhage.

- Galantamine may also cause abdominal pain, dyspepsia, syncope, rhinitis, sleep disturbances, dizziness, confusion, depression, headache, fatigue, anorexia, tremor, pyrexia, weight loss and, less commonly, cerebrovascular disease, tinnitus, leg cramps, cardiac arrhythmias and myocardial infarction.

- Rivastigmine may also cause dyspepsia, anorexia, abdominal pain, dizziness, headache, drowsiness, tremor, malaise, agitation, confusion, sweating, weight loss and, less commonly, gastric or duodenal ulceration, syncope, depression and insomnia.

A fourth drug for AD is memantine, which is an NMDA-receptor antagonist and therefore alters glutamate neurotransmission centrally. It may cause side-effects such as hypertension, headache, dizziness and drowsiness and, less commonly, vomiting, thrombosis, confusion, fatigue, hallucinations and changes in gait.

4.2 A nutritional approach

As with all nutritional intervention, the first place to start is with the patient's diet. Primarily, ensuring that blood sugar levels are kept stable can have a beneficial impact on mental health. Glucose is the energy source of choice for the brain, so ensuring the supply is continuous and steady is vital. A high carbohydrate diet can result in blood sugar levels peaking and troughing which can be unstable for the brain, resulting in a range of symptoms from mood swings to seizures.

4.2.1 PROTEIN

Protein is needed as a source of amino acids to form neurotransmitters. Protein input requirements can vary depending on the presenting condition. Low protein diets have been suggested for histadelia (Prousky and Lescheid 2002), and ketogenic diets, high in fat, adequate in protein and low in carbohydrates, have been found to be beneficial for epilepsy for over 80 years (West 2008).

4.2.2 CALCIUM AND MAGNESIUM

Magnesium and calcium interact in a complex and interdependent way to influence neuromuscular activity. With respect to neurotransmitters, magnesium has been found to act as a relaxant and an enabler to sleep. An open study on hyperexcitable children found that magnesium supplementation (along with vitamin B6) helped to increase their intracellular magnesium levels and improve their abnormal behaviour (Mousain-Bosc *et al.* 2004). Calcium is required for the release of neurotransmitter receptors; it is needed for the electrical signals of the nervous system and acts as a secondary messenger.

When there are sleep problems, dosages of up to 600mg of calcium and 250–500mg of magnesium have been suggested taken 45 minutes before going to bed.

4.2.3 ZINC

Zinc is the most prevalent trace element in the brain (Tuormaa 1995), and as such its deficiency has been associated with a variety of mental and behavioural changes, such as schizophrenia and anorexia. Zinc is used in treating histadelia as it can raise histamine levels. Zinc supplementation is used in cases of pyrroluria alongside vitamin B6 and is usually effective in producing a remission. It is normally recommended that B6 should be taken to a level where dream recall occurs; however, this may not be practical to determine, thus dosages of around 100mg twice per day is suggested. In cases of suspected pyrroluria, zinc supplementation levels of 10–30g twice daily is suggested. A randomised controlled trial of 14mg per day zinc supplementation in subjects with anorexia nervosa resulted in the BMI of those individuals increasing at double the rate of the control group; its actions are believed to be on the production of GABA, which is abnormal in anorexia (Birmingham and Gritzner 2006). In Brazil, links between zinc deficiency and low birth weights, deficits in mental development, and behaviour have been explored, and zinc supplementation at a rate of 5mg per day for 8 weeks starting at birth appeared to reverse poor behaviours and responsiveness when reviewed at 6 and 12 months (Ashworth *et al.* 1998).

4.2.4 B VITAMINS

Niacin (vitamin B3) is required for the formation of nicotinamide-adenine dinucleotide (NAD) and much of the brain's chemistry requires adequate NAD. When histamine levels are in excess, the enzyme nicotinamide-adenosine dinucleotidase (NADase) installs a histamine molecule onto NAD, making it inert; thus excess histamine can result in depletion of NAD (Prousky and Lescheid 2002). Supplementation of vitamin B3 can therefore be beneficial in quenching excess histamine.

Vitamin B6 is used in the metabolism of all amino acids as well as being a cofactor in the production of dopamine, noradrenaline, GABA, serotonin, acetylcholine and MAO. In the case of pyrroluria, it has been found that supplementation with B6 automatically reduced excretion of zinc (Pfeiffer *et al.* 1974). Vitamin B6 is essential for the conversion of tryptophan to niacin, and is itself dependent on vitamins B2 and B3 for its own activation to pyridoxal–5–phosphate (P-5-P).

Folic acid, B6 and vitamin B12 are some of the co-factors needed in the metabolism of methionine (Miller 2003) which then facilitates methylation processes, required for the synthesis of most neurotransmitters and phospholipids and for the deactivation of histamine. When folic acid, B12 and B6 levels are low, then homocysteine may be raised. A study of homocysteine, folate and monoamine metabolism in patients with severe depression concluded that measuring total plasma homocysteine was a useful measure of impaired methylation (Bottiglieri *et al.* 2000). When either B12 or methionine levels are low, folic acid can get trapped in the 5-methyl-tetrahydrofolate (5-mTHF) form, and so consideration should always be given to supplementing B12 with folic acid.

Note that supplementation is contraindicated in the case of histadelia (Edelman 2001). Daily levels of around 15mg of vitamin B6, 200mcg vitamin B12 and 275mg folic acid has been recommended to support methionine metabolism.

4.2.5 VITAMIN C

Schizophrenia patients appear to have impaired ascorbic acid (vitamin C) metabolism (Prousky and Lescheid 2002). Vitamin C at a dose of 2g per day has been shown to lower blood histamine, and so vitamin C supplementation may in theory be beneficial to lower histamine levels.

4.2.6 VITAMIN D

The occurrence of seasonal affective disorder (SAD) during periods of low sunlight has led to interest in vitamin D and its role in depression. A study of 1282 residents in the Netherlands, aged between 65 and 95 years old, found a correlation between serum vitamin D levels (25(OH)vit D) and depression, with lower levels of vitamin D resulting in more severe depression (Witte *et al.* 2008). The exact role of Vitamin D on brain activity is not yet understood, however it could well be as a result of its ability to stimulate the absorption of calcium, which itself plays a vital role in neurotransmitter receptors.

4.2.7 AMINO ACIDS

Tyrosine and tryptophan compete for absorption across the BBB, and so if both are being used as supplements, they are best given several hours apart from each other.

4.2.8 TYROSINE AND PHENYLALANINE

Tyrosine is beneficial for dopamine-dependent depression (DDD). By increasing dopamine and noradrenaline, a reward and anti-craving effect is achieved and this may be useful as a potentiator to stop addictions (Braverman 2003).

The National Academy of Sciences estimates minimum requirements for both tyrosine and phenylalanine to be 16mg/kg bodyweight; therapeutically, recommendations range between 1 and 2g per day. It should be noted that high doses may suppress appetite, while low doses can stimulate appetite; also be aware that dopamine is increased in certain pathways in schizophrenia, and some antipsychotic drugs work by acting as antidopaminergic agents.

A review of the benefits of tyrosine supplementation and its precursor DL phenylalanine (DLPA) concluded that supplementing DLPA at high doses (up to 14g per day) may be helpful in cases of depression where low noradrenaline activity was involved (Myers 2000). Supplementing tyrosine itself was not found to be beneficial; however, there have been very few studies in this area.

4.2.9 TRYPTOPHAN

Tryptophan is the precursor to serotonin and melatonin. It is useful in the treatment of insomnia, monopolar depression, SAD and carbohydrate cravings. During the ban of tryptophan from 1989 to 2005, 5-HTP, an intermediate metabolite in the tryptophan pathway, was introduced as an alternative.

Since 2005 tryptophan supplementation to a maximum of 220mg per day has been permitted by the Food Standards Agency (2006).

4.2.10 METHIONINE

Methionine can be useful in histadelia, as it is able to donate a methyl group so that histidine can be conjugated, detoxified and eliminated, thereby lowering histamine levels.

1.5g per day of DL-methionine has been found to significantly lower blood histamine levels.

Methionine is also valuable with its ability to donate methyl groups for methylation of neurotransmitters.

Literature suggests taking between 1000 and 2000mg per day in 500mg doses.

4.2.11 THEANINE

Theanine (N-ethyl L-glutamine) is an amino acid found in tea which is believed to increase the production of GABA. GABA is an inhibitory neurotransmitter in the brain which achieves a sedative and calming effect by switching off excess adrenaline and increasing serotonin. To date there is very little research, and most of what has been completed has been on rats; however, it has been found to consistently increase alpha wave production, and it appears to counteract the effects of caffeine (Kelly *et al.* 2008).

Theanine is available in dosages between 100 and 200mg, and a dosage of 200mg two to three times per day is recommended for relaxation (Thorne 2005).

4.2.12 FATTY ACIDS

There appears to be a correlation between blood levels of histamine and prostaglandin E1 (PGE1) such that blood levels of the two appear to move in the same direction under the same stimulus. Heleniak and Lamola (1999) have compared these two substances, particularly in relation to schizophrenia, and hypothesise that if GLA and EPA can increase PGE1, they may also lower histamine levels.

There is general agreement on the benefit of omega-3 long-chain PUFAs for the treatment of depression for both children (Nemets *et al.* 2006) and adults (Hakkarainen *et al.* 2004). At this time, there is no established clinically appropriate dose of omega-3 fatty acids for depression.

However, review of data indicates that 1g daily of EPA appears to give successful outcomes (Logan 2003).

Research in 1997 found that severity of depression correlated negatively with both the red blood cell membrane levels and dietary intake of omega-3 fatty acids. Although the study was small – involving only 10 depressed patients and 14 matched control subjects – confounding factors were well controlled and the results were significant (Edwards *et al.* 1998).

When looking at healthy individuals, researchers in the Netherlands found that omega-3 fatty acid supplementation appears to have a selective effect on risky decision making, with the supplemented group making fewer risk-adverse decisions than the placebo group. No consistent effects on mood were observed; however, there was no history of depression in any of the individuals (Antypa *et al.* 2009).

4.2.13 PHOSPHATIDYLCHOLINE

Acetylcholine is derived from phosphatidylcholine, found in egg yolks, organ meats and fish. As a supplement phosphatidylcholine is in high concentrations in lecithin (manufactured from eggs or soy) or as a soluble salt. The enzyme acetyl transferase is required to combine choline with an acetyl group and in some cases of AD this enzyme can be lacking, and so supplementation with choline sources may not have a beneficial effect.

Supplementation with phosphatidylcholine has been found to be beneficial in cases of bipolar depression and it is thought that the success of lithium as a treatment for bipolar disorder may be related to its ability to promote increased brain acetylcholine (Jope *et al.* 1985).

Sufferers of bipolar depression appear to gain good results from dosages of 5000–10,000mg three times per day (Murray 1996).

5. Case studies

For the nutritional therapist, having a client fill in a comprehensive health questionnaire and then engage in a consultation that can last between one and two hours, gives a great opportunity to get to the cause of a presenting problem. The following two case studies of depression revealed very different causes and therefore very different solutions.

5.1 Case study 1

A 35-year-old male presented wanting to lose weight. He was from an all male family, with a family history of depression, he had hay fever, was a light sleeper and had little body hair – all classic symptoms of histadelia. His doctor had just given him a diagnosis of bipolar disorder, and he admitted to feeling suicidal most of the time with very low self-worth and an inability to form relationships. He had been recommended antidepressants, however he had made a decision in conjunction with his doctor to stop taking them as he thought they had made him feel worse. He was seeking a natural approach.

His diet was adjusted to ensure regular eating – three meals and two snacks per day, with an increase in protein content. Supplementation included 500mg of methionine twice per day, and a male-oriented multivitamin, giving 400mg of calcium and 400mg of magnesium alongside 1g of fish oil. One month on he was already much improved, and within six months he was in a new relationship, losing weight and very happy.

5.2 Case study 2

A 55-year-old female presented wanting to lose weight. The consultation revealed poor gut health with a mix of constipation, diarrhoea and chronic bloating, all of which she had suffered for decades. She had gingivitis, athlete's foot and had suffered severe depression for most of her adult life. Her diet during childhood and early adult life had consisted primarily of simple carbohydrates and sugary snacks, though she now ate balanced, home-cooked meals.

A saliva test revealed that the client had an overgrowth of *Candida albicans* and so a protocol which improved her own immunity against *Candida*, killed off the *Candida* and supported her liver during the die-off was introduced. Her mood started to lift within a couple of weeks and continued to improve over the following weeks as the treatment progressed. It took some months for the *Candida* to be killed off and for her gut to heal; however, with that she was able to lose weight.

References

American Psychiatric Association (2000) *Diagnostic and Statistical Manual of Mental Disorders: Fourth Edition. Text Revised.DSM-IV-TR.* Washington, DC: American Psychiatric Association.

Antypa, N., Van der Does, A.J.W., Smelt, A.H.M. and Rogers, R.D. (2009) 'Omega-3 fatty acids (fish oil) and depression-related cognition in healthy volunteers.' *Journal of Psychopharmacology 23*, 7, 831–840.

Arehart-Treichel, J. (2001) 'The gut is said to have a mind of its own.' *Psychiatric News 36*, 14, 14.

Ashworth, A., Morris, S.S., Lira, P.I. and Grantham-McGregor, S.M. (1998) 'Zinc supplementation, mental development and behaviour in low birth weight term infants in northeast Brazil.' *European Journal of Clinical Nutrition 52*, 3, 223–227.

Bingham, M. (2008) *Autism and the Human Gut Flora.* Available at www.ei-resource.org/articles/autism-articles/autism-and-the-human-gut-flora, accessed on 21 February 2010.

Biolab (2009) *Urinary Kryptopyrroles.* London: Biolab. Available at www.biolab.co.uk/docs/kp.pdf, accessed on 10 November 2009.

Birmingham, L. and Gritzner, S. (2006) 'How does zinc supplementation benefit anorexia nervosa?' *Eating and Weight Disorders 11*, 4, e109–111.

Bottiglieri, G., Laundy, M., Crellin, R., Toone, B.K., Carney, M.W.O. and Reynolds, E.H. (2000) 'Homocysteine, folate, methylation and monoamine metabolism in depression.' *Journal of Neurology, Neurosurgery and Psychiatry 69*, 228–232.

Bralley, J.A. and Lord, R.S. (2002) 'Organic Acids in Urine.' In *Laboratory Evaluations in Molecular Medicine, Nutrients, Toxicants and Cell Regulators*. Georgia: Metametrix.

Braverman, E.R. (2003) *The Healing Nutrients Within*, 3rd edn. New Jersey: Basic Health Publications.

Campbell-McBride, N. (2006) *Gut and Psychology Syndrome*. Amersham: Halstan.

Deutch, A.Y. and Roth, R.H. (2008) 'Neurotransmitters.' In L.R. Squire *et al. Fundamental Neuroscience*. Burlington, MA: Academic Press.

Edelman, E. (2001) *Natural Healing for Schizophrenia*. Oregon: Borage Books.

Edwards, R., Peet, M., Shay, J. and Horrobin, D. (1998) 'Saturated fatty acid levels in the diet and in red blood cell membranes of depressed patients.' *Journal of Affective Disorders 48*, 149–155.

Food Standards Agency (2006) *Tryptophan Letter*. Available at www.food.gov.uk/multimedia/pdfs/tryptophanipletter.pdf, accessed on 10 November 2009.

Goyer, R.A. (1995) 'Nutrition and metal toxicity.' *American Journal of Clinical Nutrition 61*, 646S–650S.

Hakkarainen, R., Partonen, T., Haukka, J., Virtamo, J., Albanes, D. and Lonnqvist, J. (2004) 'Is low dietary intake of omega 3 fatty acids associated with depression?' *American Journal of Psychiatry 161*, 567–569.

Hehme, N., Engelmann, H., Kuenzel, W., Neumeier, E. and Saenger, R. (2004) 'Immunogenicity of a monovalent, aluminium-adjuvanted influenza whole virus vaccine for pandemic use.' *Virus Research 103*, 1–2, 163–171.

Heleniak, E.P. and Lamola, S.W. (1999) 'Histamine and prostaglandins in schizophrenia.' *Journal of Orthomolecular Psychiatry 14*, 3, 162–177.

Horrobin, D.F. and Bennett, C.N. (2003) 'Phospholipid Metabolism and the Pathophysiology of Psychiatric and Neurological Disorders.' In M. Peet, I. Glen and D.F. Horrobin (eds) *Phospholipid Spectrum Disorders in Psychiatry and Neurology*. Lancaster: Marius Press.

Jope, R.S., Tolbert, L.C., Wright, S.M. and Walter-Ryan, W. (1985) 'Biochemical RBC abnormalities in drug-free and lithium-treated manic patients.' *American Journal of Psychiatry 142*, 356–358.

Kelly, S.P., Ramirez, G.M., Montesi, J.L. and Foxe, J.L. (2008) 'L-Theanine and caffeine in combination affect human cognition as evidenced by oscillatory alpha-band activity and attention task performance.' *Journal of Nutrition 138*, 1572S–1577S.

Krieger, D.T. and Hughes, J.C. (1990) *Neuroendocrinology*. Sunderland: Sinauer.

Logan, A. (2003) 'Neurobehavioral aspects of omega-3 fatty acids: Possible mechanisms and therapeutic value in major depression.' *Alternative Medicine Review 8*, 4, 410–425.

McCann, D., Barrett, A., Cooper, A., Crumpler, D. *et al.* (2007) 'Food additives and hyperactive behaviour in 3 year old and 8/9 year old children in the community: A randomised, double blinded placebo-controlled trial.' *Lancet 370*, 9598, 1560–1567.

Miller, A.L. (2003) 'The methionine-homocysteine cycle and its effects on cognitive diseases.' *Alternative Medicine Review 8*, 1, 7–19.

Mousain-Bosc, M., Roche, M., Rapin, J. and Bali, J-P. (2004) 'Magnesium and vitamin B6 intake reduces central nervous system hyperexcitability in children.' *Journal of the American College of Nutrition 23*, 5, 545s–548s.

Murray, M.T. (1996) *Encyclopaedia of Nutritional Supplements*, 1st edn. New York: Three Rivers Press.

Myers, S. (2000) 'Use of neurotransmitter precursors for treatment of depression.' *Alternative Medicine Review 5*, 1, 64–71.

Nemets, H., Nemets, B., Apter, A., Bracha, Z. and Belmaker, R.H. (2006) 'Omega 3 treatment of childhood depression: A controlled, double blind pilot study.' *American Journal of Psychiatry 163*, 1098–1100.

Pfeiffer, C. (1975) *Mental and Elemental Nutrients*. New Canaan, CT: Keats Publishing.

Pfeiffer, C.C., Sohler, A., Jenney, C.H. and Iliev, V. (1974) 'Treatment of pyroluric schizophrenia (malvaria) with large doses of pyridoxine and a dietary supplement of zinc.' *Orthomolecular Psychiatry 3*, 4, 292–300.

Prousky, J.E. and Lescheid, D.W. (2002) 'Vitamin B3 and C: Their role in the treatment of histadelia.' *Journal of Orthomolecular Medicine 17*, 1, 17–21.

Puri, B.K. (2008) *Saunders' Pocket Essentials of Psychiatry*, 3rd edn. London: Saunders.

Puri, B.K., Hirsch, S.R., Easton, T. and Richardson, A.J. (2002) 'A volumetric biochemical niacin flush-based index that noninvasively detects fatty acid deficiency in schizophrenia.' *Progress in Neuropsychopharmacology and Biological Psychiatry 26*, 1, 49–52.

Puri, B.K., Tsaluchidu, S. and Treasaden, I.H. (2009) 'Serial structural MRI analysis and proton and 31PMR spectroscopy in the investigation of cerebral fatty acids in major depressive disorder, Huntington's disease, myalgic encephalomyelitis and in forensic schizophrenic patients.' *World Review of Nutrition and Diet 99*, 31–45.

Quig, D. and Urek, B.S. (2001) 'Trace element analysis in hair: Factors determining accuracy, precision and reliability.' *Alternative Medicine Review 6*, 5, 472–481.

Richardson, A.J. and Puri, B.K. (2000) 'The potential role of fatty acids in attention-deficit/hyperactivity disorder.' *Prostaglandins, Leukotrienes and Essential Fatty Acids 63*, 1–2, 79–87.

Rogers, M.A. and Simon, D.G. (1999) 'A preliminary study of dietary aluminium intake and risk of Alzheimer's disease.' *Age and Ageing 28*, 205–209.

Seidel, S., Kreutzer, R., Smith, D., McNeel, S. and Gillis, D. (2001) 'Assessment of commercial laboratories performing hair mineral analysis.' *Journal of the American Medical Association 285*, 67–72.

Siblerud, R.S., Motl, J. and Kienholz, E. (1999) 'Psychometric evidence that dental amalgam mercury may be an etiological factor in schizophrenia.' *Journal of Orthomolecular Medicine 14*, 4, 201–209.

Thorne Research Inc. (2005) 'L-Theanine.' *Alternative Medicine Review 10*, 2, 136–138.

Truss, O.C. (1984) 'Metabolic abnormalities in patients with chronic candidiasis, the acetaldehyde hypothesis.' *Journal of Orthomolecular Psychiatry 13*, 2, 66–93.

Tuormaa, T.E. (1995) 'Adverse effects of zinc deficiency: A review from the literature.' *Journal of Orthomolecular Medicine 10*, 3/4, 149–164.

Walker, R. and Lupein, J.R. (2000) 'The safety evaluation of monosodium glutamate.' *Journal of Nutrition 130*, 1049S–1052S.

West, H. (2008) 'The ketogenic diet.' *Nutrition Practitioner 9*, 2.

Whiteley, P., Rodgers, J., Savery, D. and Shattock, P. (1999) 'A gluten free diet as an intervention for autism and associated spectrum disorders: Preliminary findings.' *Autism 3*, 1, 45–65.

Witt, M.R. and Nielsen, M. (1994) 'Characterisation of the influence of unsaturated free fatty acids on brain GABA/benzodiazepine receptor binding in vitro.' *Journal of Neurochemistry 62*, 4, 1432–9.

Witte, J.G., Hoogendijk, W.J., Lips, P., Dik, M.G. *et al.* (2008) 'Depression is associated with decreased 25-hydroxyvitamin D and increased parathyroid hormone levels in older adults.' *Archives of General Psychiatry 65*, 5, 508–512.

Chapter *11*

PUTTING KNOWLEDGE INTO PRACTICE: A CASE STUDY

Lorraine Nicolle and Kate Neil

Introduction

This chapter comprises a detailed case study, in order to bring to life some of the key themes discussed in this book and to show how the technical information can be put into practice. Importantly, the case demonstrates an approach that treats the individual, rather than the disease. It illustrates the inter-relationships of body systems and thus the need to treat the whole person.

While reading the case example, the reader is encouraged to refer back to the preceding chapters, where appropriate, for more detailed discussions of the relevant biochemical processes and the evidence for the corresponding nutritional interventions.

Some other points to consider while reading this chapter are as follows:

- There is no single 'correct' intervention programme for a given situation. In the real world, specific interpretations and prescriptions differ between practitioners presented with the same case. Each practitioner is influenced by his/her unique set of experiences and spheres of knowledge.

- Because so much of the available scientific literature is controversial, incomplete and often contradictory, the authors hope to illustrate that it is only through painstaking analysis and synthesis of large quantities of data (in terms of an extensive case history, the results of laboratory tests, relevant published studies and reflection on one's own and others' clinical experiences) that one can gradually build a picture that can usefully inform one's treatment decisions. Such an approach may bring to light the possible existence of biochemical imbalances that may not otherwise have been considered.

- Reflexivity is a crucial part of the clinician's practice. The nutrition practitioner (NP) in this study returned to her case many times, reflecting on the information she had gathered and the decisions she had made.

- The role of the practitioner is to provide accessible information to the patient, so that he/she is able to make an informed choice about his/her treatment options. Using the approach outlined here, the practitioner can help the patient to understand the various different imbalances that may exist, and the ways in which they could be related (directly or indirectly) to his/her symptoms. The patient should involve his/her medical advisor, where appropriate, including and especially in all decisions that involve medical drugs.

- A full exploration of every imbalance that may exist for this patient is beyond the scope of this chapter. But many links have been made which should encourage the reader to further investigate those areas in which he/she is particularly interested.

- Finally, while this approach is evidence-informed, there may be some interventions for which strong evidence does not exist. The authors nevertheless consider such interventions valid where there is enough expert clinical opinion to believe that they could be effective and are unlikely to be harmful.

1. Case presentation

Marie is a 41-year-old white Caucasian, a full-time secondary school teacher, married with two children aged 11 and 9. Following the completion of a comprehensive health questionnaire, she went to see a NP for nutrition support in addressing her main health concerns, which were:

- rheumatoid arthritis (RA) diagnosed 18 months prior, with progressively worsening pain and swelling

- severe fatigue, weakness and slow cognition

- irritable bowel syndrome (IBS) diagnosed 9 years ago.

Implementing a functional approach to case assessment, the NP explored Marie's current and long-term health history, taking into account her family history, physical, psychological and emotional wellbeing, as well as her short- and long-term diet and lifestyle practices, using the previously completed questionnaire as a basis for discussion. The reader will need to refer throughout to Marie's timeline, Figure 11.1 on page 367 (which summarises the key events over her lifetime), and the general dietary trends that the NP obtained during the consultation, given below as Table 11.1.

Table 11.1 Marie's dietary trends

Carbohydrates

Sugars	*Refined*	*Wholegrain*	*Fruit/veg*
Daily commercial breakfast cereals, sauces and salad dressings, fruit juices and squashes, cereal bars (1–2/day), fruit yoghurts and chocolate (3/week)	White rice/pasta 5/week; breakfast cereals daily; bagels	Wheat only (2–4 slices bread daily)	2–3 portions veg daily; no salad; 2 fruit daily

Fats

Saturated	*Essential*	*Trans-*	*Oxidised*
Processed red meat 4/week; other red meat 4/week; milk, cheese and yogurt daily	Tinned tuna 1/week; no nuts or seeds	Margarine and commercially prepared foods daily	Frying/grilling in sunflower oil 5/week

Protein

Animal	*Vegetable*
Meat, dairy and tinned tuna as above; no other fish; 8 eggs/week	No pulses, beans, nuts or seeds

Other

Gluten	*Salt*	*Caffeine*	*Water*
Bread, pasta and processed foods as above. Client also adds wheatbran 2–3/week for constipation	Does not add salt to food but eats processed foods	4 teas/day	Approx. 500ml/day

2. Clinical investigations

Based on the consultation, the NP recommended the investigations given in Table 11.2 to help inform treatment options.

Table 11.2 Recommended investigations

Test Name	Rationale
Urine test for organic acids, amino acids and markers for oxidative stress	A comprehensive test offering the practitioner target areas for nutrition support, including: digestion, absorption, detoxification, mitochondrial efficiency, neurotransmission, methylation, hormonal implications and specific co-factor needs for biochemical pathways. As this test is not widely offered in conventional medicine (except to identify genetic inborn errors of metabolism in infants), the reader may be interested in Lord and Bralley (2008), chapter 1, for information on issues of reliability and quality assurance
Serum 25-hydroxy-vitamin D	Sub-optimal levels have been associated with autoimmune inflammatory conditions (Cantorna *et al.* 2004; Merlino *et al.* 2004)
Full gluten sensitivity test, including gliadin IgA and IgG, tissue transglutaminase IgA, reticulin IgA and endomysial IgA	Arthritis is commonly found in patients with coeliac disease; and autoimmune diseases occur 3–10 times more frequently in coeliacs (Lee and Green 2006)
Red cell membrane fatty acids	To be considered if necessary in three months. The ratio of membrane fatty acids influences the extent of inflammation in the body (see 5.2.3 below and Chapter 4)

Marie informed the NP that medical tests had shown high levels of inflammatory markers but that all other markers on her full blood count and biochemistry profile had been normal, including thyroid markers. The NP asked permission to write to Marie's GP requesting a copy of the results and to ask the GP to run a full gluten intolerance profile and the vitamin D test, to help reduce Marie's costs.

3. Test results

The test results in Table 11.3 demonstrated the following markers to be outside the laboratory's reference limits.

Table 11.3 Marie's test results

Test	Result	NP considerations in context of client history1
Organic acids		
Dihydroxyphenylpropionic acid (DHPPA)	High	Possible gastro-intestinal (GI) overgrowth of *Clostridia* and/or *Pseudomonas* bacteria
Vanilmandelic acid (VMA)	Low	Sub-optimal methylation, low phenylalanine and/or tyrosine, low cofactors (certain B vitamins and minerals) and/or low noradrenaline
3-methyl-4-OH-phenylglycol	Low	As for VMA
Formimino-glutamate (FIGlu)	High	Low functional folate and/or B12, supporting the possibility of sub-optimal methylation
Citric acid	High	Low co-factors (iron, glutathione (GSH)), toxic metals or high amounts of dietary citric acid
Cis-aconitic acid	High	As for citric acid
Alpha-ketoglutaric acid (AKA)	High	Low co-factors (B vitamins, magnesium (Mg), lipoic acid) or toxic metals
Pyroglutamic acid	High	Deficient GSH. Low Mg (GSH co-factor) and/or amino acid components (cysteine, glycine, glutamic acid)
Kynurenic acid	High	Low B6
Lipid peroxides	High	Oxidative stress
Amino acids		
Taurine	Low	Poor fat digestion and absorption. Low B6 (pyridoxyl-5-phosphate – P5P) (regarding conversion from cysteine), oxidative stress
Threonine	Low	Poor digestion and absorption
Cysteine	High	Low cofactors (Mg for conversion to GSH, P5P for conversion to taurine and molybdenum, B2 and/or iron for conversion to sulphate)
Glutamic acid	Low	Low GSH. Poor digestion and absorption
Glutamine	Low	Poor absorption, increased intestinal permeability
Glycine	Low	Poor digestion and absorption
Methionine	High	Co-factor deficiency (Mg) required for conversion to SAMe via methylation
Histidine	Low	Gastric hypochlorhydria

continued

Table 11.3 Marie's test results *cont.*

Test	Result	NP considerations in context of client history[1]
Organic acids		
Dietary peptides (anserine and carnosine)	High	Poor digestion and absorption
Serum 25-hydroxyvitamin D	Low	Vitamin D3 deficiency
Gluten intolerance profile		
Tissue transglutaminase IgA	Positive	Possible presence of coeliac disease. GP has recommended an intestinal biopsy to confirm

1. While many other interpretations could be relevant for this client and in general, this column lists the NP's most relevant interpretations, based on this particular case history, for informing her treatment decisions. Supporting data for the organic acids and amino acids tests is taken from Lord and Bralley (2008): Chapters 4 and 6; and Anon (2009). For further data on the evidence base for the indications relating to the individual markers (both in the table above and the text below), the reader is referred to the laboratories that are licensed to distribute these tests in the UK, such as: Genova Diagnostics (www.GDXUK.net) and Metametrix (www.metametrix.com).

When working with his/her own patients, the reader is recommended to use laboratory interpretations for individual markers, in combination with literature searches for clinical applications related to the particular client history.

4. Outputs (and consequential nutritional advice)

4.1 Digestion, elimination and detoxification

Compromised digestion, elimination and detoxification may be contributing to Marie's IBS. As there is a higher incidence of RA in people with IBS than in the general population, (although this may be partly genetic) (Svedberg *et al.* 2002), the NP thought it reasonable to see whether an improvement in Marie's IBS could help to reduce the RA activity.

4.1.1 DYSBIOSIS

IBS and RA have both been linked to alterations in intestinal microflora (Hawrelak and Myers 2004). Marie's excessive urinary levels of DHPPA indicated a possible overgrowth of *Clostridia* and/or *Pseudomonas* bacteria. Given that dysbiosis can lead to the release of inflammatory cytokines that have a systemic effect (see Chapter 8), this could be a factor in Marie's RA symptoms. She was recommended to supplement with the probiotic yeast *Saccharomyces boulardii,* which may be effective against *Clostridia* species (Guarino, Lo Vecchio and Canani 2009 and see Chapter 2). (As allergic reactions to this yeast are occasionally seen, Marie was advised to contact the NP should she experience any unusual skin rashes, wheezing or excess mucus.)

Gluten avoidance was also suggested (after the biopsy, in order to avoid a false negative result), as her probable intolerance could be contributing to malabsorption of the amino acid substrates for these problematic bacteria.

The presence of dysbiosis is unsurprising, given that chronic stress, antibiotics, excessive sugars and animal protein, as well as long-term use of the contraceptive pill (see timeline), have all been shown to contribute to the condition (Hawrelak and Myers 2004). At this point, it is worth noting that many of Marie's urinary amino acid levels are low (see section 3), despite her high protein intake. This is supportive of the NP's conclusion that Marie has some problems with digestion and absorption. The test results also show that the occasional amino acid is at excessive levels. However, this could be due to an insufficiency of co-factors hindering the efficient use of these amino acids, leading to their excretion. In some instances, excess urinary loss of an amino acid may indicate an inherited trait. The NP explained to the patient that she would consider this possibility following repeat test results after a six-month trial of the programme.

Marie was therefore recommended to:

- reduce her stress levels (see 5.3.1)

- minimise the use of antibiotics (after discussing her options with her GP)

- reduce alcohol to four units a week

- replace sugars and refined carbohydrates with (gluten-free) whole grains and increased amounts of vegetables

- take two teaspoons of psyllium husk in a pint of warm water, on rising

- reduce animal protein to once daily, avoiding processed varieties, and increasing well-chewed nuts, seeds, (gluten-free) whole grains, split peas and lentils (starting with small amounts of these foods and gradually increasing to full portion sizes, to aid digestion)

- increase total fluid intake to two litres/day (regarding her constipation and the potentially dehydrating effects of diarrhoea).

4.1.2 HYPOCHLORHYDRIA AND/OR LOW DIGESTIVE ENZYME STATUS

Marie's IBS symptoms, her history of stress and the presence of dysbiosis led the NP to suspect inadequate levels of hydrochloric acid (HCl) and/or digestive enzymes (see Chapter 2). Anecdotally, there may be a higher frequency of hypochlorhydria in RA, although research in this area is sparse.

In addition Marie had low histidine and low functional folate (elevated FIGlu) markers, both of which are vital nutrients for HCl synthesis, as is zinc. While the test results were not specific for zinc, there is an increased likelihood of zinc malabsorption with her digestive issues and particularly if hypochlorhydria is present (Sturniolo *et al.* 1991).

To improve digestive secretions, it was agreed that supplementation of betaine hydrochloride and/or digestive enzymes would be considered at the next consultation, providing Marie's non-steroidal anti-inflammatory drug (NSAID) intake had significantly reduced by then. (She was advised to speak with her GP to reduce NSAIDs by 50 per cent during the course of the next month.) Regular use of NSAIDs increases the risk of GI mucosal injury (Hippesley-Cox, Coupland and Logan 2005), in the presence of which the use of such digestive aids is contraindicated. In the meantime, Marie was recommended to:

- eat a bitter leaf salad (such as rocket, watercress, chicory, dandelion) prior to each meal (anecdotally, bitter leaves may stimulate digestive secretions)
- eat in non-stressful situations, wherever possible
- eat slowly, chew well
- leave the table prior to being completely full
- refrain from drinking fluids during meals.

4.1.3 LIVER DETOXIFICATION

One reason for the excessive urinary levels of the three energy and mitochondrial function markers (citric acid, cis-aconitic acid and alpha-ketoglutaric acid) could be a high toxic load (Schauss 2005). (See the toxic load box on Marie's timeline.) Marie was therefore advised to:

- replace processed foods and fats with whole foods and cold-pressed olive and seed oils
- avoid gluten (after the biopsy via the GP)
- reduce stress
- address the dysbiosis. Dysbiosis can increase the toxic load via the fermentation and putrefaction of bowel contents, disruption of bowel transit time and the production of enzymes that release toxic metabolites from their phase II conjugates (Hawrelak and Myers 2004)
- reduce NSAIDs by 50 per cent, with her GP's approval
- increase filtered water to 2 litres a day
- optimise liver detoxification pathways.

The latter point is vital in ensuring that toxins are transformed and excreted (as described in Chapter 3), before they have an opportunity to interfere with the body's biochemical processes, leading, in Marie's case, to fatigue and other symptoms. For example, toxins from the GI tract may be hyperstimulating the adaptive immune system (see 5.2.2), which may be contributing to Marie's RA symptoms.

The liver detoxification pathways that seemed to need most consideration in Marie's case were:

Glutathione pathways

- Marie's elevated urinary pyroglutamic acid reading indicated a likely impairment in its recycling to GSH, ultimately leaving Marie with suboptimal GSH levels. GSH is vital for phases I and II of liver detoxification.

- Interestingly, two components of the GSH tripeptide, namely glycine and glutamate, appeared at low levels in Marie's test results. (Glycine is also an independent phase II amino acid conjugate.) The NP's strategy for improving Marie's glycine and glutamic acid status was to improve her digestion and absorption (by tackling dysbiosis and low digestive secretions, as described above), thus enabling better amino acid uptake.

- Recycling pyroglutamic acid to GSH requires the cofactor magnesium. Given the elevated alpha-ketoglutaric acid, methionine and cysteine readings (see below), all of which also require magnesium to convert on (see Figure 7.2 in Chapter 7), Marie was advised to increase food containing magnesium (such as nuts, seeds, green vegetables, buckwheat and oats) and supplement magnesium in the short-term.

- The elevated energy metabolism markers, citrate and cis-aconitate, also support the hypothesis of low GSH, since they both require GSH as a cofactor to continue their metabolism through the Krebs cycle. It should also be noted that, alongside GSH, iron is required in this reaction. Hypochlorhydria and gluten enteropathy are two major considerations for iron-deficiency anaemia. The reader is recommended to review the literature on iron status and RA. By supporting digestive processes, the NP aimed to improve iron status over time.

Methylation

- Low levels of two noradrenaline metabolites (vanilmandelic acid and 3-methyl-4-OH-phenylglycol) in Marie's test results may indicate a problem with methylation. This could also be due to low precursors (such as phenylalanine and tyrosine) and/or co-factors (certain B vitamins and minerals). (Figure 7.2 in Chapter 7 includes methylation.)

- Sub-optimal methylation is consistent with the elevated levels of the histidine metabolite formimino-glutamic acid, as this occurs in situations of low functional folate. (Note that although this could also be due to a B12 deficiency, as B12 is needed in the recycling of folate, the marker that is more indicative of B12 status (methylmalonic acid) was normal in this case.)

- Marie was advised to eat three good portions of leafy greens daily for folate and to take a multivitamin and mineral supplement. It was made clear that the priority for intervention was to focus on the diet and to support digestion, in order to maximise nutrient absorption. Although there could be genetic polymorphisms on the folic acid and/or methylation pathways, the NP focused on the diet initially because it was so obviously deficient.

- The amino acid test indicated elevated methionine, another possible indicator of poor methylation, implying impaired metabolism to S-adenosylmethionine (SAMe). As mentioned under the GSH section above, this could be due to low levels of the necessary co-factor magnesium. This was therefore increased through magnesium-containing foods and short-term supplementation.

- The NP also considered that, although the serotonin metabolite 5-hydroxy-indoleacetic acid (5HIA) was within the normal range, poor methylation (if this is present) may be affecting Marie's melatonin synthesis. Melatonin is a methylation product of serotonin, for which process magnesium is again required. Melatonin is an important antioxidant and hormone required for a good night's sleep. Marie had not reported sleep problems but she did feel exhausted on waking in the morning.

  There is conflicting data on the role of melatonin in RA, with some suggesting that it may have a disease-promoting effect (Maestroni *et al.* 2005). However, this view is now being challenged and recent research suggests that melatonin may be helpful in the treatment of RA, especially given its anti-inflammatory (Korkmaz 2008) and anti-proliferative properties (Nah *et al.* 2009).

  In the light of this, the NP felt it important to optimise conditions for normalising Marie's melatonin synthesis, primarily by increasing natural light exposure during the daytime and having a fully darkened room at night, and improving methylation.

- Serotonin's precursor amino acid is tryptophan. Most dietary tryptophan is converted via the kynurenine pathway to niacin and nicotinamide adenine dinucleotide (NAD). Raised urinary kynurenine suggests a block in this conversion. Pyridoxal-5-phosphate (P5P) is needed as a co-factor. It is worth noting that disturbed tryptophan metabolism is an important area of research in RA (Penberthy 2007). The NP ensured that Marie's multi-vitamin and mineral supplement included vitamins B6 (as P5P) and B3.

Sulphation

- If functional B6 is low (which is a possibility, indicated by the elevated kynurenic acid and other markers previously discussed), trans-sulphuration may also be low, compromising the sulphation detoxification pathway. There is an increased prevalence of poor sulphation in patients with IBS (Moss and Waring 2003) and RA (Emery *et al.* 1992). Sulphation is required to synthesise glycosaminoglycans (GAGs) (Sagawa *et al.* 1998) that are important components of cartilage in musculoskeletal joints and gut membrane integrity (Murch *et al.* 1993).

- Another reason to suspect poor sulphation is Marie's high urinary level of cysteine. This may indicate low co-factors to metabolise it to sulphate (molybdenum and iron), or indeed to GSH (magnesium, as mentioned above) and/or taurine (P5P) (see Figure 7.2, Chapter 7). Interestingly, low taurine also showed up on Marie's amino acid test result. Of further relevance here is taurine's role in the synthesis of bile acids to eliminate fat-soluble toxins from the liver. The reader is also recommended to explore taurine's role in immune defence.

- To help normalise these pathways, the NP ensured that the multi-supplement included these co-factors. Marie was also advised to take Epsom salt baths three times a week to increase her sulphur status (Moss and Waring 2003; Waring 2004). This is because high-sulphur foods were not heavily promoted, due to the possible creation of hydrogen sulphide in the gut (Magee *et al.* 2004), which may worsen her IBS symptoms. Sulphur-containing foods are primarily eggs and other animal proteins (over 75% of sulphate is formed from the oxidation of cysteine (Waring 2001)) and vegetables containing organosulphur compounds (onions, garlic and brassicas). Anecdotally, the baths may also help with pain relief.

Oestrogen metabolism pathways

- The issues discussed above indicate that Marie's capacity for detoxifying fat-soluble compounds may be significantly compromised. Of further note is that methylation, sulphation and good GSH status are needed specifically for oestrogen detoxification. Bland (2006) claims that certain oestrogen metabolites (16-alpha-hydroxylated oestrone and 4-hydroxyoestrone) can contribute to the development of autoimmune diseases. Indeed, these metabolites have been found to be significantly elevated in cases of RA (Cutolo 2004; Weidler *et al.* 2004). Thus it is worth seeing whether improving these three aspects of liver detoxification may help the situation. (As seen in Chapter 7, sulphur also helps to keep oestrogen in its bound state.)

- Although high-sulphur foods were not heavily promoted (see above), cruciferous vegetables were allowed in moderation. This is because they contain glucosinolates that are converted to indole-3-carbinol, which has been found to shift oestrogen metabolism towards metabolites with less oestrogenic action (McAlindon *et al.* 2001). Marie was advised that once her GI health has improved, she should be eating cruciferous vegetables daily. It was agreed to consider testing her oestrogen metabolism in six months' time, if her symptoms have not improved.

4.2 Immunity (reducing inflammation)

4.2.1 INTESTINAL PERMEABILITY (IP)

Many RA patients have increased intestinal permeability (IP), especially in times of symptom flare-ups (Cordain *et al.* 2000). In IP, a lack of non-inflammatory secretory IgA

(SIgA) results in an over-reactivity of the *adaptive* immune response, which can become systemic (see Chapter 8). Hence, a 'leaky gut' is a probable contributory factor in many autoimmune diseases (Watts *et al.* 2005).

The test results that indicate an increased likelihood of IP include:

- low levels of some amino acids, especially threonine, suggesting that malabsorption may be an issue, and glutamine, required for enterocyte health

- dysbiosis, as problematic bacterial loads can degrade tight junctions in the gut epithelia and also cause gut inflammation (Berkes *et al.* 2003)

- poor sulphation (see 5.1.3), as this is needed for the synthesis of membrane structural components like GAGs (Sagawa *et al.* 1998), which are an important part of intestinal tissue (Murch *et al.* 1993)

- possible gluten sensitivity: gliadin has been shown to increase zonulin, a protein that opens the tight junctions in the small intestine enterocytes, leading to increased IP in coeliac sufferers (Drago *et al.* 2006). Gluten grains have also been found to inhibit the action of the anti-inflammatory nutrient vitamin D (see 5.2.2), even in the absence of a hypersensitivity effect (Cordain 2006).

The NP recommended the '4R programme' (Lukaczer 2005, pp.462–468), comprising:

- **Removal** of the likely causes:

  o reduce dysbiosis

  o reduce stress (Kelly 1999)

  o reduce NSAID intake by 50 per cent initially (with GP's approval), with the aim of avoidance in the long term

  o avoid gluten (after the biopsy), due to the sensitivity test results. Avoid cow's milk products in the short-term, as these may cause sensitivity reactions in individuals with autoimmune diseases (Bland 2006).

    RA symptoms have been found to diminish with a gluten-free vegan diet (Hafstrom *et al.* 2001), as well as with fasting followed by a gluten-free vegetarian diet (Kjeldsen-Kragh 1999). Despite these studies, regular fish consumption was kept in Marie's diet for blood sugar control and because she was eating in a family situation. Also, fish contains essential amino and fatty acids and there is evidence that disease activity in RA may decrease in (fish-inclusive) Mediterranean diets (Skoldstam, Hagfars and Johansson 2003). A significantly reduced amount of organic, unprocessed eggs and meat was also allowed, for essential amino acids and to maximise dietary compliance. Fasting and veganism will be considered in future, if appropriate. Fasting in the modern world should not be undertaken lightly, due to the potential liberation of many stored toxins.

- **Replacement** of digestive aids (in some weeks' time): elevated urinary levels of dietary peptide markers indicate probable sub-optimal enzyme levels. Digestive enzymes can reduce the immunological burden by digesting residual food matter (Ash 2006 and see Chapter 8), degrading immune complexes (often found in RA) and reducing prostaglandin E2 (PGE2) (Brien *et al.* 2004) and pro-inflammatory cytokines (Leipner and Saller 2000). In addition, as mentioned above, the low histidine and low functional folate markers indicate possible hypochlorhydria. However, due to Marie's high intake of NSAIDs, the NP advised dietary ways of improving digestive secretions in the short term (see 5.1.2), with a view to supplementing enzymes and/or hydrochloric acid at the follow-up consultation, only providing NSAIDs have been reduced as planned.

- **Re-inoculation** of the gut with beneficial bacteria. There is growing evidence that certain *Lactobacilli* spp. can reduce subjective symptoms of RA (Hatakka *et al.* 2003; Nenonen *et al.* 1998). Thus this was supplemented, as was *S. boulardii*, which has been shown to increase SIgA (see Chapter 8).

- **Repair** of the lining of the GI tract. Marie was advised to:

  o chew all food well because saliva contains epidermal growth factor (EGF) that repairs epithelial tissue (Frey, Golovin and Polk 2004)

  o eat oily fish for EPA and DHA to help reduce any GI tract inflammation that may prevent healing (Simopoulos 2008 and see Chapter 4)

  o eat more soluble fibre to increase n-butyrate for colonocyte health (Daly *et al.* 2005). Replace wheatbran with psyllium husks

  o supplement l-glutamine in order to support the health of the enterocytes (De Souza and Green 2005). The glutamine marker was also low in the amino acids test.

The multi-vitamin and mineral supplement prescribed above included vitamin A for the health of the mucous membranes (Elli *et al.* 2009) and vitamins B5 and C for general healing (Lukaczer 2005, p.468).

4.2.2 ADAPTIVE IMMUNE SYSTEM

Nuclear factor kappa B (NFκB) is a major driver of the adaptive immune (inflammatory) response in RA (Feldmann *et al.* 2002) and it works through the transcription of genes that produce inflammatory cytokines and influence cyclo-oxygenase 2 (COX2). These cytokines may also be worsening the patient's fatigue, by slowing the central nervous system ('sickness syndrome') (Ash 2006).

Phytochemicals like resveratrol (Bharti and Aggarwal 2002) and quercetin (Nair *et al.* 2006) have been found to down-regulate NFκB. Quercetin may also help to stabilise cell membranes, reducing the release of inflammatory mediators such as histamine (Amella *et al.* 1985). Marie was therefore advised to eat berries and eight portions of brightly coloured vegetables every day. (Supplementation of these nutrients was rejected for cost reasons.) Although these foods are high in phenolic compounds, which compete for the sulphation pathway, the strategies recommended for improving sulphation (see 5.1.3) should allow Marie to increase them without detrimental effect.

Curcumin was supplemented (600mg x 3/day), as this has been found not only to inhibit COX2 and PGE2 while reducing levels of tumour necrosis factor alpha (TNF-α) and NFκB (Bharti and Aggarwal 2002; Chan 1995), but also to reduce symptoms of RA in a double-blind trial (Deodhar, Sethi and Srimal 1980). It is also a potent antioxidant (Sreejayan Rao 1994).

Vitamin D3 deficiency is associated with many conditions of pain, inflammation and autoimmunity, including RA (Cantorna *et al.* 2004; Merlino *et al.* 2004). Supplementation may help to reduce inflammatory interleukin 6 (IL-6), C-reactive protein (CRP) and NFκB (Cohen-Lahav *et al.* 2006; D'Ambrosio *et al.* 1998), as well as matrix metallopeptidase 9 (MMP9) (Timms *et al.* 2002), a protease found in RA that breaks down collagen. Given Marie's low serum vitamin D levels, and a difficulty in her guaranteeing an hour's sun exposure daily, the author prescribed 2000 iu vitamin D3/day and a follow-up test in three months' time. (Vitamin D is also an important antioxidant.) See Chapter 8 for more information on vitamin D's role in the immune system.

4.2.3 EICOSANOID SYNTHESIS

The NP was concerned that Marie's intake of dietary fats may be contributing to an eicosanoid imbalance in favour of the inflammatory pathway. People with RA have been reported to eat more animal fat than those without the disease (Jacobsson *et al.* 1990) and have been found to improve on diets low in arachidonic acid (Adam *et al.* 2003). In addition, an excessively high omega-6:3 ratio can be pro-inflammatory, as seen in Chapter 4.

In contrast numerous studies show EPA to reduce symptoms in RA (Calder 2008; Stamp, James and Cleland 2005). Mechanisms may include the suppression of NFκB and the competition with arachidonic acid as a substrate for COX.

Olive oil (omega-9) has been found to reduce RA symptoms (Linos *et al.* 1999) and, although it is of the omega-6 family, GLA has also been effective in some trials (Belch and Hill 2000; Zurier *et al.* 1996).

Marie was advised to:

- reduce animal fats (meat reduction and dairy avoidance, as above)
- avoid refined vegetable and seed oils, *trans* and hydrogenated fats
- steam, slow-cook or bake foods, rather than frying or grilling in oil
- eat oily fish three times a week
- swap the commercial salad dressings for cold pressed mixed seed oils and olive oil.

The NP felt that it would not be best practice to consider EPA, DHA and/or GLA supplementation until the patient's diet, and thus her antioxidant status, had improved and a red cell membrane fatty acid test had been undertaken. It was agreed to consider such a test in three months' time.

4.2.4 JOINT TISSUE REPAIR

Chronic inflammation causes damage to the affected tissue, especially when coupled with high levels of stress (as is apparent from Marie's timeline). By following the recommendations given above, Marie will be increasing her intake of the nutrients necessary for tissue repair, while also addressing the biochemical imbalances that are preventing the healing process. Improving sulphation, for example, will be important in optimising GAG synthesis for healthy cartilage (Murch *et al.* 1993; Sagawa *et al.* 1998).

It was therefore agreed that any further specific action regarding joint tissue repair should be postponed until the next review. In particular, the inflammation needs to be better controlled before healing can take place.

4.3 Communication

4.3.1 ADRENAL GLAND FUNCTION

The low urinary noradrenaline metabolites (VMA and 3-methyl-4-OH-phenylglycol) could be due to low levels of this hormone, which many suggest some element of sub-optimal adrenal function. This could be contributing to her fatigue, as seen in Chapter 6.

If this is the case, there may also be low cortisol, especially given Marie's long history of stress and fatigue. As cortisol inhibits the release of arachidonic acid from the cell membrane (Chrousos 1995), its absence leaves the body vulnerable to escalating inflammation (Ash 2006). Long-term IBS, her RA symptoms and her current and historic levels of emotional stress (such as the building work at home and returning to work with two young children) may have significantly taxed her adrenal glands (Kelly 1999). Thus part of the NP's programme was to support adrenal function.

The NP referred Marie to a stress counsellor. She also recommended:

- outdoor walking for 30 minutes daily

- 30 minutes of 'quiet time' alone every evening

- going to bed by 10pm

- eating breakfast by 10am

- discussing with her head teacher the issues she is experiencing at work

- doing things that make her smile and laugh as often as possible

- eating a low-glycaemic load, nutrient-dense diet of small and frequent protein-containing meals, to address any dysglycaemia, which is stressful to the body. (Sugar, refined and processed foods, tea, coffee, alcohol and carbohydrate-only meals were to be minimised or avoided.) High insulin also up-regulates the delta-5-desaturase enzyme (as described in Chapters 4 and 5), which could lead to an increase in arachidonic acid secretion. Chapter 5 comprises a fuller discussion of dysglycaemia and its links to chronic diseases

- taking the multi-nutrient supplement that included vitamin C, pantothenic acid, B6, zinc and magnesium, all of which are needed for steroid synthesis and secretion (Kelly 1999).

See Chapter 6 for a discussion on the importance of adrenal gland health.

4.3.2 NEURONAL ISSUES

The low VMA and 3-methyl-4-OH-phenylglycol readings could indicate not only low noradrenaline (as above), but also low dopamine. This could lead to problems with neuronal communication function, further contributing to Marie's severe fatigue and slow mental cognition.

Other markers to consider here are the low glycine and taurine, as these are both inhibitory neurotransmitters (see Chapter 10). For example, an important role of taurine in the central nervous system is that of exerting anti-anxiety effects (Zhang and Kim 2007).

Glutamate, an excitatory neurotransmitter, is also low. The NP considered that this could be affecting Marie's slow cognition because glutamate is believed to be involved in learning and memory. It is also a precursor for gamma-aminobutyric acid (GABA), which has a relaxing, anti-anxiety effect (Kemp 2006).

At excessive levels, excitatory neurotransmitters can become neurotoxic. Thus a marker of concern here is the patient's elevated cysteine levels. Cysteine has been described as an excitoxin that evokes neuronal degeneration (Janaky *et al.* 2000).

Thus the NP felt that Marie's programme needed to include advice for helping to balance neurotransmission. This advice comprised the recommendations for improving digestion and absorption (for amino acid neurotransmitter precursors), and for optimising methylation (for neurotransmitter synthesis) and co-factor status (for neurotransmitter synthesis and cysteine metabolism).

The benefits of balanced neurotransmission are further discussed in Chapter 10.

4.4 Mitochondrial function and oxidative stress

A number of the test results are pertinent here:

- high levels of lipid peroxides
- low levels of the antioxidants (AOs) taurine and GSH (see 5.1.3). Taurine has been shown to reduce lipid peroxidation (Di Leo *et al.* 2002)
- diminished mitochondrial output (shown in the elevated Krebs cycle intermediates citric acid, cis-aconitic acid and alpha-ketoglutaric acid), which could be contributing to the patient's fatigue. Elevations of these markers may imply either Krebs cycle co-factor deficiency (for example, GSH, certain B

vitamins and/ or magnesium) and/ or a heavy toxic load (Schauss 2005) (see 5.1.3). Marie has a highly processed diet and has had significant toxin exposure throughout her life (see the toxic load box on the timeline). See Chapter 9 for a discussion on the role of oxidative stress in diminishing mitochondrial function.

AOs are crucial to the functioning of the immune system and to defend cells from oxidative damage, especially in the face of the excessive release of free oxidising radicals (FORs) that occurs during chronic inflammation. AOs also help neutralise the FORs produced during phase I hepatic biotransformation (Liska, Lyon and Jones 2005, p.278) of agents that may be triggering the immune system. In addition, deficiencies of the AOs selenium and zinc have been found in autoimmune disease (Honkanen *et al.* 1991).

Marie was advised to:

- improve methylation and trans-sulphuration for GSH (see 5.1.3)

- improve taurine status by generally improving digestion and absorption (as there is no evidence that her diet is deficient) and by lessening her requirement for this amino acid, by reducing her toxic load. This included altering her intake of fats, to reduce the high levels of lipid peroxides, and improving her detoxification capacity (see 5.1.3)

- eat a wide range of brightly coloured fruits and vegetables to improve AO intake

- take magnesium and the multi-supplement for co-factors for the Krebs intermediates and for a broad spectrum of antioxidants.

5. Summary of Marie's nutrition programme following this consultation

5.1 Diet

- A wholefood diet: low-glycaemic, nutrient-dense, vegan foods and a portion a day of either fish (oily fish to be eaten three times per week), eggs or meat (organic or wild).

- Avoidance of:

  o gluten grains (after the GP-referred biopsy)

  o dairy products

  o sugar and refined carbohydrates

  o *trans*, hydrogenated and oxidised fats

  o processed foods (including processed meats).

- High-sulphur foods (eggs and other animal proteins, onions, garlic, brassicas) to be eaten only in moderation, with a view to eating brassicas daily, once digestive function is improved.

- The diet to be rich in olive oil and omega-3 fats (oily fish and flax seeds and oil), with some omega-6 from seeds and salad oils.

- A wide range of brightly coloured fruits and vegetables, some raw. A bitter leaf salad as a starter for lunch and dinner. In total, eat nine to ten portions of vegetables a day (start with four portions and gradually increase).

- Small, regular meals (breakfast by 10am), eaten slowly and chewed well.

- Each meal to include a protein food.

- 2 litres of water, taken between meals (up to half an hour before, and two hours after, a meal) (may be taken in herbal teas).

- No coffee or black tea.

- Alcohol reduced to four units a week.

- Foods to be steamed or slow-baked, rather than fried or grilled with oil.

5.2 Supplements

- A broad-spectrum multi-vitamin and mineral that comprises the more bio-available nutrient forms.

- *Lactobacillus rhamnosus GG* 5 billion x 2/day (dose to be increased if necessary, following a review in six weeks' time).

- *Saccharomyces boulardii* 500mg x 3/day.

- Curcumin 600mg x 3/day.

- Vitamin D3 2,000iu/day.

- L-glutamine 500mg x 3/day.

- Psyllium husk: 2 teaspoons in a pint of warm water, on rising.

- Magnesium 350mg/day (as citrate).

5.3 Lifestyle

- Epsom salt baths, using a good mugful of the salt, three times a week.

- Reduce NSAID intake by 50 per cent (with the GP's approval).

- Avoid antibiotics unless really necessary (with the GP's guidance).

- See the stress counsellor to which Marie was referred.

- Eat only when not stressed, eat slowly, chew well, leave the table before being completely full.

Figure 11.1 Marie's timeline

Age	Event
0–4	Hospitalised with tropical disease.
18	Started Pill. University life included high alcohol intake, poor diet and smoking. Bloating and flatulence starts.
22	Haemorrhoids diagnosed (re. constipation). Frequent headaches.
24	Found parents' divorce v upsetting. Chicken-pox. Gave up smoking.
30	First child. (Stopped Pill aged 29). Returned to work after 6 months.
32	Second child. Post-natal fatigue. Thyroid tests normal. ?Compromised adrenals. Colonoscopy. Irritable bowel syndrome (IBS) diagnosed.
37–8	Returned to full-time work. Found it a 'shock to the system'. Stressful life event: building work on house ('like living on a building site'). Fatigue better but IBS remains. Intermittent joint pain starts.
39	Fatigue returns. IBS remains. Thyroid test normal. RA diagnosis.
41	Continuing fatigue, anxiety and feeling of being unable to cope with life. 2 weeks off work re. above. Seeks help via nutritional therapy.

Timeline axis points: 0   4   18   22   24   30   32   37–8   39   41

Childhood and teens:

High dose antibiotics aged 4 following contraction of unnamed tropical disease → hospitalisation and parenteral feeding for 2 weeks, followed by oral medication for many weeks.

Generally constipated.

Passive smoker (both parents smoked).

Period pain.

Family history (English ancestry):
No apparent FH of autoimmune (AI) diseases.

Mother: hypertension.

Father: osteoarthritis, gastritis re: H. Pylori and non-fatal MI aged 60 (?inflammation, ?poor gut mucosal integrity, ?immuno-compromised).

Paternal grandmother: died of colorectal cancer age 76 (?as for father + ?poor detoxification).

Paternal grandfather: stroke (? inflammation).

Throughout 20s:

Moved to Central London (pollution). Fast-paced life, alcohol, smoking (10/day), no exercise, stressful job as teacher. High intake wheat bran (for constipation).

Non-steroidal anti-inflammatory drugs (NSAIDs) 2–3/week for headaches.

Toxic load across years:
- Smoking (active and passive).
- Low water intake.
- Diet (see text): toxic fats, sugar, potential allergens, additives, nutrient deficiencies.
- Heavy alcohol use prior to having children.
- Excess cortisol (prior to adrenal fatigue).
- Dysbiosis.
- NSAIDs, contraceptive Pill.
- Childhood antibiotics.
- Stress and blood sugar imbalance most of adult life.
- Pollution.
- Living in a house with major building work taking place.

Early to mid-30s:

Frequent colds.

Occasional thrush. (?immuno-compromised?)

Colonoscopy was 'clear' but revealed some 'minor' inflammation only visible under a microscope.

Two young children → lack of sleep. Headaches when over-tired. NSAIDs 3/week.

IBS. Constipation and diarrhoea. Haemorrhoids injected mid-30s.

Mid-30s to current:

Finding it increasingly hard to deal with the pressures of a difficult job and looking after the family. Worried about money. Dislikes being the primary regular breadwinner (husband = free-lance illustrator) but feels guilty about leaving so much of the childcare to her husband. Feels she has no control over her life.

No exercise (lack of time and motivation).
- Blood pressure 98/60.
- Feels dizzy on standing.
- Cravings for salty and sugary foods.
- Feeling low, tearful and unable to cope with life.
- Headaches (2/7).
- Dry, flaky skin and scalp.
- IBS: believes she is 'allergic' to many foods.
- PMS.

NSAIDs 3–4/week re headaches and RA.

No dietary restrictions. Shares cooking with husband. Family have said they will also make dietary changes (within reason) to support her.

Favourite foods: Bread, Marmite, bagels, cake, cheese, dried fruit.

Current BMI: 22 (pretty stable).

- Walk outside in daylight for at least 30 minutes daily.
- Have 30 minutes of 'quiet time' alone every evening (the bath times can be included).
- Go to bed by 10pm.
- Seek help from the head teacher in resolving the workplace issues.
- Laugh!

6. Next steps

Marie was given meal planners and recipes at the consultation and she was advised to have her supplement programme approved by her medical consultant prior to starting the treatment. It was agreed that Marie would return for a review of her progress in six weeks' time, alerting the NP in the meantime, should she experience any problems.

While a discussion of the progress of the patient is beyond the scope of this chapter, the reader may be interested to know that compliance was high and that, at the six week follow-up appointment, improvements were seen in Marie's subjective experience of joint pain, IBS and fatigue.

References

Adam, O., Beringer, C., Kless, T., Lemmen, C. *et al.* (2003) 'Anti-inflammatory effects of a low arachidonic acid diet and fish oil in patients with rheumatoid arthritis.' *Rheumatology International 23*, 27–36.

Amella, M., Bronner, C., Briancon, F., Haag, M., Anton, R. and Landry, Y. (1985) 'Inhibition of mast cell histamine release by flavonoids and bioflavonoids.' *Planta Medica 51*, 16–20.

Anon (2009) *Optimal Nutrition Evaluation Commentary Guide.* New Malden: Genova Diagnostics. Available from Genova Diagnostics Europe, Parkgate House, 356 West Barnes Lane, New Malden, Surrey KT3 6NB.

Ash, M. (2006) 'Resolving and reducing inflammation and pain using natural interventions.' Paper delivered at Royal Society of Medicine lecture, 11 March.

Belch, J. and Hill, A. (2000) 'EPO and borage oil in rheumatologic conditions.' *American Journal of Clinical Nutrition 71*(Suppl), 352S–6S.

Berkes, J., Viswanathan, V.K., Savkovic, S.C. and Hecht, G. (2003) 'Intestinal epithelial responses to enteric pathogens: Effects on the tight junction barrier, ion transport and inflammation.' *Gut 52*, 3, 439–451.

Bharti, A.C. and Aggarwal, B.B. (2002) 'Chemopreventive agents induce suppression of nuclear factor-kappaB leading to chemosensitization.' *Annals of the New York Academy of Sciences 973*, 392–395.

Bland, J. (2006) 'Understanding the origins and applying advanced nutritional strategies for autoimmune diseases.' Annual Nutri lecture for complementary therapists, London, 14 October.

Brien, S., Lewith, G., Walker, A., Hicks, S.M. and Middleton, D. (2004) 'Bromelain as a treatment for osteoarthritis: A review of clinical studies.' *Evidence Based Complementary and Alternative Medicine 1*, 3, 251–257.

Calder, P.C. (2008) 'Session 3: Joint Nutrition Society and Irish Nutrition and Dietetic Institute Symposium on nutrition and autoimmune disease PFA, inflammatory processes and RA.' *Proceedings of the Nutrition Society 67*, 4, 409–418.

Cantorna, M.T., Zhu, Y., Fruicu, M. and Wittke, A. (2004) 'Vitamin D status, 1,25-dihydroxyvitamin D3 and the immune system.' *American Journal of Clinical Nutrition 80*, suppl., 1717S–1720S.

Chan, M.M.Y. (1995) 'Inhibition of tumour necrosis factor by curcumin, a phytochemical.' *Biochemistry and Pharmacology 49*, 1551–1556.

Chrousos, G.P. (1995) 'The hypothalamic-pituitary-adrenal axis and immune-mediated inflammation.' *New England Journal of Medicine 332*, 20, 1351–1362.

Cohen-Lahav, M., Shany, S., Tobvin, D., Chaimovitz, C. and Douvdevani, A. (2006) 'Vitamin D decreases NFkappaB activity by increasing IkappaBalpha levels.' *Nephrology Dialysis Transplantation 21*, 4, 889–897.

Cordain, L. (2006) 'Solved: The 10,000-year-old riddle of bread and milk.' *The Paleo Diet Newsletter 2*, 1, 1–5. Available at www.thepaleodiet.com/newsletter/back_issues.shtml, accessed 1 October 2009

Cordain, L., Toohey, L., Smith, M.J. and Hickey, M.S. (2000) 'Modulation of immune function by dietary lectins in rheumatoid arthritis.' *British Journal of Nutrition 83*, 3, 207–217.

Cutolo, M. (2004) 'Estrogen metabolites: Increasing evidence for their role in rheumatoid arthritis and systemic lupus erythematosus.' *Journal of Rheumatology 31*, 3, 419–421.

Daly, K., Cuff, M.A., Fung, F. and Shirazi-Beechey, S.P. (2005) 'The importance of colonic butyrate transport to the regulation of genes associated with colonic tissue homeostasis.' *Biochemical Society Transactions 33*, 4, 733–735.

D'Ambrosio, D., Cippitelli, M., Cocciolo, M.G., Mazzeo, D. *et al.* (1998) 'Inhibition of IL-12 production by 1,25-dihydroxyvitamin D3. Involvement of NF-kappaB downregulation in transcriptional repression of the p40 gene.' *Journal of Clinical Investigation 101*, 1, 252–262.

Deodhar, S.D., Sethi, R. and Srimal, R.C. (1980) 'Preliminary study on antirheumatic activity of curcumin.' *Indian Journal of Medical Research 71*, 632–634.

De Souza, D.A. and Greene, L.J. (2005) 'Intestinal permeability and systemic infections in critically ill patients: Effect of glutamine.' *Critical Care Medicine 33*, 5, 1175–1178.

Di Leo, M.A., Santini, S.A., Cercone, S., Lepore, D. *et al.* (2002) 'Chronic taurine supplementation ameliorates oxidative stress and Na+ K+ ATPase impairment in the retina of diabetic rats.' *Amino Acids 23*, 4, 401–406.

Drago, S., El Asmar, R., Di Pierro, M., Grazia Clemente, M. *et al.* (2006) 'Gliadin, zonulin and gut permeability: Effects on celiac and non-celiac intestinal mucosa and intestinal cell lines.' *Scandinavian Journal of Gastroenterology 41*, 4, 408–419.

Elli, M., Aydin, O., Bilge, S., Bozkurt, A. *et al.* (2009) 'Protective effect of vitamin A on ARA-C induced intestinal damage in mice.' *Tumori 95*, 1, 87–90.

Emery, P., Bradley, H., Gough, A., Arthur, V. and Waring, R. (1992) 'Increased prevalence of poor sulphoxidation in patients with RA: Effect of changes in the acute phase response and second line drug treatment.' *Annals of the Rheumatic Diseases 51*, 318–320.

Feldmann, M., Andreakos, E., Smith, C., Bondeson, J. *et al.* (2002) 'Is NF-kappaB a useful therapeutic target in rheumatoid arthritis?' *Annals of the Rheumatic Diseases 61*, suppl. 2, ii13–8.

Frey, M.R., Golovin, A. and Polk, D.B. (2004) 'Epidermal growth factor-stimulated intestinal epithelial cell migration requires Src family kinase-depended p38 MAPK signalling.' *Journal of Biological Chemistry 279*, 43, 44513–44521.

Guarino, A., Lo Vecchio, A. and Canani, R.B. (2009) 'Probiotics as prevention and treatment for diarrhoea.' *Current Opinion in Gastroenterology 25*, 1, 18–23.

Hafstrom, I., Ringertz, B., Spangberg, A., von Zweigbergk, L. *et al.* (2001) 'A vegan diet free of gluten improves the signs and symptoms of rheumatoid arthritis: The effects on arthritis correlate with a reduction in antibodies to food antigens.' *Rheumatology 40*, 1175–1179.

Hatakka, K., Martio, J., Korpela, M., Herranen, M. *et al.* (2003) 'Effects of probiotic therapy on the activity and activation of mild rheumatoid arthritis – a pilot study.' *Scandinavian Journal of Rheumatology 32*, 4, 211–215.

Hawrelak, J.A. and Myers, S.P. (2004) 'The causes of intestinal dysbiosis: A review.' *Alternative Medicine Review 9*, 2, 180–197.

Hippisley-Cox, J., Coupland, C. and Logan, R. (2005) 'Risk of adverse GI outcomes in patients taking cyclo-oxygenase-2 inhibitors or conventional non-steroidal anti-inflammatory drugs: Population based nested case-control analysis.' *British Medical Journal 331*, 7528, 1310–1316.

Honkanen, V., Konttinen, Y.T., Sorsa, T., Hukkanen, M. *et al.* (1991) 'Serum zinc, copper and selenium in rheumatoid arthritis.' *Journal of Trace Elements and Electrolytes in Health and Disease 5*, 4, 261–263.

Jacobsson, L., Lindgarde, F., Manthorpe, R. and Akesson, B. (1990) 'Correlation of fatty acid composition of adipose tissue lipids and serum phosphatidylcholine and serum concentrations of micronutrients with disease duration in rheumatoid arthritis.' *Annals of the Rheumatic Diseases 49*, 11, 901–905.

Janaky, R., Varga, V., Hermann, A., Saransaari, P. and Oja, S.S. (2000) 'Mechanisms of L-cysteine neurotoxicity.' *Neurochemical Research 25*, 9–10, 1397–1405.

Kelly, G.S. (1999) 'Nutritional and botanical adaptations to assist with the adaptation to stress.' *Alternative Medicine Review 4*, 4, 249–265.

Kemp, J.A. (2006) 'Glutamate- and GABA-based CNS therapeutics.' *Current Opinion in Pharmacology 6*, 1, 7–17.

Kjeldsen-Kragh, J. (1999) 'RA treated with vegetarian diets.' *American Journal of Clinical Nutrition 71*, 5, 1211–1213.

Korkmaz, A. (2008) 'Melatonin as an adjuvant therapy in patients with rheumatoid arthritis.' *British Journal of Clinical Pharmacology 66*, 2, 316–317.

Lee, S.K. and Green, P.H. (2006) 'Celiac sprue (the great modern-day imposter).' *Current Opinion in Rheumatology 18*, 1, 101–107.

Leipner, J. and Saller, R. (2000) 'Systemic enzyme therapy in oncology: Effect and mode of action.' *Drugs 59*, 4, 769–780.

Linos, A., Kaklamani, V., Kaklamani, E., Koumantaki, Y. *et al.* (1999) 'Dietary factors in relation to rheumatoid arthritis: A role for olive oil and cooked vegetables?' *American Journal of Clinical Nutrition 70*, 6, 1077–1082.

Liska, D., Lyon, M. and Jones, D. (2005) 'Detoxification and Biotransformational Imbalances.' In D. Jones (ed.) *The Textbook of Functional Medicine.* Gig Harbour, WA: Institute for Functional Medicine.

Lord, R. and Bralley, J. (2008) *Laboratory Evaluations for Integrative and FM*, 2nd edn. Georgia: Metametrix Institute.

Lukaczer, D. (2005) 'The '4R' Program.' In D. Jones (ed.) *The Textbook of Functional Medicine.* Gig Harbour, WA: Institute for Functional Medicine.

Maestroni, G.J., Cardinali, D.P., Esquifino, A.I. and Pandi-Perumal, S.R. (2005) 'Does melatonin play a disease promoting role in rheumatoid arthritis?' *Journal of Neuroimmunology 158*, 1–2, 106–111.

Magee, E.A., Curno, R., Edmond, L.M. and Cummings, J.H. (2004) 'Contribution of dietary protein and inorganic sulphur to urinary sulphate: Toward a biomarker of inorganic sulphur intake.' *American Journal of Clinical Nutrition 80*, 137–142.

McAlindon, T.E., Fulin, J., Chen, T., Klug, T., Lahita, R. and Nuite, M. (2001) 'Indole-3-carbinol in women with SLE: effect on estrogen metabolism and disease activity.' *Lupus 10*, 11, 779–783.

Merlino, L.A., Curtis, J., Mikuls, T.R., Cerhan, J.R., Criswell, L.A. and Saag, K.G. (2004) 'Vitamin D intake is inversely associated with RA: Results from the Iowa Women's Health Study.' *Arthritis and Rheumatism 50*, 1, 72–77.

Moss, M. and Waring, R. (2003) 'The plasma cysteine/sulphate ratio: a possible clinical biomarker.' *Journal of Nutritional and Environmental Medicine 13*, 4, 215–229.

Murch, S.H., MacDonald, T.T., Walker-Smith, J.A., Levin, M., Lionetti, P. and Klein, N.J. (1993) 'Disruption of sulphated glycosaminoglycans in intestinal inflammation.' *Lancet 341*, 8847, 711–714.

Nah, S.S., Won, H.J., Park, H.J., Ha, E. *et al.* (2009) 'Melatonin inhibits human fibroblast-like synoviocyte proliferation via extracellular signal-regulated protein kinase/P21^{CIP1}/P27^{KIP1} pathways.' *Journal of Pineal Research 47*, 1, 70–74.

Nair, M.P., Mahajan, S., Reynolds, J.L., Aalinkeel, R. *et al.* (2006) 'The flavonoid quercetin inhibits proinflammatory cytokine (tumour necrosis factor alpha) gene expression in normal peripheral blood mononuclear cells via modulation of the NF-{kappa} {beta} system.' *Clinical Vaccine and Immunology* 13, 319–328.

Nenonen, M.T., Helve, T.A., Rauma, A.L. and Hanninen, O.O. (1998) 'Uncooked, lactobacilli-rich, vegan food and rheumatoid arthritis.' *British Journal of Rheumatology 37*, 3, 273–281.

Penberthy, W.T. (2007) 'Pharmacological targeting of IDO-mediated tolerance for treating autoimmune disease.' *Current Drug Metabolism 8*, 3, 245–266.

Sagawa, K., DuBois, D., Almon, R., Murer, H. and Morris, M.E. (1998) 'Cellular mechanisms of renal adaptation of sodium dependent sulphate cotransport to altered dietary sulphate in rats.' *Pharmacology 287*, 3, 1056–1062.

Schauss, M. (2005) *Toxins and the Citric Acid Cycle.* Carbon Based Corporation. Available at www.carbonbased.com/modules/mydownloads/, accessed on 10 November 2009.

Simopoulos, A.P. (2008) 'The importance of the omega-6/omega-3 fatty acid ratio in cardiovascular disease and other chronic diseases.' *Experimental Biology and Medicine 233*, 6, 674–688.

Skoldstam, L., Hagfars, L. and Johansson, G. (2003) 'An experimental study of a Mediterranean diet intervention for patients with rheumatoid arthritis.' *Annals of the Rheumatic Diseases 62*, 208–214.

Sreejayan Rao, M.N.A. (1994) 'Curcuminoids as potent inhibitors of lipid peroxidation.' *Journal of Pharmacy and Pharmacology 46*, 12, 1013–1016.

Stamp, L.K., James, M.J. and Cleland, L.G. (2005) 'Diet and RA: A review of the literature.' *Seminars on Arthritis and Rheumatism 35*, 2, 77–94.

Sturniolo, G.C., Montino, M.C., Rossetto, L. and Martin, A. (1991) 'Inhibition of gastric acid secretion reduces zinc absorption in man.' *Journal of American College of Nutrition 10*, 372–375.

Svedberg, P., Johansson, S., Wallander, M.A., Hamelin, B. and Pedersen, N.L. (2002) 'Extra-intestinal manifestations associated with irritable bowel syndrome: A twin study.' *Alimentary Pharmacology and Therapeutics 16*, 5, 975–983.

Timms, P.M., Mannan, N., Hitman, G.A., Noonan. K. *et al.* (2002) 'Circulating MMP9, vitamin D and variation in the TIMP-1 response with VDR genotype: Mechanisms for inflammatory damage in chronic disorders?' *Quarterly Journal of Medicine 95*, 12, 787–796.

Waring, R. (2001) 'Autism and ADHD: Could diet affect the symptoms?' *Nutrition Practitioner 3*, 3, 8–10.

Waring, R.H. (2004) 'Report on absorption of magnesium sulfate (Epsom salts) across the skin.' Magnesium Online Library. Available at www.mgwater.com/transdermal.shtml, accessed on 10 November 2009.

Watts, T., Berti, I., Sapone, A., Gerarduzzi, T. *et al.* (2005) 'Role of the intestinal tight junction modulator zonulin in the pathogenesis of type 1 diabetes in diabetic-prone rats.' *Proceedings of the National Academy of Sciences USA 102*, 8, 2916–2921.

Weidler, C., Harle, P., Schedel, J., Schmidt, M., Scholmerich, J. and Straub, R.H. (2004) 'Patients with rheumatoid arthritis and systemic lupus erythematosus have increased renal excretion of mitogenic estrogens in relation to endogenous antiestrogens.' *Journal of Rheumatology 31*, 3, 419–421.

Zhang, C.G. and Kim, S.J. (2007) 'Taurine induces anti-anxiety by activating strychnine-sensitive glycine receptor in vivo.' *Annals of Nutrition and Metabolism 51*, 4, 379–386.

Zurier, R.B., Rossetti, R.G., Jacobson, E.W., DeMarco, D.M. *et al.* (1996) 'GLA treatment of RA. A randomized, placebo-controlled trial.' *Arthritis and Rheumatism 39*, 11, 1808–1817.

CONTRIBUTORS

Lorraine Nicolle MSc, BA (Hons), Dip. BCNH, Dip. CIM, NTCC, MBANT is a nutritional therapist with a regular clinic at a London-based natural health centre (www.greenwichnaturalhealth.co.uk).

Lorraine is also a lecturer at Thames Valley University in London, teaching on the BSc (Hons) Nutritional Therapy; and leading the development of other nutrition-related degree programmes at both undergraduate and postgraduate level.

In addition, she undertakes nutrition consultancy and training for various organisations in the healthcare, educational and business consultancy sectors, including as part of employee welfare programmes.

Her relevant qualifications include a Masters degree in Nutrition and Chronic Disease. She is registered with the government-backed CNHC (Complementary and Natural Healthcare Council).

Ann Woodriff Beirne BSc, MSc, DipRaworth has degrees in Food Science and Applied Immunology. She worked for ten years in haematology and blood transfusion laboratories before training in complementary medicine, including dietary therapy.

Ann worked at CNELM (Centre for Nutrition Education and Lifestyle Management) for eight years, lecturing on the BSc Nutritional Therapy and Masters courses. In addition, she wrote for and sub-edited the professional journal, *The Nutrition Practitioner*, for three years.

During this time, Ann also ran a busy clinic, specialising in deep tissue therapeutic massage, aromatherapy and reflexology. She is trained as a Master NLP (Neuro-Linguistic Programming) Practitioner and uses this in conjunction with other therapies.

Michael Ash BSc (Hons), DO, ND, FDipION is an osteopath, naturopath and nutritional therapist, in private practice since 1982.

He has developed a special interest in the mucosal immune system and its relevance to health, with a particular emphasis on the gastro-intestinal tract and its effect on the brain and other tissues. Musculoskeletal medicine, nutritional medicine and immunology are the three cornerstones of clinical care in his practice and research life. He has contributed chapters to text books related to immunology, written many articles, presented at conferences internationally and is the Editor of www.nleducation.co.uk.

Justine Bold BA (Hons), Dip. BCNH, NTCC, MBANT is a nutritional therapy practitioner and lectures on the BSc Human Nutrition and the Masters in Nutritional Therapy at the University of Worcester. She is currently researching for an MPhil/

PhD on the dietary management of inflammatory bowel disease and irritable bowel syndrome. She presented related areas of work at the International Coeliac Symposium in April 2009.

She has worked in practice since 2003 and has also worked in the community, including running workshops on healthy eating/cookery in south Kilburn in London. She has also worked on many corporate wellness projects and written for national and consumer press.

Michael Culp MA, NMD is a naturopathic medical doctor and is currently the Director of The Natural Health and Wellness Centre in London (www.nhwc.co.uk), an innovative multi-disciplinary medical clinic specialising in the treatment of chronic diseases and the promotion of optimal wellness.

Dr Culp received his medical degree from Bastyr University in Seattle, Washington, where he was later appointed to the faculty to teach medical nutrition and nutritional biochemistry while practising as a family general practitioner at the University Health Clinic in Seattle. For six years, he was the Director of Medical Education for Genova Diagnostics Laboratory, before moving to the UK.

Ada Hallam BSc (Hons), Dip. NT trained in nutritional therapy at Raworth International College and then went on to gain a first class honours degree at the University of Westminster.

Ada has lectured and provided clinical supervision at universities internationally and focuses on the evidence-based use of nutritional therapy to counterbalance the stressors of today, and to help individuals maximise their own health potential. Ada firmly believes that many chronic and sub-clinical health conditions can be positively impacted by the integrative and collaborative approach of nutritional therapy and is currently in the process of setting up private practice in the US.

Smita Hanciles MSc, BSc (Hons) is a nutritionist who has had diverse research and teaching roles, including programme leader/lecturer of a Nutritional Therapy degree programme. She delivers training on child nutrition for various organisations and is currently involved with infant and child nutrition projects within the NHS.

Helen Lynam BSc (Hons), NTCC, MBANT spent 18 years as an engineer with British Airways, rising to Senior Manager before leaving to study nutritional therapy. After gaining a first class degree in Nutritional Therapy at the CNELM, Helen went on to gain her Master NLP Practitioner and has established herself as a nutritional therapist specialising in eating disorders. She sees clients in two practices, one in Ascot and one in Wokingham. Helen is a supervisor and module leader at the CNELM and is also joint Sub-editor of *The Nutrition Practitioner* journal.

Angelette Müller MSc, PGDip, MBANT is Director of CREATE, School of Food and Health, a community interest company that offers integrated culinary and health education for the community and schools. This includes teacher training to encourage cross-curricular health promotion.

She is a specialist in delivering food and health education for children and adolescents; and acted as a nutrition advisor for an Ealing-based documentary about nutrition, exams and teenagers. She also works part-time as a senior lecturer in Nutritional Therapy at Thames Valley University in London, where she is involved with programme development and delivery, module leadership and student clinic supervision.

Kate Neil MSc, FRSM, FRSA, MBANT, NTCC is Director of the Centre for Nutrition Education and Lifestyle Management, which teaches nutrition degrees and postgraduate courses validated by Middlesex University. She is Programme Leader for the degrees and teaches on the courses.

Kate is Editor of *The Nutrition Practitioner* professional journal. She regularly writes for a number of publications and speaks at external conferences and seminars.

Kate has an MSc in Nutritional Medicine and has practised as a nutritional therapist for over 20 years, specialising in women's health and children with learning and behavioural difficulties. Kate received the 2004 CAM Award for her contribution to the nutritional therapy community.

Jane Nodder is a practising nutritional therapist and Senior Lecturer and Clinic Supervisor for the BSc (Hons) Health Sciences: Nutritional Therapy at the University of Westminster, London. Her special interests include nutritional approaches to weight management, eating disorders and endocrine modulation.

Jane has attended the Institute for Functional Medicine intensive five-day training programme 'Applying Functional Medicine in Clinical Practice', and is completing the MSc in Nutritional Medicine at the University of Surrey, Guildford, where her research is focusing on dietary practices amongst club level marathon runners. Jane sits on the Ethics Committee of the British Association for Applied Nutrition and Nutritional Therapy (BANT).

Zeller Pimlott BA (Hons), BSc (Hons), MBANT, NTCC is a practising nutritional therapist and a lecturer in Nutritional Therapy at Thames Valley University in London.

Zeller's early career was in science, including research in molecular biology. This was followed by a period working in financial information systems. After taking a gap from work to start her family, Zeller decided to retrain. She completed a certificate in psychotherapy and counselling, but decided to focus on nutrition.

Since completing a degree in Nutritional Therapy in 2005, Zeller has run a private practice in London and also runs short courses in nutrition. She is registered with the CNHC.

Surinder Phull BA (Hons), BSc (Hons), MBANT is a lecturer in Nutritional Therapy at Thames Valley University in London and is also a practising nutritional therapist. She runs a London-based nutrition consultancy, running seminars and lectures for both the private and public sector. She has a strong presence in the media and is a regular contributor to many popular health publications and BBC radio programmes. Her specialist interests include variations in ethnic eating patterns, and the biochemical, genetic, familial and cultural factors that influence eating behaviours.

Professor Basant K. Puri MA (Cantab), PhD, MB, BChir, BSc (Hons) MathSci, MRCPsych, DipStat, PG Cert Maths, MMath is Professor and Honorary Consultant at Hammersmith Hospital and Imperial College London.

Professor Puri has primary and postgraduate degrees in Medicine from the University of Cambridge, post-doctoral work in Molecular Genetics at the University of Cambridge and in Imaging at the Royal Postgraduate Medical School. He has researched the effects of lipids on brain structure and chemistry and has directed a clinical programme studying the effects of lipids on major neurological and psychiatric disorders.

Laurence Trueman PhD is a senior lecturer at the University of Worcester and a founding member of the Masters in Nutritional Therapy and the BSc in Human Nutrition.

He graduated from the University of Durham with a degree in Molecular Biology and Biochemistry and went on to obtain a doctorate in the same discipline from the University of Manchester Institute of Science and Technology (UMIST). His teaching areas include: human biochemistry, genetics (including nutrigenomics and epigenomics), the molecular basis of disease and nutritional medicine.

Dr Christabelle Yeoh MBBS, MRCP, MSc qualified from St George's Hospital Medical School, London, in 1999. She trained in acute medicine and became a Member of the Royal College of Physicians. She worked in Gastroenterology at the Royal London Hospital and later obtained a Masters in Nutrition from King's College London.

After more time in general medicine, she joined Breakspear Hospital in 2006. She became a member of the British Society of Ecological Medicine, the American Academy of Environmental Medicine and has been registered as a Defeat Autism Now! practitioner. She treats patients with fatigue syndromes, chronic infections, neuro-behavioural disorders, allergies and chemical sensitivity.

SUBJECT INDEX

AUTHOR INDEX

Aaseth, J. 90
Abdelghani, M.B. 42
Abdennour, C. 86
Adam, O. 362
Aderem, A. 264
Advisory Committee on the
    Microbiological Safety of
    Food 41
Aggarwal, B.B. 243, 361, 362
Agrawal, A. 262
Ajjan, R.A. 201
Akerberg, A.K. 158
Aktuna, D. 203
Al Somal, N. 41
Albanes, D. 144, 314
Albarracin, C. 161
Allan, S. 274
Allison, A.C. 283
Allison, D.B. 149
Amella, M. 361
American Association of
    Clinical Endocrinologists
    (AACE) 174, 181, 188,
    191, 192,
American College of Physicians
    15
American Psychiatric
    Association (APA) 132,
    330, 331
Ames, B.N. 304
Amici, D. 30
Anderson, B.M. 107, 113, 120
Anderson, E.J. 146
Anderson, K.V. 264
Anderson, O. 90
Anderson, R.A. 155, 160,
    161, 162
Anderson, R.J. 206
Andersson, A. 150
Andersson, R. 52
Andrès, E. 42
Angstwurm, M.W. 89
Anon 354
Antinoro, L. 153
Antonio, J. 208
Antonopoulos, D.A. 282
Antypa, N. 345
Aon, M.A. 256
Aouacheri, W. 86
Appel, L.J. 112, 153
Appleton, K.M. 135
Aprill, B.S. 208
Arehart-Treichel, J. 334
Arem, R. 177, 179, 182, 185, 187,
    188, 189, 191, 199, 207
Argmann, C. 151
Arlt, W. 210

Armstrong, D. 285
Arnaud, M. 58
Arthur, J.R. 175, 180, 202,
    203, 204, 205
Arts, M.J. 313
Asa, S.L. 176
Aschner, M. 205
Ash, M. 361, 363
Ashworth, A. 342
Assumpcao, C.R. 146
Athyros, V.G. 110
Atisook, K. 280
Atkinson, C. 244
Atkinson, W. 52, 55, 56
Attia, N. 143
Auborn, K. 83
Auwerx, J. 151
Avila, J.R. 89
Awasthi, A. 283

Bablis, P. 44
Bach, J.F. 260, 268, 282
Baillie-Hamilton, P. 225
BaisierW.V. 182, 186
Baker, B.P. 83
Baker, S.M. 304
Balk, E.M. 112
Ballor, D.L. 150
Balz, F. 312
Bandyopadhyay, D. 298
Banerjee, R. 40
Bangert, S.K. 177, 180, 182,
    183, 185, 190
Bannenberg, G. 158
Bantle, J.P. 148
Baranwal, A. 48
Barbagallo, M. 160, 210
Barbara, G. 53
Barnes, B.O. 186
Baroni, S.S. 154
Barre, D.E. 113
Barrett, K.E. 43
Barrett-Connor, E.L. 208
Barroso-Aranda, J. 81
Bartlett, J. 48
Bartsch, H. 303
Baschetti, R. 197
Baskaran, K. 163
Bass, E. 314
Bassaganya-Riera, J. 288
Bassey, J.E. 117
Bates, D. 116
Batten, M. 286
Baur, J.A. 151
Bayoumi, R.A. 245
Beal, F. 298
Beastall, G.H. 182

Bebakar, W.M. 144
Béchamp, A. 24, 25
Beckett, G.J. 175, 180, 185,
    202, 203, 204, 205
Beck-Nielsen, H. 147
Bekhof, J. 210
Bekkali, N. 57
Belch, J.J. 116, 362
Belchetz, P.E. 185
Belin, R.J. 159
Bell, D.S. 206
Ben Amotz, A. 314
Benard, A. 280
Bender, D.A. 244
Bennet, P. 87
Bennett, C.N. 328, 329
Benninga, M.A. 56
Benvenga, S. 208
Benzie, I.F. 309
Bercik, P. 52, 53
Berger, W. 158
Berkes, J. 360
Berk-Planken, I.I.L. 242
Bermejo-Fenoll, A. 40
Bernard, C. 25
Bernardo, A. 130
Berquin, I.M. 114, 115, 120
Bertuglia, S. 302
Bettelli, E. 266
Bevan, M.J. 284
Bhardwaj, S.B. 53
Bharti, A.C. 361, 362
Bhattacharyya, A. 183
Biassi, F. 109
Bingham, M. 334
Bingham, S.A. 45, 157
Biolab 338
Biondi, B. 188, 201
Bird, C. 30
Birdsall, T.C. 198
Birmingham, L. 342
Biswas, S.K. 89
Bjelakovic, G. 314
Bjorck, I.M. 158
Bland, J.S. 33, 82, 202, 206,
    227, 229, 236, 243, 359,
    360
Blaxill, M.K. 77
Blomhoff, R. 310
Bloomfield, S. 268
Bode, J.C. 44
Boden, G. 141
Bohnet, H.G. 204
Bollinger, R.R. 278
Bolton, J.L. 228, 229, 233
Bonello, R. 44
Bonnesen, C. 230

Borghesi, L.A. 70
Borkman, M. 155
Bosi, E. 279
Bosma, P.J. 92
Bosmans, E. 267
Bottiglieri, G. 343
Bougle, D. 159
Bourre, J.M. 115
Boxshall, G. 82
Bradfield, C.A. 273
Bradshaw, H.B. 129
Brady, J. 83
Bralley, J. 75, 101, 107, 108,
    110, 113, 118, 224, 236,
    338, 352, 354
Brand-Miller, J.B. 147
Braverman, E.R. 343
Brazier, J. 48
Brenna, T. 118
Brien, S. 361
British Dietetic Association
    (BDA) 201
British Medical Journal (BMJ)
    57
British Nutrition Foundation
    (BNF) 47, 201
British Thyroid Foundation (BTF)
    179, 184, 188, 189, 192
Broadhurst, C.L. 161
Brosnan, J. 236
Brown, A. 282
Broyer, P.A. 204
Bruewer, M. 280
Bryan, C.S. 21
Bryden, N.A. 160
Buchinger, W. 203
Buddington, R. 82
Bueld, J.E. 158
Buettner, G.R. 146
Buhler, D.R. 308, 311
Bulló, M. 105
Bulun, S.E. 222
Bunevicius, R. 181, 188
Burmeister, S. 48
Burnet, F.M. 258

Cadbury, D. 221,
Cain, J.R. 43, 44
Calcinaro, F.D.S. 287
Calder, P.C. 102, 106, 107,
    109, 116, 362
Callard, R.E. 93
Calviello, G. 114
Camilo, M.E. 89
Campbell, N.R. 207
Campbell-McBride, N. 334
Campieri, M. 277

CPI Antony Rowe
Eastbourne, UK
November 03, 2023